Kanagas

Sajeesh K

Leonard G

Jorge Cuadros

Editors

Teleophthalmology

Kanagasingam Yogesan
Sajeesh Kumar
Leonard Goldschmidt
Jorge Cuadros
Editors

Teleophthalmology

With 116 Figures, mostly in Color

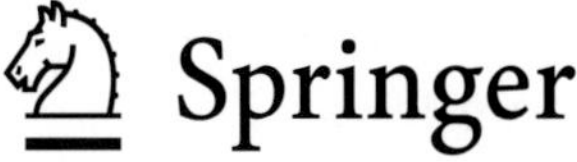

Kanagasingam Yogesan, PhD
Professor in Ophthalmology
Director, Center of Excellence in E-Medicine
University of Western Australia
Lions Eye Institute
Nedlands 6009 WA
Australia

Sajeesh Kumar, PhD
Center of Excellence in E-Medicine
University of Western Australia
Lions Eye Institute
Nedlands 6009 WA
Australia

Leonard Goldschmidt, MD, PhD
Medical Director, Telehealth and
Medical Informatics
Department of Veterans Affairs
Palo Alto Health Care System
Palo Alto, California 94304,
USA

Jorge Cuadros, OD, PhD
University of California
School of Optometry
Berkeley 94720-2020,
USA

2nd Printing 2008
1st Edition 2006

ISBN 978-3-540-70515-4
e-ISBN 978-3-540-33714-0

Library of Congress Control Number: 2005937529

Cover design: Frido Steinen-Broo, eStudio, Calamar, Spain

Printed on acid-free paper
9 8 7 6 5 4 3 2 1
springer.com

Foreword

The import of communication and digital technology into the field of health has opened new vistas in patient care (diagnostics and treatment), distance learning for health personnel, and health education for patients. The discipline of ophthalmology lends itself admirably to application in all these domains. Moreover it is a means of achieving equity in specialist service delivery with acceptable levels of care that is evidence based, even in situations where trained specialist personnel and infrastructure resources are limited. However the cost/benefit issues of such intervention in various situations and their acceptance in different socio-economic and cultural settings must still be generally established. There is increasing evidence from pilot studies, some described in this publication, that are encouraging provided that further containment of capital and recurring costs occur. There is also a need to develop and adopt more user friendly technologies such as those that have already revolutionized global communication.

Technological interventions such as teleophthalmology in health care are a means to an end and not end products themselves. The product it helps to deliver is eye health. It is important, therefore, as we continue to improve on our technologies, that we continue to measure and assess their impact on the outcomes of care. In the final analysis the value of any new health technology based on innovation and research must be seen against the benefit that it brings to our patients.

This multiauthor source book is a collection of articles from a range of countries that not only describe what is already available but also postulates what the future holds for teleophthalmology. In this context it is necessary to "think outside the box" and, as late Sir John Wilson said, "I believe that to constrain our horizon to the current state of awareness and knowledge is to destroy the possibility of unexpected novelty and success in improving the human condition."

Dr. Ramachandra Pararajasegaram
Consultant
Prevention of Blindness and Deafness
World Health Organization
Geneva, Switzerland

Foreword

Ophthalmic disease is characterized by pathology made visible and therefore able to be imaged due to the essential transparent nature of the internal eye structures. Not only can the disease process be readily imaged, but in western and developed countries, most blindness is caused by a small number of very prevalent conditions namely cataract, macular degeneration, glaucoma with optic disc cupping, diabetic retinopathy and other vascular diseases. In addition, these diseases tend to be relatively slow in onset and therefore asymptomatic in the early stages and increasingly treatable if detected before vision is lost. The number of people visually impaired across the world from these major conditions is increasing as the population ages and adopts a more sedentary lifestyle.

The exciting and rapidly developing field of teleophthalmology encompasses high-resolution digital imaging, image storage and transmission to expert disease monitoring centers, image compression, data security and intelligent systems. Teleophthalmology in the future offers the opportunity to maintain image data banks of whole populations and the possibility of detecting the vast majority of blinding eye disease very early.

In developing countries where the prevalence of blindness is much higher, and where the disease spectrum causing it includes infections of the ocular surface and injuries in addition to cataract, diabetic retinopathy and glaucoma, teleophthalmology offers the chance to develop very cheap methods of screening for eye disease with portable digital imaging equipment operated by less expensive and ubiquitous health workers throughout the community.

Before all this can happen, further technological breakthroughs are required. Cheap, easy to operate, and portable digital slit lamps and digital ophthalmoscopes need to be developed with a precision matching expensive optical equipment already available in ophthalmic specialist offices today. Secure transmission, storage and analysis needs to be developed specifically for this type of program. For widespread use, teleophthalmic systems need to develop economic reality through a reimbursement formula from government health and insurance agencies so that health workers everywhere can take on these responsibilities in addition to their often already stretched work loads. A wholesome program of community awareness on the nature and dangers of eye disease needs to be carried out to induce the whole population to participate in screenings even if they think their eyes are normal. Ophthalmologists and optometrists need to be convinced that teleophthalmology will be a powerful addition to their medical and optical expertise rather than a faceless competitor.

This book encapsulates global efforts in the development of teleophthalmology with contributions from many international experts with first-hand experience. Their contributions in the not-too-distant future will be seen as major developments in eye health care.

Professor Ian Constable
Director – Lions Eye Institute
Centre for Ophthalmology and Visual Science
University of Western Australia

Preface

If a group of ophthalmologists, nurses, computer scientists, or scientists from other disciplines were asked the question, "What is teleophthalmology?" the response would certainly not be unanimous. Some might point out examples of applications in the area of ophthalmic service delivery. Others would highlight the technology itself. These replies portray the tip of the iceberg, since developments in teleophthalmology are progressing at great speed. As a consequence, there is a need for a broad overview of the field. This first-ever book on teleophthalmology is presented in a way that should make it accessible to anyone, independent of their knowledge of technology. This book is designed to be used by *all*, including clinicians, nurses, allied health professionals and students.

In a very short time, the field of teleophthalmology has become too extensive to be covered by only a small number of experts. Consequently, this *book* has been written with contributions from a host of renowned international authorities in the field. Our guiding hope during this task was that as editors of multiple chapters we could still write with a single voice and keep the content coherent and simple. We hope that the clarity of this book makes up for any limitations in its comprehensiveness.

The editors took much care that this *book* would not be merely a collection of separate chapters, but rather offer a consistent and structured overview of the field. We are aware that there is still considerable room for improvement and that certain elements of teleophthalmology are not fully covered, such as legal and reimbursement policy. The editors invite readers to send comments and feedback (suggestions, remarks, corrections, demonstrations, questions and answers, etc.) to further improve and expand future editions of this *book*.

This *book* has been organized systematically. The 33 chapters are grouped into four main sections. The book starts with foundational chapters explaining the concepts that are the mainstay to teleophthalmology and subsequent chapters are built upon those foundations. The first section covers the basic concepts of teleophthalmology, current issues and technology used. The chapters on cost evaluation and legal issues are deliberately placed in the first section of the book to emphasize the fundamental importance of these topics.

The second section covers the current state of the art in disease-specific screening systems. The predominant paradigms of each disease-specific screening are discussed. This section provides a justification for the clinical services described in the following section on global efforts.

The third section covers the major threads of services, research and development in various nations in an effort to provide better eye care delivery. Throughout this section, a theme of implementation and feasibility are sustained. Considerable focus is given on works being done in developing countries. The final section covers the current, ongoing experiments and future directions of teleophthalmology.

Appendix 1 lists information on some of the educational and training opportunities available. Nevertheless this list is not inclusive, since opportunities are progressively arising in this domain. Appendix 2-7 illustrates samples of various administrative tools necessary for any teleophthalmology trials.

We would like to thank all authors for making this book possible through their contributions. This book would not have been possible without the assistances of various people. We acknowledge and appreciate the assistance of Ms. Kitty Drok, editorial assistant from Western Australia and the reviewers Prof. Ian J. Constable, Dr. Antonio Guibilato and Dr. Nitin Verma. We are indebted to Prof. Ian J. Constable and Dr Para Rajasegaram for their warm and constant support and endowing foreword to this book.

Kanagasingam Yogesan
Sajeesh Kumar
Leonard Goldschmidt
Jorge Cuadros

Contents

Chapter 9
Cost-Effectiveness of Teleophthalmology in Diabetic Retinopathy Screening
I-van Ho, Nitin Verma

Chapter 10
Economic Evaluations in Teleophthalmology
Johanna Lamminen, Heikki Lamminen, Ville Voipio

Part II
Looking for Problems and Solutions – Telescreening

Chapter 11
Teleophthalmology Assessment of Diabetic Retinopathy
Ingrid E. Zimmer-Galler

Chapter 12
Diabetic Retinopathy Screening: What Model is Appropriate?
Chris J. Barry, Ian L. McAllister, Ian J. Constable, Kanagasingam Yogesan

Chapter 25
Teleophthalmology in Spain
Francisco Gonzalez, Adrian F. Castro

Chapter 26
Telemedicine to Improve the Quality and Cost Efficiency of Providing Eye Care
Vladimir Kazinov

Chapter 27
Cataract and Refractive Surgery Post-operative Care – Teleophthalmology's Challenge in Argentina
Giselle Ricur, Roberto Zaldivar, Maria Gabriela Batiz

Chapter 28
Teleophthalmology in the United States Army
Michael J. Mines, Kraig S. Bower, Thomas P. Ward

Acronyms

3G	Third generation
7SF	Seven 30° field, stereoscopic
AIDS	Acquired immunodeficiency syndrome
AMD	Age-related macular degeneration
ANSI	American national standards institute
AREDS	Age-related eye disease study
ASP	Active server pages
ATM	Asynchronous transfer mode
AUD	Australian dollar
AVR	Arteriovenous ratio
BIO	Binocular indirect ophthalmoscopy
CAN	Canadian dollar
CCD	Charged coupled device
CD	Compact disc
CDA	Clinical document architecture
COM	Component object model
CRAE	Central retinal artery equivalent
CRT	Cathode ray tube
CRVE	Central retinal vein equivalent
CSME	Clinically significant macular edema
DICOM	Digital imaging and communications in medicine
DPI	Dots per inch
DSL	Digital subscriber line
ETDRS	Early treatment of diabetic retinopathy study
EUR	Euro
FEH	Flying Eye hospital
GBP	Great Britain pound
GIF	Graphic interface file
GPRS	General packet radio service
GSM	Global system for mobile commu nication
HBP	Hospital based programs
HL7	Health level 7
HTML	Hypertext markup language
IOD	Image object definition
IOP	Intraocular pressure
IP	Internet protocol
IRR	Internal rate of return
ISDN	Integrated services digital network
ISO	International organization for standardization
ISRO	Indian space research organization
IT	Information technology
JPEG	Joint photographic experts group
LAN	Local area network
LASIK	Laser-assisted in situ keratomileusis
LCD	Liquid crystal display
MPEG	Motion pictures experts group
NASA	National aeronautics and space administration
NICU	Neonatal intensive care units
NPDR	Non-proliferative diabetic retinopathy
NPV	Net present value
PACS	Picture archiving and communiction systems
PCC	Primary health care center
PNG	Portable network graphic
POTS	Plain old telephone service
RGB	Red, green, blue
ROI	Region of interest
ROP	Retinopathy of prematurity
SLR	Single lens reflex
SQL	Structured query language
T1	Transmission 1
TCP/IP	Transmission control protocol/ internet protocol
TIFF	Tagged image file format
USB	Universal serial bus
USD	United States dollar
VF	Volunteer faculty
VPN	Virtual private network
VSAT	Very small aperture terminal

WFIDS Web-based fundus image database system

WRAMC Walter Reed Army medical center

WRESP Warfighter refractive eye surgery program

XML Extensible markup language

List of Contributors

Rafat R. Ansari
Vision Research and Human Health
Diagnostics Laboratory
NASA Glenn Research Center
21000 Brookpark Road
Cleveland, OH 44135
USA
Rafat.R.Ansari@nasa.gov

Tariq Aslam
Royal Manchester Eye Hospital
Oxford Road
Manchester
United Kingdom
TAslam@aol.com

S.S. Badrinath
Sankara Nethralaya
18 College Road, Nungambakkam
Chennai 600006, Tamil Nadu
India
drssb_sn@yahoo.com

Chris J. Barry
Lions Eye Institute
University of Western Australia
2, Verdun Street
Nedlands, 6009 WA
Western Australia
Australia
cjbarry@cyllene.uwa.edu.au

Valerijus Barzdziukas
Institute for Biomedical Research
Telemedicine Center
of Kaunas University of Medicine
Eiveniu 4, 50009 Kaunas
Lithuania
vb@tmc.kmu.lt

María Gabriela Batiz
Instituto Zaldivar
Emilio Civit 685
M5502GVG, Mendoza
Argentina
mbatiz@institutozaldivar.com

Rubens Belfort Jr.
Vision Institute/Ophthalmology
Department, Federal University of São Paulo
(UNIFESP)
Rua Botucatu 820
04023-062 São Paulo–SP
Brazil

Neera Bhatia
School of Legal Studies
University of Wolverhampton
Molineux Street
Wolverhampton, WV1 1SB
England
n.bhatia2@wlv.ac.uk

Marie Carole Boucher
Department of Ophthalmology
University of Montreal
3455 Vendome
Montreal, Quebec H4A 3M6
Canada

Kraig S. Bower
Ophthalmology Service
Department of Surgery
Walter Reed Army Medical Center
6900 Georgia Ave, NW
Washington, DC 20307
USA
Kraig.Bower@na.amedd.army.mil

Adrian F. Castro
Department of Physiology
School of Medicine
University of Santiago de Compostela
15782 Santiago de Compostela
Spain
fsadrian@usc.es

Opas Chutatape
School of Electrical and Electronic Engineering
Nanyang Technological University
Singapore 639798
eopas@ntu.edu.sg

Ian J. Constable
Lions Eye Institute
University of Western Australia
2, Verdun Street
Nedlands, 6009 WA
Western Australia
Australia
ijc@cyllene.uwa.edu.au

Jorge Cuadros
Clinical Research Center
Optometric Eye Center
University of California, Berkeley
Berkeley, CA 94720
USA
jac@eyepacs.org

Heike Elflein
Department of Pediatric Ophthalmology
Strabismology and Ophthalmogenics Klinikum
University of Regensburg
93042 Regensburg
Germany
heike.elflein@gmx.de

Luciano Peixoto Finamor
Vision Institute/Ophthalmology
Department, Federal University of São Paulo
(UNIFESP)
Rua Botucatu 820
04023-062 São Paulo–SP
Brazil

Nikica Gabrić
Poliklinika "Svjetlost"
Bukovačka 27
10000 Zagreb
Croatia
Nikica.Gabric@svjetlost.hr

Leonard Goldschmidt
Medical Director, Telehealth and Medical
Informatics
Department of Veterans Affairs Palo Alto Health
Care System
Palo Alto, California 94304
USA
Leonard.Goldschmidt@va.gov

Francisco Gonzalez
Department of Physiology
School of Medicine
University of Santiago de Compostela
15782 Santiago de Compostela
Spain
francisco.gonzalez@usc.es

Eugene M. Helveston
ORBIS Telemedicine
702 Rotary Circle
Indianapolis, IN 46202
USA
ehelveston@msn.com
ehelveston@ny.orbis.org

P. Lloyd Hildebrand
608 Stanton L. Young Boulevard
Department of Ophthalmology
University of Oklahoma
Oklahoma City, OK 73104
USA
lloyd-hildebrand@ouhsc.edu

I-van Ho
Hobart Eye Surgeons
P.O. Box 97, North Hobart 7002
Tasmania, Australia
ivanho73@bigpond.net.au

Beth Hudson
Carnarvon Regional Hospital
Cleaver Street
Carnarvon
Australia
Beth.Hudson@health.wa.gov.au

Randy T. Jose
University of Houston College of Optometry (UHCO)
University Eye Institute
505 J. Davis Armistead Bldg
Houston, TX 77204-2020
USA
RJose@UH.EDU

Vladimir Kazinov
DiViSy Group, Stchelkovskoe
Shosse 77
107497 Moscow
Russia
inf@divisy.com
Kazinov@mail.ru

R. Kim
Aravind Eye Hospitals &
Postgraduate Institute of Ophthalmology
1, Anna Nagar
Madurai 625020
India
kim@aravind.org

Sajeesh Kumar
Centre of Excellence in e-Medicine
Lions Eye Institute
University of Western Australia
2, Verdun Street
Nedlands, 6009 WA
Western Australia
Sajeesh@cyllene.uwa.edu.au

R. Vasantha Kumar
Lions Aravind Institute of Community Ophthalmology
72, Kurvikaran Salai
Gandhi Nagar
Madurai 625020
India
vasanth@aravind.org

Skaidra Kurapkienė
Institute of Biomedical Research
Telemedicine Center
of Kaunas University of Medicine
Eiveniu 4, 50009 LT, Kaunas
Lithuania
sk@tmc.kmu.lt

Heikki Lamminen
Tampere University of Technology
Korkeakoulunkatu 10
33101 Tampere
Finland
Heikki.Lamminen@uta.fi

Johanna Lamminen
CFO, Evli Bank,
Aleksanterinkatu 19
00100 HELSINKI
johanna.lamminen@evli.com

Paulo Lopes
Health Informatics Department
Federal University of São Paulo (UNIFESP)
Rua Pedro de Toledo 781
04039-032 São Paulo–SP
Brazil

Birgit Lorenz
Department of Pediatric Ophthalmology
Strabismology and Ophthalmogenics Klinikum
University of Regensburg
93042 Regensburg
Germany
birgit.lorenz@klinik.uni-regensburg.de

David Maberley
Department of Ophthalmology
University of British Columbia
2550 Willow St. Vancouver, BC
V5Z 3N9
Canada

Ilias Maglogiannis
University of Aegean
Department of Information and Communications Systems Engineering
83200 Karlovasi, Samos
Greece
imaglo@aegean.gr

Jacques Marescaux
IRCAD – European Institute of Telesurgery
1 Place de l'Hospital
67091 Strasbourg
France
Jacques.Marescaux@ircad.u-strasbg.fr

Ian L. McAllister
Lions Eye Institute
University of Western Australia
2 Verdun Street
Nedlands, 6009 WA
Western Australia
Australia

Lawrence M. Merin
Vanderbilt Ophthalmic Imaging Center
Vanderbilt Eye Institute
333 Commerce Street
Nashville, TN 37201
USA
Lawrence.merin@vanderbilt.edu

Michael J. Mines
Ophthalmology Service
Department of Surgery
Walter Reed Army Medical Center
6900 Georgia Ave, NW
Washington, DC 20307
USA
Michael.Mines@na.amedd.army.mil

Christina Muccioli
Vision Institute/Ophthalmology
Department, Federal University of São Paulo
(UNIFESP)
Rua Botucatu 820
04023-062 São Paulo–SP
Brazil
murali@snmail.org

V. Murali
Sankara Nethralaya
18 College Road, Nungambakkam
Chennai 600006, Tamil Nadu
India

Niall Patton
Princess Alexandra Eye Pavilion
Chalmers Street
Edinburgh EH3 9HA
United Kingdom
niallpatton@hotmail.com

Alvydas Paunksnis
Institute fo Biomedical Research
Telemedicine Center
of Kaunas University of Medicine
Eiveniu 4, 50009 LT, Kaunas
Lithuania
apaun@medi.lt

Sotiris Pavlopoulos
National Technical University of Athens
School of Electrical and Computer Engineering
Biomedical Engineering Laboratory
Zografou Campus
9 Iroon Polytechniou Street
15773 Zagrafou
Greece
spav@biomed.ntua.gr

Ivan Torres Pisa
Health Informatics Department
Federal University of São Paulo (UNIFESP)
Rua Pedro de Toledo 781
04039-032 São Paulo–SP
Brazil

Rajiv Raman
Sankara Nethralaya
18 College Road, Nungambakkam
Chennai 600006, Tamil Nadu
India

Petar Raštegorac
Dom zdravlja zagrebačke županije
Dom zdravlja "Samobor"
Gajeva 36
10430 Samobor
Croatia
oftalmologija@comping.hr

Giselle Ricur
Instituto Zaldivar
Emilio Civit 685
M5502GVG, Mendoza
Argentina
gricur@institutozaldivar.com

Francesco Rubino
IRCAD – European Institute of Telesurgery
1 Place de l'Hospital
87091 Strasbourg
France

Chris J. Rudnisky
Department of Ophthalmology
University of Alberta
Royal Alexandra Hospital
10240 Kingsway Avenue
Edmonton, Alberta, T5H 3V9
Canada
crudnisk@ualberta.ca

Patrick J. Saine
Dartmouth Hitchcock Medical Center
1 Medical Center Drive
Lebanon, NH 03766
USA
Patrick.J.Saine@hitchcock.org

S. Sanjay
Sankara Nethralaya
18 College Road, Nungambakkam
Chennai 600006, Tamil Nadu
India
ss72@rediffmail.com

K. M. Sasipriya
Lions Aravind Institute of Community Ophthalmology
72, Kurvikaran Salai
Gandhi Nagar
Madurai 625020
India
sashi@aravind.org

Jade S. Schiffman
University Eye Institute at the University of Houston
#635-2476 Bolsover St.
Houston, TX 77005
USA
neurooph@msn.com

J. Sebag
Department of Clinacal Ophthalmology
University of Southern California
VMR Institute
7677 Center Avenue
Huntington, CA 92647
USA
jsebag@vmrinstitute.com

Daniel Sigulem
Vision Institute/Ophthalmology Department, Federal University of São Paulo (UNIFESP)
Rua Botucatu 820
04023-062 São Paulo–SP
Brazil

Luci Meire P. Silva
Federal University of São Paulo (UNIFESP)
Vision Institute/Ophthalmology Department
Rua Botucatu 820
04023-062 São Paulo–SP
Brazil

Lynda M. Smallwood
ORBIS Telemedicine
702 Rotary Circle
Indianapolis, IN 46202
USA

Rosa A. Tang
University of Texas Medical Branch
Department of Ophthalmology and Visual Sciences
Galveston., TX 77550
USA
rtangmd@hotmail.com

Mei-Ling Tay-Kearney
Lions Eye Institute
University of Western Australia
2, Verdun Street
Nedlands, 6009 WA
Western Australia
Australia
kearny@cyllene.uwa.edu.au

Matthew T. S. Tennant
Department of Ophthalmology
Royal Alexandra Hospital
10240 Kingsway Avenue
Edmonton, AB T5H 3V9
Canada
mtennant@alberta-retina.com

Mohan J. Thazhathu
ORBIS Telemedicine
702 Rotary Circle
Indianapolis, IN 46202
USA

R. D. Thulasiraj
Aravind Eye Hospitals &
Postgraduate Institute of Ophthalmology
1 Anna Nagar
Madurai 625020
India
thulsi@aravind.org

Nitin Verma
Hobart Eye Surgeons
P.O. Box 97, North Hobart 7002
Tasmania, Australia
nver3888@bigpond.net.au

Ville Voipio Ville
Novametor Oy
Sarastuspolku 5 B 14
01670 Vantaa
Finland
ville.voipio@iki.fi

Thomas P. Ward
Ophthalmology Service
Department of Surgery
Walter Reed Army Medical Center
6900 Georgia Ave, NW
Washington, DC 20307
USA

Gina G. Wong
University of Houston College of Optometry
Veterans Affairs Northern California Health Care System
10535 Hospital Way 112/I
Mather, CA 95655-1200
USA
gwong10998@aol.com

Kanagasingam Yogesan
Centre of Excellence in e-Medicine
Lions Eye Institute
University of Western Australia
2, Verdun Street
Nedlands, 6009 WA
Western Australia
Yogesan@cyllene.uwa.edu.au

Akitoshi Yoshida
Asahikawa Medical College
Telemedicine Center
Midorigaoka Higashi 2-1-1-1
Asahikawa, 078-8510
Japan
ayoshida@asahikawa-med.ac.jp

Roberto Zaldivar
Instituto Zaldivar
Emilio Civit 685
M5502GVG, Mendoza
Argentina
rzaldivar@institutozaldivar.com

Ingrid E. Zimmer-Galler
Wilmer Eye Institute
Ophthalmology
Johns Hopkins University
600 N. Wolfe Street
Baltimore, MD 21287
USA
izimmerg@jhmi.edu

Part I

The Current View – Issues and Technology

Chapter 1

Overview of Teleophthalmology

1

Sajeesh Kumar, Kanagasingam Yogesan

This chapter addresses the following

Key Concepts:

- All patients should have access to ophthalmic and other medical specialists, regardless of a patient's geographical location.
- Ophthalmic specialists are not available in many areas.
- Using a computer, digital camera, specialized software, and telecommunications technology, clinical data can be transferred between remote sites, regardless of the location of ophthalmic specialists and their patients.
- Teleophthalmology can include real-time transmission between consulting parties, and/or store-and-forward transmission.
- Today's teleophthalmology, which encompasses access to eye care specialists for remotely located patients, includes ophthalmic disease screening, monitoring, diagnosing, management, sharing of medical resources, collaboration on research and clinical trials, distance learning, and continuing education.

1.1 Indroduction

"Watson, come here. I want you," said Alexander Graham Bell on 10 March 1876, when he accidentally spilled battery acid on himself while making the world's first telephone call [1]. Little did Bell realize at the time that he was transmitting the world's first telemedical consultation. The field of telemedical communications has come a long way since then; not only is *telesurgery commonplace,* telemedicine has made it possible to bring state-of-the-art ophthalmic care to patients in rural and other hard-to-reach areas.

Prior to the development of telemedical communications, ophthalmic expertise was not available in several areas of the world. This was due to the higher concentration of eye care specialists in large, urban cities, with fewer in suburban and rural areas. To compensate, patients often were referred elsewhere at considerable expense – even though, in many cases, treatment could have been carried out by a local physician had advice been available from a specialist. All this has changed with the development of technology ranging from personal computers and digital cameras to appropriate software and telecommunications. Locale is no longer a limitation in receiving quality eye care, for the emerging field of *teleophthalmology* has made it possible to transfer clinical data from any part of the world to any other part.

1.2 What is Teleophthalmology?

Tele is a Greek word meaning "distance," and *ophthalmology* is the branch of medicine that deals with the anatomy, functions, pathology, and treatment of the eye.

Teleophthalmology is a method by which patients' eye-related problems can be examined, investigated, monitored, and treated, even though the eye care specialist and patient are located in different geographical areas. Though initially considered futuristic and experimental, teleoph-

1

thalmology has evolved into a specialty that is allowing quality eye care to reach patients worldwide.

One of the first applications of telemedicine to ophthalmology was tested in 1987 as part of a project to monitor retinal vessels during space flights. To ascertain its efficacy, the Johnson Space Center in Houston, Texas, developed a system for real-time transmission of retinal images that were acquired by a portable video funduscope. Tested on the space shuttle Columbia during mission STS-50 [2], the device used state-of-the-art telecommunication tools to provide ophthalmic advice remotely; today, such technology is an integral part of eye care services in several parts of the world. Image acquisition, image storage, image display and processing, and image transfer represent the basis of teleophthalmology. Such technology is making it possible to bring high quality eye care services to patients in hard-to-reach areas, rather than having to transport patients to a distant eye care center. Because of this application, two major goals of teleophthalmology are to (1) eliminate unnecessary traveling for patients and their caretakers, and (2) enable eye hospitals to treat patients from all over the world without concern about geographical limitations.

1.2.1 Scope of Teleophthalmology

Teleophthalmology covers a wide range of activities: the transferring of high-resolution ophthalmic images, ultrasound, electrooculography and electroretinography results. Today, the applications of teleophthalmology encompass:

- Access to eye specialists for patients in rural or remote areas
- Ophthalmic disease screening, diagnosis, monitoring, and management
- Linking and sharing of diverse medical resources
- Research and clinical trial collaborations
- Distant learning and continuing education

1.3 Teleophthalmology Around the World

Because of the high prevalence of eye disease in South Africa and the country could not afford the level of ophthalmic specialization achieved in the United Kingdom, a dedicated Internet site was set up by the UK's Moorfields Eye Hospital. This system offers teleophthalmology service to African countries including Ghana, Gambia, Tanzania and South Africa [3].

The Middle East Ophthalmology Network (MEON) is a unique network among ophthalmologists working in major ophthalmology centers in Israel, Jordan, Morocco, Tunisia and the Palestinian Authority [4], because the project offered some 50 physicians across the Middle East the opportunity to benefit from sharing clinical consultation for diagnosis and management decisions beyond physical and political boundaries. The system also overcame some of the constraints imposed by the uneven distribution of medical resources and expertise in the region, reduced professional isolation, encouraged more collaboration between physicians, and offered peace dividends based on cooperation between physicians across the political divide [4].

In the Azerbaijan Republic, the quickest and most cost-effective way to improve medical care was reported to be through telemedicine [5]. The first Internet and telemedicine station in Azerbaijan was started in 1997. Since then, ophthalmology- and surgery-based telemedicine consultations have been carried out with clinics in Moscow.

In 1998, using an integrated services digital network (ISDN) line conveying information at a rate of 128 kb/s, an endoscopic laser-assisted dacryocystorhinostomy procedure was transmitted in real time from the Saint Francis Medical Center in Honolulu, Hawaii, to ophthalmologists at the Makati Medical Center in Manila, Philippines, more than 5000 miles away [6]. Live surgical and endoscopic images were sent in real time with explanations by the surgeon and with interactive questions and answers during and after the procedure. It was the first time telemedicine technology was used to support real-time surgical telementoring to remove an orbital tumor, and it opened the door to further use and development of telementoring technology to disseminate surgical skills to distant sites.

1.4 Anatomy of a Teleophthalmology Consultation

Specific teleophthalmology and communication devices all are key components of the teleophthalmology infrastructure. They include specialized application software, data storage devices, database management software, medical devices capable of electronic data collection, and storage and transmission. In turn, these devices are enhanced through the use of telecommunications technology, network computing, video conferencing systems, and modems.

Teleophthalmology customarily uses two methods to transmit images data and sound – either live, real-time transmission wherein the consulting health care professional participates in the examination of the patient while diagnostic information is collected and transmitted; or store-and-forward transmission is used, wherein the consulting professional reviews data simultaneously with its collection. Ideally, the real-time assessment should be coupled with high-resolution, digitally still images for documentation purposes and ongoing follow-up care.

1.5 Equipment Used for Teleophthalmology Consultations

Digitally still and video cameras are used for conducting the external portion of the general eye exam in store-and-forward or real-time mode. The image quality of these cameras are usually sufficient to adequately detect gross ocular adnexal pathology, ocular motility, and alignment abnormalities (i.e. esotropia, exotropia, hypertropias, head-tilts, etc.). However, the pupillary assessment, which is usually obtained from the recorded findings of a trained examiner, utilizes sophisticated video camera systems.

For reporting the refractive status of the eyes, autorefractors are used in teleophthalmology. Many of these autorefractors have high levels of accuracy and require minimal training to use. Any of the ancillary health care personnel at remote sites can use this equipment.

The portability of devices are ideal for teleophthalmology. For instance, at remote telemedicine sites visual field testing is done through portable automated perimeters. The Humphrey Frequency Doubling Technology (HFDT) Perimeter and Dicon FieldView Perimeter are two examples of user-friendly visual field testers. They require only a short testing time, while at the same time they produce field reports in digital format that can be easily forwarded to the consulting ophthalmologist.

Intraocular pressure is measured using Keeler's non-contact, air-puff tonometer, assuming appropriately trained personnel are present at the remote site. Hand-held tonometers, such as the Tono-Pen XL or the Clarke/Perkins tonometer, are also ideal for telemedicine applications, since they are portable and require minimal training.

Non-mydriatic digital fundus cameras are widely used to assess posterior segment pathology via teleophthalmology. The Heidelberg Retina Tomograph II, Panoramic200TM scanning laser ophthalmoscope and the Topographic Scanning System (TopSS) are also used in teleophthalmology. Refractive surgery patients are followed up teleophthalmologically, with the use of a slit lamp video imaging system and a corneal topography unit.

High magnification images of the optic nerve and fovea can be obtained by direct video ophthalmoscope, however it allows a very limited view of the fundus. Currently available digital indirect ophthalmoscopes may not be a practical device for most teleophthalmology applications, since they require someone who is well-trained in indirect ophthalmoscopy at the remote site. Additionally, two people are generally required to capture images using this device: an observer who watches the video monitor, while at the same time, the examiner is attempting to bring the retina into focus. Once the image is in focus on the monitor, the observer needs to instruct the examiner to capture the image.

1.6 Teleophthalmology Considerations

In an ideal world, everyone would have immediate access to the appropriate specialist for medical consultation. However, the current status of health services is such that total primary medical care cannot be provided in many rural areas. Even secondary and tertiary medical care is not uniformly available in suburban and urban areas. Incentives to entice specialists to practice in suburban or rural areas have failed in many nations.

For decades, research has revealed that communities most likely to benefit from teleophthalmology are those least likely to afford it, or to have the requisite communication infrastructure. However, this may no longer be accurate. In contrast to the challenge of providing quality care to patients in rural and hard-to-reach areas, Internet connections and computer literacy are becoming more affordable, and therefore, easier to obtain and utilize [7] for healthcare and other purposes.

Theoretically, it is far easier to set up an excellent telecommunication infrastructure in suburban and rural areas than to place hundreds of medical specialists in these places. The world has realized that the future of telecommunications lies in satellite-based technology and fiber-optic cables. More and more, providing health care in remote areas through the use of high technology is manifesting; for instance, there has been a phenomenal explosion in the use of computers in Indian villages [7].

1.6.1 Challenges

Immediate or widespread implementation of teleophthalmology often is hindered by many factors [8]: lack of a telecommunication infrastructure; affordability of programs; cost of equipment; accuracy of the medical and non-medical devices used; training of appropriate personnel; lack of guidelines and protocols; sustaining projects; reimbursement for teleophthalmology consultations; regulations regarding sharing of information; legal liability; privacy; and security.

To expedite the use of teleophthalmology, financial planning for it should include the costs of creating and sustaining a telecommunication and information technology infrastructure and medical devices, as well as costs such as personnel training, monthly network access fees, maintenance, telephone bills, and other operational expenses [9].

Once the objectives of a program are identified, technology support personnel should be consulted to clarify technical equipment specifications and facility requirements. Protocols and guidelines must be developed to provide clear direction for how to utilize teleophthalmology most effectively. The training of remote operators is especially critical in telediagnosis of eye conditions that require hands-on examination [8]. The reliability of a program is also related to the consulting ophthalmologists' experience with telemedicine technology, and their awareness of both its strengths and limitations.

Another challenge is many nations do not have explicit policies to pay for teleophthalmology services therefore, establishing a teleophthalmology payment policy is crucial [10]. In this regard, several telemedicine services are being integrated into regular health care systems in the United States and the Scandinavian countries that include reimbursement and payment options [11, 12].

Additionally, studies need to be conducted about implementing, monitoring, evaluating, and refining the teleophthalmology payment process. In this regard, it should be noted that teleophthalmology licensure and indemnity laws may also need to be formulated. This issue however, remains a cloudy region for health care strategists and has implications for consulting ophthalmologists and rural/remote practitioners who practice across state or country lines.

It has been observed that successful teleophthalmology programs are often the product of careful planning, sound management, dedicated professionals and support staff, and a commitment to appropriate funding to support capital purchases and on-going operations. Clearly, implementing an effective system reflects a commitment to teamwork, and to linking technical and operational complexities into a fully integrated and efficiently functioning program. Teleophthalmology service providers, health insurance agencies, and all concerned institutions should convene to create a workable model for teleophthalmology service improvements. The eye care professional communities would also benefit by creating teleophthalmology service guidelines, which would pave the way for consensus on several challenging issues, such as technical and clinical service standardization for teleophthalmology.

1.6.2 Rewards

Worldwide, there is difficulty in retaining eye care and other specialists in non-urban areas. Once the virtual presence of a specialist is acknowledged through teleophthalmology, a patient can access resources in a tertiary eye care center without being limited by distance. Teleophthalmology also ensures maximum utilization of suburban or rural hospitals. General practitioners in rural and suburban areas often feel that they may lose their patients to a city consultant. With teleophthalmology, the community doctor continues to primarily treat the patient, under the guidance of a specialist. Teleophthalmology also avoids unnecessary travel and expense for patients, their families and caregivers; and it improves health outcomes.

It is also personally and professionally rewarding for health practitioners to know they have played a role in increasing access to eye care services and to improving quality of care. Few moments are as rewarding as receiving an anxious look from a patient in need, and giving reassurances that access to the best medical care is only a moment away.

References

1. Connected Earth (2005) Galleries: telecommunications age, http://www.connected-earth.com/Journeys/Telecommunicationsage/Firststeps.htm, cited 14 June 2005
2. Hunter N, Caputo M, Billica R (1993) Portable dynamic fundus instrument: uses in telemedicine and research. Seventh Annual Workshop on Space Operations Applications and Research (SOAR) 2:555–256
3. Johnston K, Kennedy C, Murdoch I, Taylor P, Cook C (2004) The cost-effectiveness of technology transfer using telemedicine. Health Policy Plan 19(5):302–309
4. Shanit D, Striebel W, Michelson G, Ayed S, Al Assi S, Belfair N, Ben-Simon G, Hamida F, Kanawati C, Lifshitz T, Madia G, Rafi M, Tahat A, Treister G, Tucktuck K, Zaghloul K (2002) Telemedicine in the service of peace. J Telemed Telecare 8(Suppl 2):76–77
5. Samedov RN (1998) An Internet station for telemedicine in the Azerbaijan Republic. J Telemed Telecare 4(Suppl 1):42–43
6. Camara JG, Rodriguez RE (1998) Real-time telementoring in ophthalmology. Telemed J 4(4):375–377
7. Ganapathy K (2005) Telemedicine in India – the Apollo experience. In: Neurosurgery on the web. www.thamburaj.com/telemedicine.htm, cited 14 June 2005
8. Sajeesh KR, Yogesan K, Constable IJ (2003) Teleophthalmology in India. Is it here to stay? Indian J Ophthalmol 51(4):295–296
9. Sajeesh KR, Mei-LingTay-Kearney, Constable IJ, Yogesan K (2005) Internet based ophthalmology service: impact assessment. Br J Ophthalmol, in press
10. Jakobsen KR (2002) Space-age medicine, stone-age government: how Medicare reimbursement of telemedicine services is depriving the elderly of quality medical treatment. Health Care Law 274:9–37
11. Gutierrez G (2001) Medicine, Medicare, the Internet, and the future of telemedicine. Crit Care Med 9(8 Suppl):N144–150
12. Health Care Financing Administration. Revision of Medicare reimbursement for Telehealth Services (AB-01-69), www.hcfa.gov/pubforms/transmit/memos/comm_date_dsc.htm, cited 14 June 2005

Chapter 2

Ophthalmic Imaging Essentials for Telemedicine

2

Patrick J. Saine

This chapter addresses the following

Key Concepts:

- In the digital realm of ophthalmic imaging, an image is worth a million words.
- The greater the number of pixels – on which digital photographs are usually based – the finer the detail.
- Designating each picture element (pixel) to one of three additive primary colors – red, green, or blue – creates a color digital image.
- In telemedicine applications, large files that contain fine clinical details must be balanced with transmission requirements that favor more compact files.
- There is a strong relationship between the amount and type of image compression and the quality of the information that is transferred.
- Ophthalmic imaging encompasses a wide range of photographic modalities, each of which is designed to capture a specific type of visual information.

2.1 Introduction

Whoever coined the timeless expression, "a picture is worth a thousand words," must surely have had the application of ophthalmic photography to telemedicine in mind. For while ophthalmic specialists can describe their patients with words and numbers, nothing tells the story of a patient's ophthalmic health status as good as a fine, digital photograph (Fig. 2.1).

To appreciate the intricacies and contributions of ophthalmic imaging, consider the digital application of the word *retina*. The six letters making up this description are encoded into the computer using six different American Standard Code for Information Interchange (ASCII) characters, each of which is a specific two digit number that is represented in a single byte of memory. This means that the word *retina* uses six bytes of computer space. Therefore, multiplying the word *retina* by one million results in a six megabyte image file – a *picture* that might reasonably be said to describe the word *retina* (Fig. 2.2).

There is also a third meaning to the expression, "a picture says a thousand words," because an image is the end result of a long, multi-step imaging chain. The subject is first chosen, lit, and precisely framed. Upon the photographer's decision, the light arriving from the subject enters the camera lens, passes through the open shutter, and strikes the digital sensor. This exposure initiates an electronic signal that is processed digitally within the camera, which, in turn, is transferred to the computer. The digital image's input into the computer drives a specific series of events that involve storage media, the computer hard drive, random access memory (RAM), the communication bus, and many electrons. The image is processed (digitally, not conventionally) before it is presented on the screen or printed. So the end product – a single image exposed in a fraction of a second – is, in reality, the result of a long, multi-step process.

This chapter provides an introduction to digital ophthalmic imaging for telemedicine. It be-

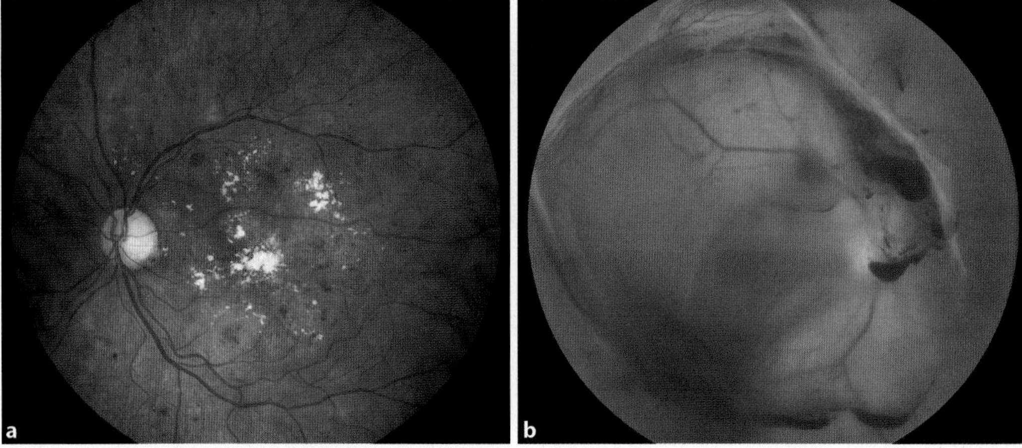

Fig. 2.1. Examples of two patients with similar demographics, similar visual acuity (20/400), and similar history (diabetes for 13 years). Retinal photography highlights the variable outcomes of their common disease process

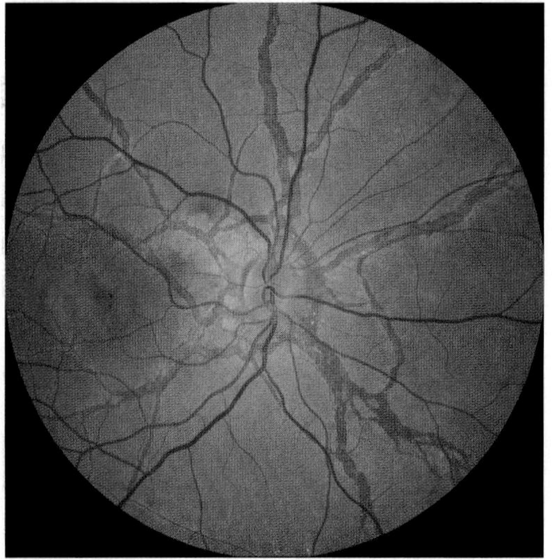

Fig. 2.2. This 24 bit color image of the retina uses 6 megabytes of computer space. The file uses 1 channel each of red, green, and blue information. It was sent to the printer as a 4.8" x 4.8" 300 DPI .tif file.

gins by explaining the essential tenets of digital imaging and concludes with a description of digital imaging instrumentation.

2.2 Digital Imaging Essentials

When a digital image is created, the image does not really exist. This is because, unlike traditional photographs, a digital image is really just an electronic description for creating an image – as opposed to an actual physical object. As descriptions, digital images use specific parameters to recreate an impression of the original object. As in art, digital images are conceptual as opposed to exact physical replications, and they consist of four key components: pixels, color, file formats, and data compression.

2.2.1 Pixels

Computer descriptions come in two basic varieties: vector based and pixel based [1]. Vector based images use mathematical equations to describe the image. These are generally compact (small file sizes), and therefore are not very efficient at conveying large amounts of small detail.

Digital photographs are usually pixel-based images. Each pixel represents a single point in a graphic image – similar to dots in halftones or in grains of film. Both the physical size of the pixels and their density on the imaging chip can affect their ability to resolve fine detail. In the simplest of examples, these pixels can be turned on or off, in which case they can be distributed to create a black and white image. Of course, the greater the number of pixels, the finer the detail that can be resolved (Fig. 2.3).

A larger computer file is required to describe a larger collection of pixels. In telemedicine applications, the quest for larger files that produce finer clinical details must be balanced with telemedicine transmission requirements that favor more compact files.

For more tonal variety, each pixel can be expressed using multiple shades of grey. The number of shades represented is called the *bit depth* of the image. If only pure black and white are used to create the image, then the bit depth is two (Fig. 2.4).

Current international computer standards define an eight-bit system with 256 (2^8) different shades of grey as possible at each pixel. More expensive 16-bit (2^{16} or 65,536 shades of grey) imaging systems are commercially available, but their expense limits their use to specialized applications. Just as black and white bit depth affects ability to represent small changes in grey scales, the bit depth of color images affects ability to distinguish subtle colors.

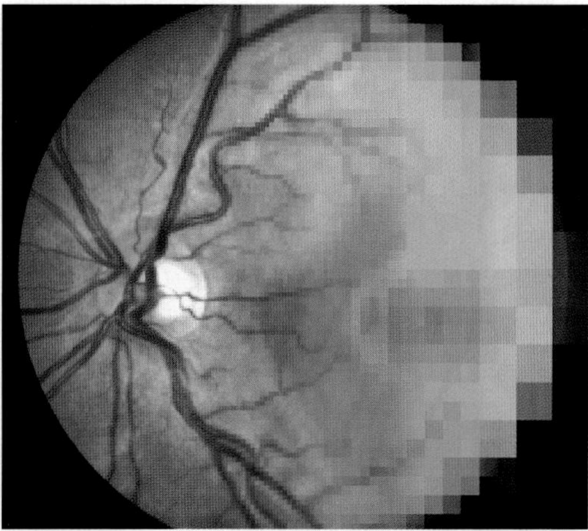

Fig. 2.3. Detail in this retinal photograph decreases from left to right as the relative size of the pixels increase, and the relative number of pixels decrease. Larger numbers of pixels usually mean greater detail

2.2.2 Color

Designating each pixel to one of three additive primary colors creates a color digital image, with the eight-bit gray scale image providing a building block for the 24-bit color image (there are eight bits each for red, blue, and green channels). This is accomplished on the digital imaging chip by overlaying a matrix of colored filters. The Bayer Mosaic (BM) describes the pattern used most often: a green pixel is alternated with either red or blue in the horizontal and the vertical direction (Figs. 2.5 and 2.6).

In most circumstances, the green channel resolves the finest detail; red contains the next largest amount of information; blue the least (Fig. 2.6). Two circumstances prevent the preponderance of green pixels from overwhelming information from the other colors in the final image. First, the information from each pixel is recorded in two ways: as an absolute value (white, light grey, dark grey, black) for that particular pixel, and also as a color driven value (white, light green, dark green, black). The camera digitally processes the image before it is output to the display device; at this point, it assigns green, red, and blue values to each and every pixel based on either the actual pixel value, or on extrapolated values obtained from information inherent in adjacent pixels. The result is a more color-balanced output to the monitor that uses evenly alternating green, red, and blue points to convey the information.

If a single color is represented in the computer by one of 16 million Red, Green, Blue (RGB) values, then the universe of these values can be defined as the "color space." The Commission Internationale d'Eclairage (CIE) color model represents a standard set of color values (referred to as the *human eye's color space*) [2] as perceived by most normal-sighted individuals. Digital imaging (and also film) is physically unable to adequately represent each and every color within this set. The two most common color spaces used in digital imaging are subsets of the larger CIE color space: Adobe RGB 1998 and sRGB.

In Fig. 2.7, notice that Adobe RGB contains additional sensitivity in the green area of the spectrum. These color spaces describe values that are available in digital color sensors and color monitors that use the RGB model; they are not

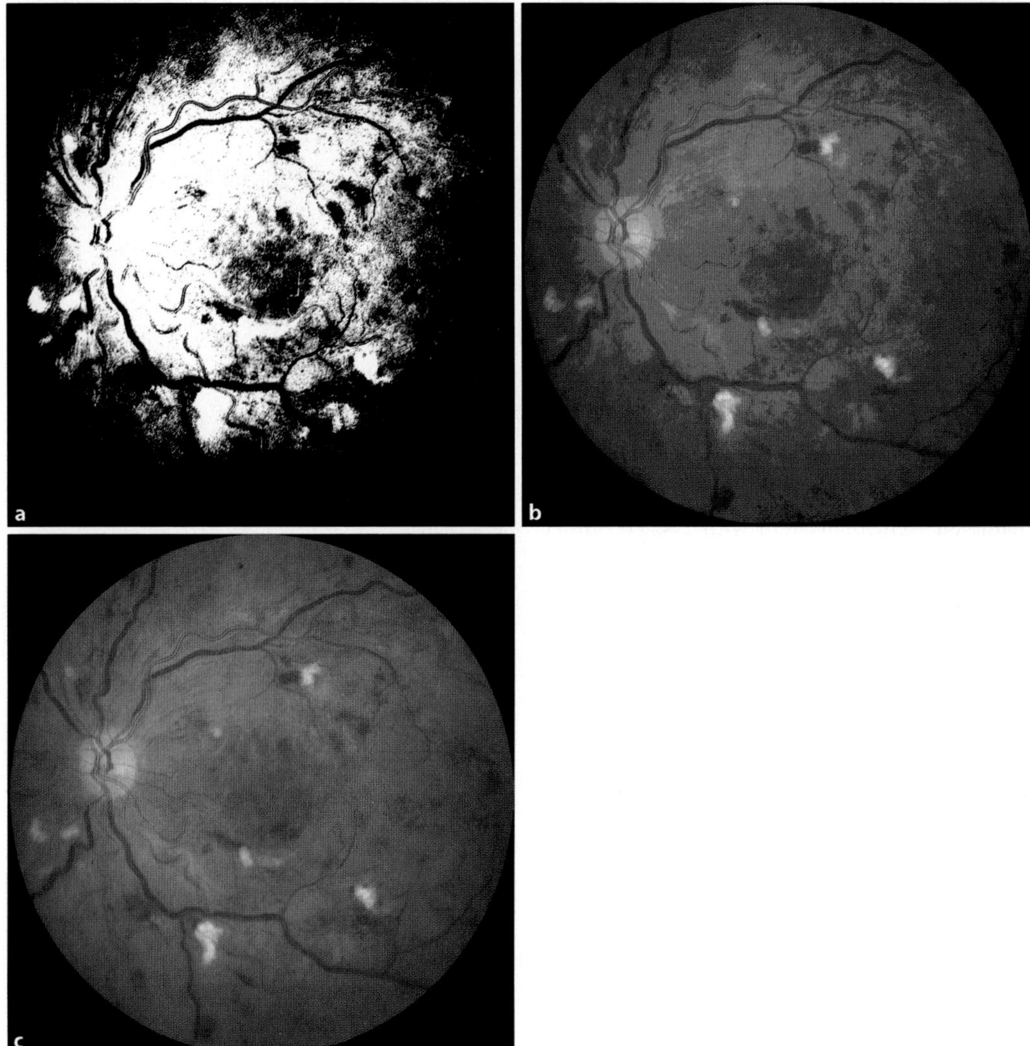

Fig. 2.4. Comparison of the ability to distinguish fine color gradations and bit depth as it increases from (**a**) two bit (pure black + pure white) to (**b**) four bit ($2^4 = 16$ colors) to (**c**) 24 bit ($2^{24} = 16\,777\,216$ different colors)

available in printed material that uses the CMYK (cyan, magenta, yellow, and black) color model.

It would seem that defining color using a numerical-based system would further our pursuit for precision and color accuracy. But different sensors and different monitors may represent the same numerical value in different ways – in the same way that different films from different manufacturers, different films from the same manufacturer, and even different emulsion batches of the same film from the same manufacturer, register colors slightly differently. Calibrating color input (camera settings) and output (monitor settings) at all telemedicine sites is an important step toward ensuring that all involved parties are making decisions based on similar visual information.

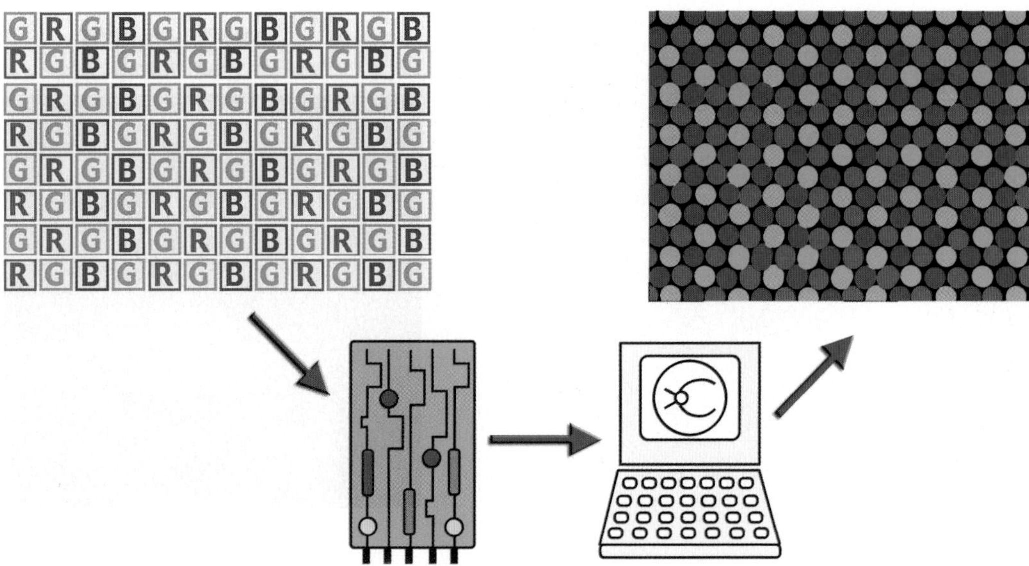

Fig. 2.5. Digital camera-based example of captured information using the Bayer pattern – a checkerboard design with 50% green, 25% red, and 25% blue filters (*left*). The computer interpolates this information and outputs it in equal parts of green (33%), red (33%), and blue (33%) (*right*)

2.2.3 File Formats

Each image, description of physical space, and set of directions for making a picture must be compiled so that the information can be easily read on multiple computers. This writing convention is defined by the *file format* of the image. There are literally hundreds of different file formats in use today. The four most popular formats are: .tif (Tagged Image File Format, TIFF); .jpg (Joint Photographic Experts Group, JPEG); .pdf (Portable Document Format, PDF), and; .gif (Graphic Interface File, GIF). Files written in the .tif format are usually large, because each separate pixel is individually described. A 300 pixels-per-inch .tif file to size is the standard requested by most high quality, glossy publications. A .jpg file is a *lossy* compressed image file, and it does not contain all of the information of the original image description. The .jpg compression standard calls for first deleting non-critical information by rounding and removing redundant information, then ordering the information using Huffman encoding, converting to sRGB color space, and sub-sampling. Artifacts can be easily seen when high .jpg compression ratios are used (Fig. 2.8).

A 72 pixels-per-inch .jpg file to size is the web publication standard, while a 1,000 pixel by 750 pixel .jpg file is the standard for PowerPoint and similar electronic presentations. A .pdf file, which is really a combination of files that was developed for the publishing industry, combines text information with .jpg images. Optical coherence tomography is an example of an ophthalmic instrument that can output information in .pdf format. A .gif is a pixel-based file format that incorporates *dithering* to make the most of its minimal eight-bit (256 colors) range. This format is widely used for small web graphics, but is rarely used to convey ophthalmic information. Table 2.1 summarizes common file formats and their uses.

2.2.4 Data Compression

An important imaging concept is the relationship between the amount and type of image compression and the quality of the information that is transferred. The speed of information transfer is called *bandwidth*. Because bandwidth is limited, telemedicine image files are often compressed,

Fig. 2.6. Three individual channels – green, red, and blue – that compose a color .tif image. Each channel contributes specific tonal information to the final image

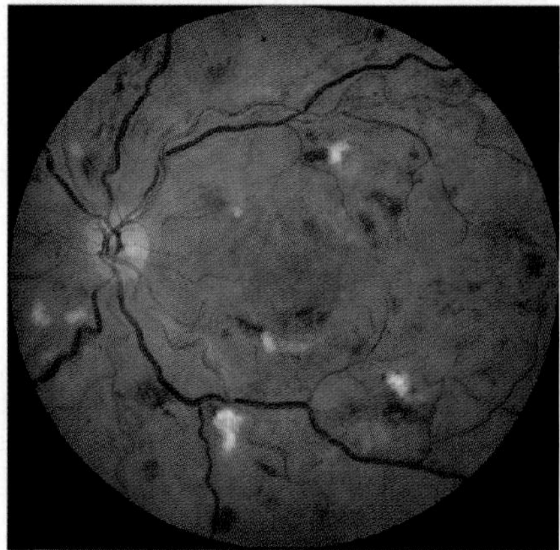

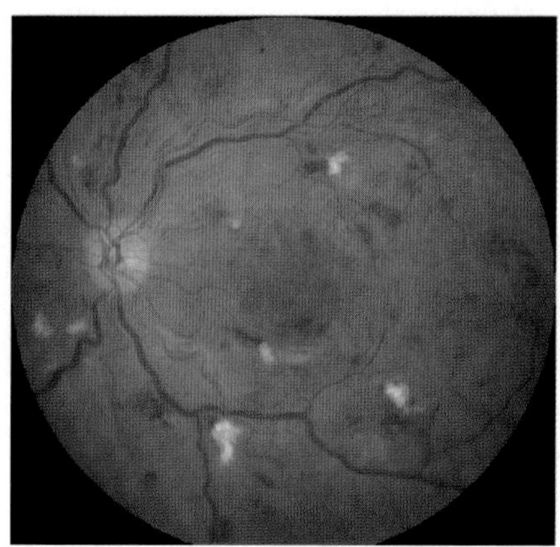

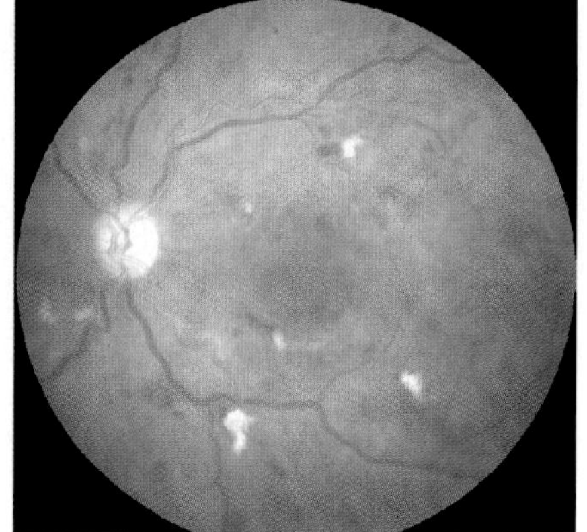

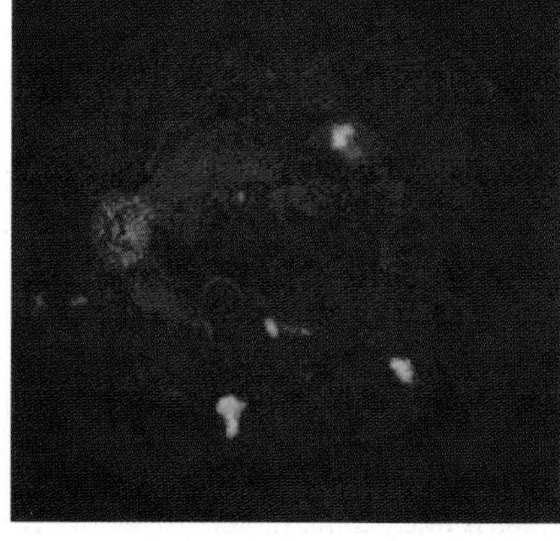

Table 2.1. Common file formats and their uses

Image type	File use	Preferred format	Comments
Continuous tone photograph	Archived master image	.tif, raw	Highest available resolution
Continuous tone photograph	Publication	.tif	300 DPI at printed size
Continuous tone photograph	Presentation (PowerPoint)	.jpg	100 DPI sized at 10 × 7.5"
Continuous tone photograph	E-mail, WWW	.jpg	72–96 DPI at screen size
Line-art/graphic	WWW	.gif	Low bit depth format
Document with text and images	Electronic distribution	.pdf	Not for archiving: uses .jpg images

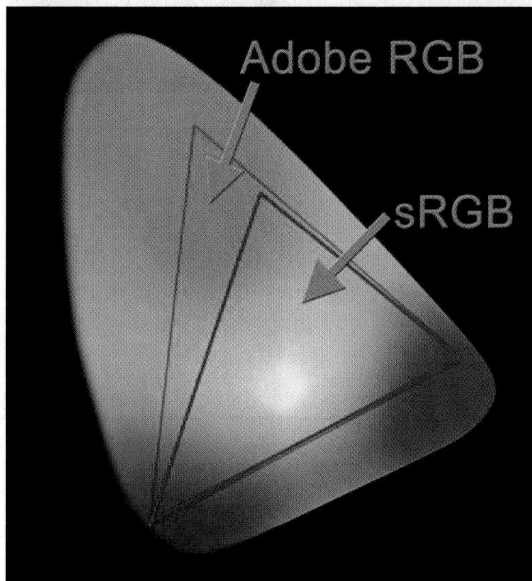

Fig. 2.7. Example of Commission Internationale de l'Eclarage (CIE) color space, which represents the full range of color seen by a standard human observer. Color digital imaging can represent a subset of these colors by implementing either the smaller sRGB color space or the larger Adobe 1998 color space

which reduces image file size. This can be accomplished in one of two ways: via *lossless* or *lossy* compression schemes. The following analogy explains the difference between the two. Imagine conveying the information contained in the image of this page of text. You could list the letters involved, include their size and order, define the space they take up as black, and then specify that the rest of the image is white. This set of directions is likely to be smaller than specifying each and every data point in a pixel based image file of the page. When the image is reconstituted, this lossless compression will convey the same information as the original image of the text page.

A second lossy method of compressing the same information might assume that the letters *i* and *l* look very similar, which makes it possible to replace each *i* with an *l*. This reduces the number of different letters involved, making the resulting file smaller. As this letter replacement compression scheme continues, the letters *n* and *m* can be paired, as can the letters *d* and *b*; *c*, *e*, and *o*; and so on. As letters are continually replaced, the meaning of the original page becomes more and more difficult to read, which is a problem that is inherent in implementing lossy compression. While ophthalmic images certainly can be compressed to very small sizes that are easy to transfer, care must be taken that the information to be conveyed is not lost in the process.

The problem of using image compression to reduce the size of medical images has been researched by a number of specialties – with varied results. For instance, Koenig studied dental lesions and concluded "JPEG compression does not impact detectability of artificial periapical lesions at low and moderate compression ratios up to and including 28:1" [3]. A recent paper by Stellingwerf concluded "the compression of the digital images seems to have some adverse effect on the detection of diabetic retinopathy" [4]. Beal's radiology study concluded "five of six radiologists had a higher diagnostic accuracy when interpreting uncompressed chest radiographs versus the same images modified by 10:1 lossy

2

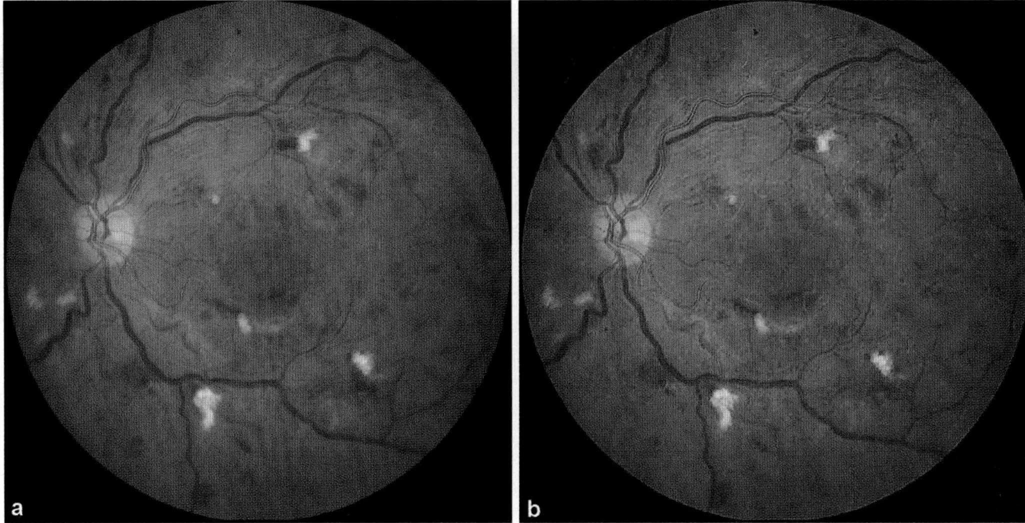

Fig. 2.8. Proper resolution fundus photograph with lost sharpness and color because: (**a**) of overcompression using a lossy file formator (**b**) multiple saves in lossy compression formats degrades images

compression, but this difference was not statistically significant" [5]. Because digital imaging compression is still an evolving technology, expert clinical judgment may be the best guide in resolving limitations.

2.3 Digital Ophthalmic Photography Instrumentation

Ophthalmic imaging encompasses a wide range of photographic modalities, each of which is designed to capture a specific type of visual information. General cameras with macro lenses are used to image oculoplastic conditions and strabismus. Slit lamp cameras illustrate the anterior segment, and fundus cameras image the posterior segment [6, 7].

2.3.1 External Photography

External ocular photography documents the external eye, lids, and ocular adnexa. Professional grade digital cameras with high quality, close focusing capabilities are required. The challenge of external photography is that it appears to be so easy. But unless careful steps are taken to accurately capture visual information such as tissue size, color, position, asymmetry, motion, and modification, photographs could display false color, distorted perspective, or insufficient information.

Preferred camera angles, magnification, and backgrounds should be standardized during the image capture process. Specific digital camera recommendations quickly become outdated as the industry continues to evolve at a rapid pace. The lowest priced digital single-lens reflex (SLR) camera that is compatible with traditional film SLR lenses is currently priced below US$1,000. These 6–14 megapixel cameras provide appropriate color reproduction and resolution for medical imaging projects. Large image files should not be a cause for concern if the computer and storage media is kept up to current specifications.

The purpose of the image also affects the choice of capture resolution. For instance, a publication quality 7"×10", 300 dots per inch (DPI) .tif file requires a six megapixel capture, while a screen resolution (web/PowerPoint use) 7"×10" 72 DPI image requires only a one megapixel capture resolution.

Inexpensive consumer cameras (1–2 megapixel) should be avoided, as their low pixel res-

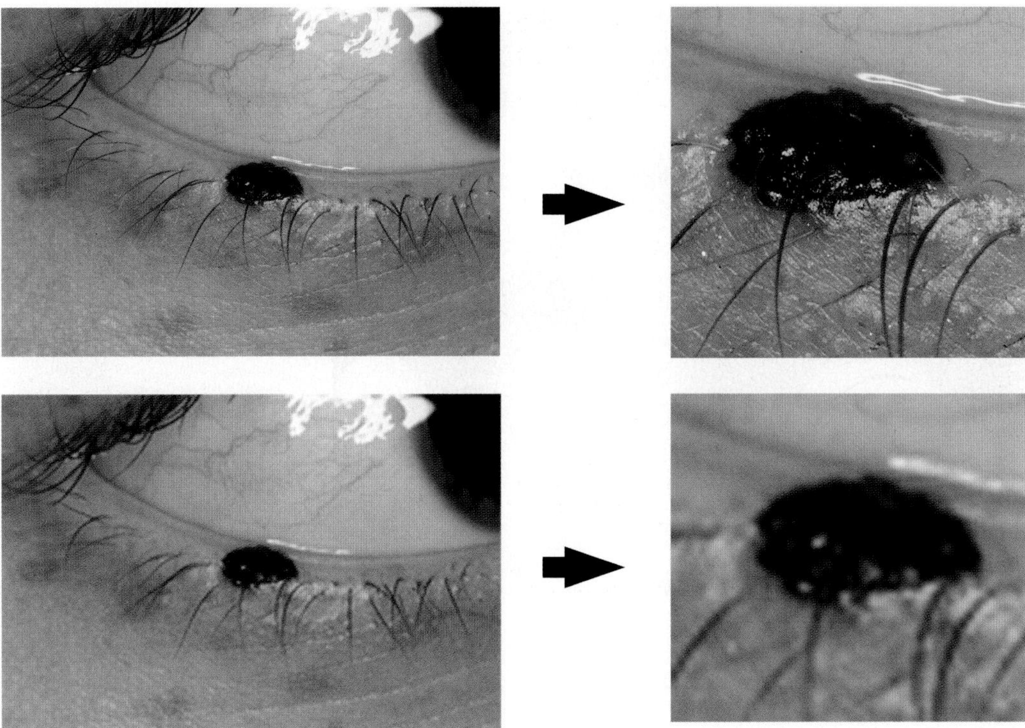

Fig. 2.9. High resolution, eight megapixel image of lid lesion loses little when enlarged (*top*), while the enlarged one megapixel image loses contrast and detail (*bottom*).

olution will not adequately capture fine detail (Fig. 2.9).

A mid- or high-range rangefinder-type consumer digital camera (4–8 or above megapixels) may be useful; however, the suitability of the camera's macro focusing function should be checked for any wide angle distortion when focusing closely. Other considerations are the electronic viewfinder of the digital camera, which can be used to overcome any parallax error that may be evident in the optical viewfinder; the ease with which settings can be changed; and the ease with which appropriate image download and transfer procedures can be planned.

2.3.2 Imaging the Anterior Segment

A photo slit lamp is required to image the anterior segment. While standard cameras may provide adequate magnification, it is effectively capturing the slit illumination that maximizes the information.

There are essential technique differences between corneal examination and slit lamp photography. The slit lamp examination is a dynamic process. As you drag the slit across the cornea, changing the illumination, magnification and angle of approach, making these and other fine adjustments – a synopsis or a *movie* of the cornea is created. The final impression gained after a slit lamp examination is not based on any single view, but is rather an accumulation of the pertinent details. Slit lamp photography, on the other hand, is by nature a detail. A slit lamp photograph is a *snapshot*. It is information from a single moment; a single frame from the movie. While this limitation can be overcome by using multiple photographs to tell a *picture story*, each single photograph is still limited to conveying a single visual statement.

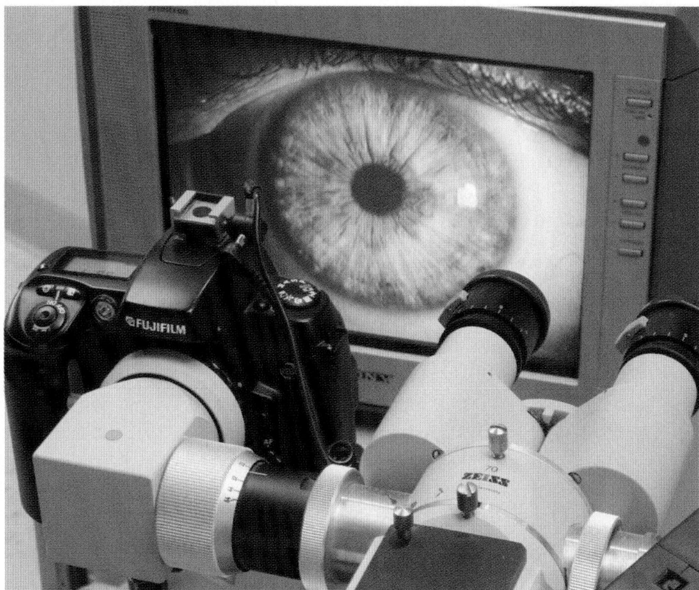

Fig. 2.10. Vintage Zeiss photo slit lamps can be converted to effective digital telemedicine tools by integrating new digital single lens reflex camera bodies

Subtle differences in color and detail exist between corneal examination and photography. The dynamic range appreciated by the examiner at the slit lamp is much greater than the dynamic range that can be captured digitally. This means that structures outside the slit beam that may be quite visible while viewing through the oculars are very dark and indistinguishable when recorded with the camera. The photo slit lamp's background illumination flash adds fill light, which helps to brighten the shadow areas of the image, creating photographs that more closely resemble the cornea during a slit lamp examination.

Multiple instruments are available for anterior segment imaging. The lowest tech solution is to adapt a digital snapshot camera to a standard slit lamp [8]. To do this, the digital camera should be focused on infinity, and aligned to the ocular; the camera's liquid crystal display (LCD) should be used to monitor the image. Note that this method may be awkward in practical terms. To compensate, an adapter may be constructed to facilitate alignment.

Another solution is to refurbish a traditional Zeiss photo slit lamp. While this unit is no longer manufactured, it was popular for years, so is still generally available (Fig. 2.10). The film SLR body can easily be replaced with a newer digital SLR body [9]. Alternately, both Haag Streit and Topcon have recently introduced digital photo slit lamps (Fig. 2.11). Video based slit lamp imaging instruments generally have too little resolution for quality work. By increasing magnification and capturing several fields it is possible to overcome limitations of resolution with video capture. For example, by setting magnification to 40× on a Haag Streit BQ slit lamp, the 640 × 480 resolution is comparable to a higher resolution image from a Haag Streit BM slit lamp; however, illumination must be increased in order to capture higher magnification images.

If only a few images are required, and image quality is not critical, the slit lamp light source should be turned to its maximum setting and photographed with a close focusing hand held digital camera. At the same time, the color balance should be set to *tungsten* to avoid yellow images. Multiple images may be required to obtain the best focus and proper composition.

2.3.3 Imaging the Fundus

The optical instrument used to visually document the retina is called a fundus camera. Fundus cameras are often described by the angle of

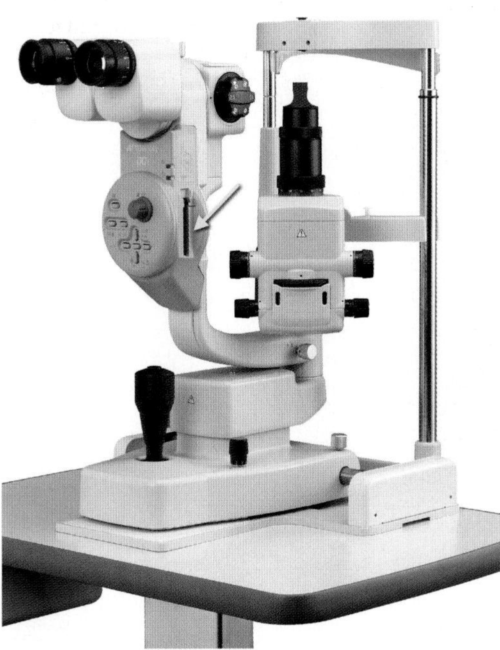

Fig. 2.11. Newer photo slit lamps, like this Topcon SL-D2, incorporate a digital camera that writes directly to a compact flash card (*arrow*) (image courtesy of Topcon America Corporation, Paramus, New Jersey)

view – the optical angle of acceptance of the lens. An angle of 30°, considered the normal angle of view, creates a film image 2.5 times larger than life. Wide-angle fundus cameras image between 45° and 140° and provide proportionately less retinal magnification. A narrow-angle fundus camera has an angle of view of 20° or less. Normal-angle cameras have smaller illuminating annuli, making them more suitable for patients with pupils of a smaller diameter. The inner diameter of the illuminating ring in wide-angle cameras is larger, which makes it harder to photograph patients with small pupils.

Fundus cameras can be described as either mydriatic and non-mydriatic. Mydriatic fundus cameras require pharmacologic dilation, while non-mydriatic fundus cameras use an infrared viewing system to exploit the patient's natural dilation in a dark room. Infrared light is used to preview the retina on a video monitor. Once the monitor's image is focused and aligned, photographic technology takes over: a flash is fired and the image is exposed. Most users describe more consistent photographs when patients have been dilated with 1% Mydriacyl (tropicamide) [10].

The non-mydriatic fundus camera was pioneered by Canon in the late 1970s, and by the mid-1980s, Canon, Kowa, Reichert, and Topcon were marketing various models. The typical angle of view of a non-mydriatic fundus camera is 45°. While traditionally used for screening purposes, newer diabetic screening devices (DSD) substitute digitally databased electronic images for traditional Polaroid and 35-mm film [11]. Currently available *non-myds* use 1–8 Mb digital chips to capture retinal images. Images are displayed on built-in LCD monitors and output to compact flash memory cards (CFMC) or a database via a universal serial bus (USB) connection. An advantage of these newer models is that their small chips function better in lower light levels than traditional film, making the flash less bright and maximal dilation less of an issue.

Still, it's a good idea to keep two spare viewing lights, flash tubes, and fuses readily available.

The fundus camera's instruction manual will contain detailed installation procedures. Fundus cameras that are used daily should have yearly inspections by factory-trained technicians. Alternately, contact the manufacturer's technical representative, and consider returning the camera to the factory for complete optical realignment and refurbishment every 5–10 years; mobile cameras may need service more often.

A medium-priced multiple-angle fundus camera offers respectable sharpness in a variety of optical angles and is suitable for a general ophthalmic practice. Built for performance first and price second, the normal-angle fundus camera is favored by the retinal specialist, because it is designed to produce sharp photographs of the macula, which it does extremely well. Its small illumination doughnut facilitates photographing through narrow pupils, and the astigmatic compensation device is useful for far peripheral views. Special-use fundus cameras include: extreme wide-angle, simultaneous stereo, and hand-held fundus cameras. If no angiography is involved, a digital non-mydriatic fundus camera is a good choice for telemedicine (Fig. 2.12).

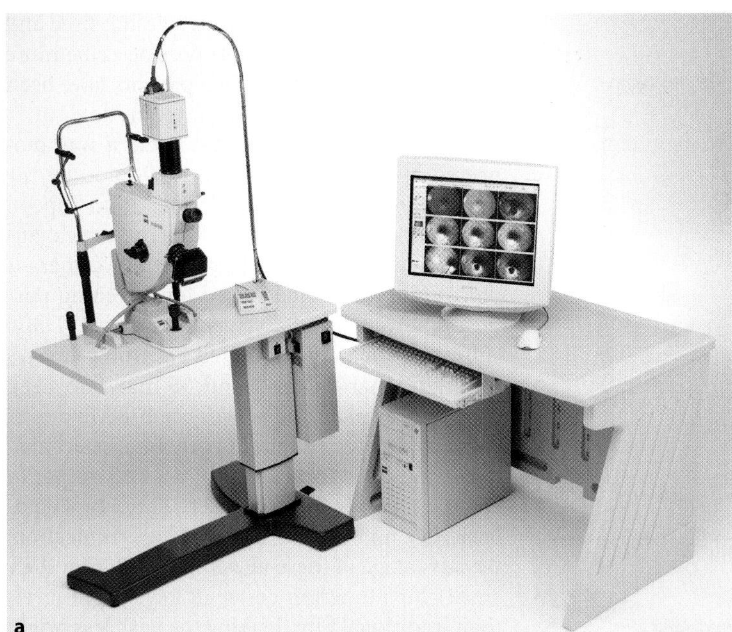

Fig. 2.12 a.

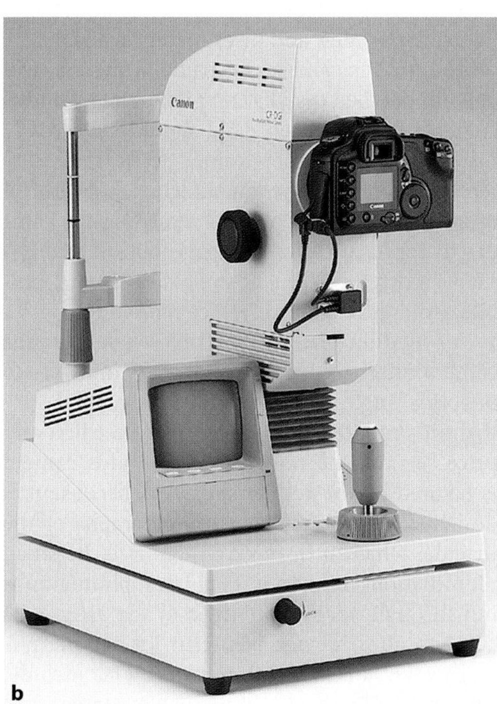

Fig. 2.12. Fundus cameras that are new, whether standard angiography models (**a**) or non-mydriatic (**b**), are available with digital output. Some models were developed specifically for telemedicine applications. Images courtesy of Carl Zeiss Meditec, Dublin, California (**a**); Canon USA, Lake Success, New York (**b**); and Topcon America Corporation, Paramus, New Jersey (**c**)

Fig. 2.12 c.

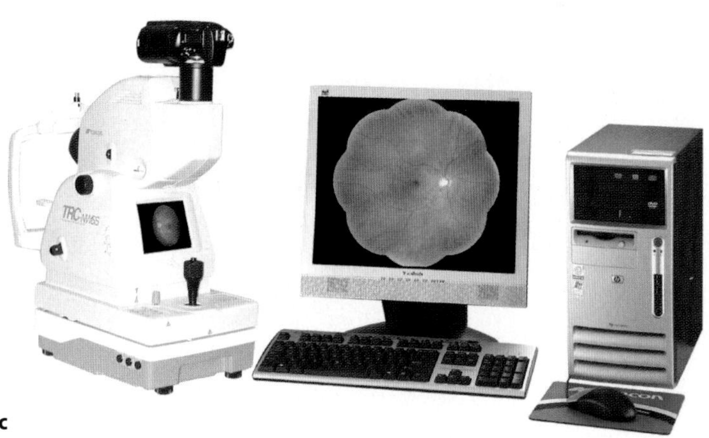

Most new fundus cameras are available as digital imaging instruments. Recent instruments (1998 or newer) and the widely available Zeiss FF series fundus camera can usually be converted from film to digital imaging [12].

References

1. Tyler ME, Saine PJ, Bennett TM (2003) Practical retinal photography and digital imaging techniques. Butterworth-Heinemann, Boston
2. Zwimpfer M (1988) Color, light, sight, sense: theory of color in pictures. Schiffer, West Chester, PA
3. Koenig L, Parks E, Analoui M, Eckert G (2004) The impact of image compression on diagnostic quality of digital images for detection of chemically-induced periapical lesions. Dentomaxillofac Radiol Suppl 33(1):37–43
4. Stellingwerf C, Hardus PL, Hooymans JM (2004) Assessing diabetic retinopathy using two-field digital photography and the influence of JPEG-compression. Doc Ophthalmol 108(3):203–209
5. Beall DP, Shelton PD, Kinsey TV, Horton MC, Fortman BJ, Achenbach S, Smirnoff V, Courneya DL, Carpenter B, Gironda JT (2000) Image compression and chest radiograph interpretation: image perception comparison between uncompressed chest radiographs and chest radiographs stored using 10:1 JPEG compression. J Digital Imaging 13(2 Suppl 1):33 –38
6. Martonyi CL, Bahn CF, Meyer RF (1985) Clinical slit lamp biomicroscopy and photo slit lamp biomicrography. Time One Ink, Ann Arbor, MI
7. Saine PJ, Tyler ME (2001) Ophthalmic photography: retinal photography, angiography and electronic imaging. Butterworth-Heinemann, Boston
8. Fogla R, Rao SK (2003) Ophthalmic photography using a digital camera. Indian J Ophthalmol 51(3):269–272
9. Tyler ME , Michalec GS (2005) Digital Stereo Slit-Lamp Imaging. J Ophthalmic Photogr 7(2), in press
10. Wade M, Barry C, McAllister I (1998) Diabetic retinopathy screening in remote Australian communities with non-mydriatic fundus cameras. J Ophthalmic Photogr 20(3):80–83
11. Bursell SE, Cavallerano JD, Cavallerano AA, et al. (2001) Stereo nonmydriatic digital-video color retinal imaging compared with early treatment diabetic retinopathy study seven standard field 35-mm stereo color photos for determining level of diabetic retinopathy. Ophthalmology 108:572–585
12. Scott JR (2002) An affordable alternative to the high cost of digital fundus photography. J Ophthalmic Photogr 24(2):55–58

Chapter 3

The DICOM Standard and Teleophthalmology– Striving for Interoperability

3

P. Lloyd Hildebrand

This chapter addresses the following

Key Concepts:

- Guidelines and rules provide standards for a common protocol that allows interconnecting processes to run smoothly.
- There is a need to adopt standards for medical informatics that facilitate remote care and interoperability across health care information systems, including telemedicine.
- The Digital Imaging and Communications in Medicine (DICOM) standard is actively supported by many professional societies throughout the world, and has been incorporated by most major diagnostic medical imaging vendors.
- DICOM is used, or will soon be used, by virtually every medical profession that uses digital imaging.

3.1 Introduction

The rapid proliferation of digital information technologies in health care has fostered a growing global momentum for the adoption of medical informatics standards that facilitate remote care and interoperability across health care information systems, including telemedicine. In the United States (US), the Health Insurance Portability and Accountability Act (HIPAA) of 1996 required the adoption of uniform standards nationwide for electronic transmission of certain administrative and financial transactions. David Brailer, National Coordinator for Health Information Technology in the US, recently emphasized the need for "immediate attention from the Federal government as well as public and private sector participants" [1] with respect to interoperability standards and policies.

The National Health Service's (NHS) National Programme for Information Technology (NPIT) in Great Britain has adopted and is deploying national medical informatics standards across its infrastructure to facilitate implementing secure electronic medical records, on-line scheduling, e-prescribing, quality and analyses systems, and image data storage and exchange [2]. Similar adoption and promulgation of standards is evident throughout the European Union (EU), Canada, Australia, New Zealand, and many other countries.

Standards provide guidelines and rules that serve as an invisible framework and common protocol, so that interconnecting processes can run smoothly. Standards evolve out of three main processes: legislative mandate; a consensus process whereby those impacted by standards join together and agree on elements of the standards; or de facto standards, whereby an overwhelming majority of users already apply a given method, making it a standard by acclamation. In addition, many medical information systems have evolved using local or regional coding system implementations, with limited ability to communicate outside their own system.

With widespread access to the Internet and wide area networks, broader standardization to facilitate information exchange is critical. In response, the industry is developing standards for both the administrative and clinical aspects of health care that address:

1. Identifier standards that universally and uniquely identify patients, providers, facilities, products, services, and supplies
2. Communication standards for facilitating, creating, and communicating messages
3. Content and structure standards that provide frameworks for electronic health records systems
4. Clinical data codes that document clinical activities
5. Standards for confidentiality, data security, and authentication
6. Standards for quality indicators, data sets, and practice guidelines

This chapter will focus on the Digital Imaging and Communications in Medicine (DICOM) digital imaging standard, and on critical and significant elements of ophthalmic telemedicine applications that have evolved since the year 2000.

3.2 Digital Imaging and Communications in Medicine (DICOM)Standard

The Digital Imaging and Communications in Medicine (DICOM) Standard Committee creates and maintains a standard for communication of biomedical diagnostic and therapeutic information in disciplines that use digital images and associated data. The goals of DICOM are to achieve compatibility and to improve workflow efficiency between imaging and other information systems in health care environments [3]. DICOM is developed through vendor and user collaboration. Most major diagnostic medical imaging vendors have incorporated standards established by DICOM; additionally, many professional societies world-wide actively support and participate in enhancing standards created by DICOM.

Seeking to create a standard method for the transmission of digital radiology images, the DICOM standard evolved out of a collaboration between the American College of Radiology (ACR) and the National Electrical Manufacturers Association (NEMA) in the late 1980s [4]. Prior to this, the communication of images was achieved by storing them in a proprietary format, then transferring files of these proprietary formats over a network, or on removable media. While the initial versions of the ACR-NEMA effort created standardized terminology, an information structure, and unsanctioned file encoding, the promise of a standard method of communicating digital image information was not fully realized until the release of version 3.0 of the Standard in 1993, which also included a name change to DICOM [5].

The new DICOM Standard [6] was composed of three critical components: Image Object Definitions (IODs), Service Classes (the semantics of commands and associated data), and a network protocol using Transmission Control Protocol/Internet Protocol (TCP/IP). The new Standard included a unique mechanism for identifying Information Objects (images, patients, studies, reports, and other data image-related data groups), and defined the operation of Service Classes beyond the simple transfer of data (e.g., printing, queries).

The Standard was also restructured as a multi-part document, designed to facilitate its extension. These enhancements permitted the transfer of medical images in a multi-vendor environment, and also facilitated the evolution and expansion of Picture Archiving and Communication Systems (PACS) with interfaces to medical information systems (MIS) [7]. In 1996, the DICOM Standards Committee was expanded beyond radiology to include all domains of biomedical imaging including ophthalmic imaging.

Today, DICOM is used – or will soon be used – by virtually every medical profession that uses digital imaging, including ophthalmology, cardiology, orthopedics, pathology, pediatrics, surgery, dentistry, and specialties using endoscopy, mammography, radiation therapy, and radiology [8]; it is even used in veterinary medical imaging applications [9]. DICOM also addresses the integration of information in the patient's electronic health record (EHR) that is produced by these various specialty applications. It also defines the network and media interchange services, allowing storage and access to these DICOM objects for electronic health record systems.

3.3 Technical Overview

The DICOM Standard supports the exchange of information by using a network model, as well as interchange media. Independent of the physical network, DICOM currently defines an upper layer protocol for use over TCP/IP messages, services, information objects, and an association negotiation mechanism. These definitions ensure that any two implementations of a compatible set of services and information objects can effectively communicate.

Independence from the underlying network technology allows DICOM to be deployed in many functional areas of application that include, but are not limited to: communication within a single site (often using various forms of Ethernet); between sites, over leased lines, or Virtual Private Networks (VPNs); within a metropolitan area (often using asynchronous transfer mode); across dial-up or other remote access connections (such as by modem, ISDN or Digital Subscriber Line (DSL)); and via satellite (with optimized protocol stacks to account for increased latency) [10].

3.3.1 Services and Information

At the application layer, services and information objects address five primary areas of functionality:

- Transmission and persistence of complete objects (images, waveforms and documents)
- Query and retrieval of these objects
- Performance of specific actions such as hardcopy output of images
- Workflow management (support of worklists and status information)
- Quality and consistency of image appearance (both for display and print)

DICOM can be considered a standard for communication that crosses "boundaries" between heterogeneous, as well as disparate applications, devices, and systems. However, it does not define an entire system architecture, nor does it specify functional requirements beyond the behavior defined for specific services. For example, storage of image objects is defined in terms of the information that must be transmitted and retained, not how images are displayed or annotated.

An additional DICOM service is available that specifies how the image must be presented with annotations for the user [11]. The services and objects that are defined in DICOM are designed to address specific, real-world applications (such as the performance of an imaging st udy on an acquisition device). As such, DICOM is not a general-purpose tool for distributed object management, because information is transferred in bulk according to a document paradigm.

3.3.2 Addressing Challenges

Currently, pressing challenges in DICOM – as indicated by the priorities of the various working groups – that need to be addressed target issues relating to new modality technology, structured and coded documents for specific clinical domains, workflow management, security, and performance. These needs are being successfully addressed using conventional, underlying DICOM technology [12].

Where there are interfaces to standards based on other technologies (such as Health Level 7 (HL7), V2.x, and 3), the focus for harmonization is on a shared information model. When specific new technology is required, such as in support of new features such as security and compression, the strategy is to adopt proven international, industry, or de facto standards. Accordingly, network confidentiality and peer authentication in DICOM are provided by the use of either Transport Layer Security (an Internet standard) or Integrated Secure Communication Layer (an International Organization for Standardization (ISO)-based standard). Similarly, rather then develop medical-image-specific compression schemes, DICOM has adopted standards developed by ISO/IEC JTC 1/SC 29/WG 1 (the International Organization for Standardization), such as the JPEG Imaging Standard, and more recently, the JPEG 2000 family of imaging standards. For interchange media, standard file systems compatible with conventional software (such as ISO 9660 and Universal Disc Format) are used.

3.4 DICOM's Relationship to Other Standards

3

Throughout the development of DICOM, much attention has been devoted to establishing working relationships with other related standard initiatives throughout the world. This is reflected in the initial version of the the DIACOM Standard, which leveraged prior work by ASTM International (formerly the American Society for Testing and Materials); then the Internet protocol TCP/IP was adopted in 1993. In the 1990s, solid cooperation with the CEN, the European Committee for Standardization, resulted in a number of jointly developed supplements. Since then, CEN has created and approved a normative reference to the DICOM standard with EN 12052, an official European Norm.

The integration of a Japanese interchange media format (IS&C) with DICOM parallels the work of CEN, which required much collaboration with JIRA, the Japan Industries Association of Radiological Systems [13]. In the USA, DICOM participated in the early coordination efforts for health care standards with the American National Standards Institute (ANSI) Health Information and Surveillance Systems Board, from which DICOM adopted a harmonized patient name structure, and started proactively to define links with HL7. These collaborative efforts entered into a very active phase in 1999 with the creation of a joint DICOM-HL7 working group: a Type A liaison with the ISO Technical Committee 215. While the ISO TC 215 has decided not to create an imaging working group, it will rely on DICOM for biomedical imaging standards, and will create and approve a standard that will reference the DICOM standard, as CEN has done.

In 2003, the DICOM Standards Committee became a member of the E-health Standardization Coordination Group, a group endorsed by the International Telecommu-nication Union with the objective to promote a stronger coordination amongst the key players in the e-health standardization area. DICOM is also focusing its attention on the evolution of standards linked to the Internet, with the intention of integrating Internet recommendations as soon as they are stable and largely disseminated in consumer commercial products [14]. In this evolution, much care is taken to ensure that the consistency of the DICOM standard is maintained with its large installed base. DICOM already uses standard health care enterprise intranets, the e-mail exchange of DICOM objects (using a Standard Multipurpose Internet Mail Extensions type) is possible, and the Web Access to DICOM Persistent Objects service has been defined in a joint effort with ISO TC215. It is clear that the use of DICOM objects and services in commonly used information technology applications will grow in the future, given the world-wide ambition in health care to create Electronic Health Records. DICOM also maintains a strong relationship with the Integrating the Healthcare Enterprise initiative, where profiles of standards are defined as solutions for health care workflow and enterprise integration challenges.

3.5 DICOM's Organizational Structure

DICOM is a standards organization administered by the NEMA Diagnostic Imaging and Therapy Systems Division. The complete bylaws of the DICOM Standards Committee are available on the NEMA web site at medical.nema.org [15]. Working groups of the DICOM Standards Committee perform the majority of work on the extension of and corrections to the Standard. Working groups are formed by the DICOM Committee to work on a particular classification of tasks. Once formed, working groups petition the DICOM Standards Committee to approve work items for which the working group will execute the plan delineated in the work item. After the output of a work item (generally a supplement or correction proposal) has been completed, it is submitted to the Base Standards Working Group (WG-06) for their review. To become a supplement to the Standard, the item is submitted to the public for comments. If approved, the DICOM Committee authorizes the supplement for letter ballot, which requires two thirds of DICOM members to vote affirmatively or negatively. Since the working groups perform the majority of work on the extension of and corrections to the Standard, the current status and future directions of the

DICOM Standard are best represented by review of each working group.

3.6 Ophthalmic Extensions of DICOM

DICOM Working Group 9 (WG-9) is dedicated to enhancing the standard for ophthalmic applications. Two important extensions of the DICOM Standard that are specifically applicable to ophthalmic digital imaging have been fully integrated: (1) the definition of "visible light image object," [16] and (2) the definition of "ophthalmic photography image object" [17].

There is also a current work item to develop an image object definition (IOD) for ophthalmic coherence tomography [18]. Additionally, in collaboration with other specialty organizations that use non x-ray/ultrasound visible light imaging (pathology, gastroenterology, dentistry), ophthalmologists are developing an extension to the DICOM Standard – an IOD for visible light imaging.

References

1. Brailer D (2005) Health Information Technology HIMSS. http://www.hhs.gov/healthit/BrailerSpch05.html. Cited 4 Oct 2005
2. Business Plan Summary 2005-2006 (2005) Connecting for Health: National Health Service.http://www.connectingforhealth.nhs.uk/publications/nhs_cfh_business_plan_summary. pdf. Cited 4 Oct 2005
3. The DICOM Standards Committee (2004) Digital imaging and communications in medicine standard, part 1: introduction and overview. National Electrical Manufacturers Association, Rosslyn, VA, pp 9–10
4. Best DE, Horii SC, Bennett W, Thomson B, Snavely D (1992) Review of the American College of Radiology–National Electrical Manufacturers Association standards activity. Comput Meth Programs Biomed 37(4):305–309
5. The DICOM Standards Committee (2004) Digital imaging and communications in medicine standard, part 1: introduction and overview. National Electrical Manufacturers Association, Rosslyn, VA, p 5
6. The DICOM Standard (2005) http://medical.nema.org/dicom/2004.html. Cited 4 Oct 2005
7. The DICOM Standards Committee (2004) Digital imaging and communications in medicine standard, part 1: introduction and overview. National Electrical Manufacturers Association, Rosslyn, VA, pp 5–6
8. Bidgood WD, Horii SC (1996) Modular extension of the ACR-NEMA DICOM standard to support new diagnostic imaging modalities and services. J Digit Imaging 9(2):67–77
9. Bernardo TM, Malinowski RP(2005) Progress in the capture, manipulation, and delivery of medical media and its impact on education, clinical care, and research. J Vet Med Educ 32(1):21–30
10. Strategic Document (2005) http://medical.nema.org/dicom/geninfo/Strategy.htm. Cited 4 Oct 2005
11. Strategic Document (2005) http://medical.nema.org/dicom/geninfo/Strategy.htm. Cited 4 Oct 2005
12. Strategic Document (2005) http://medical.nema.org/dicom/geninfo/Strategy.htm. Cited 4 Oct 2005
13. Japan Industries Association of Radiological Systems (2004) http://www.jira-net.or.jp/e/index.htm. Cited 4 Oct 2005.
14. Strategic Document (2005) http://medical.nema.org/dicom/geninfo/Strategy.htm. Cited 4 Oct 2005
15. The DICOM Standard (2004) http://medical.nema.org/dicom/2004.html. Cited 4 Oct 2005
16. The DICOM Standards Committee (2004) Digital imaging and communications in medicine standard, part 3: image object definitions. National Electrical Manufacturers Association, Rosslyn, VA, pp 145–153
17. The DICOM Standards Committee (2004) Digital imaging and communications in medicine standard, part 3: image object definitions. National Electrical Manufacturers Association, Rosslyn, VA, pp 195–198
18. Work items approved by the DICOM Standards Committee (2004) http://medical.nema.org/dicom/geninfo/Work-Items-DSC.pdf. Cited 4 Oct 2005

Chapter 4

Stereopsis in Teleophthalmology

4

Chris J. Rudnisky, Matthew T. S. Tennant

This chapter addresses the following

Key Concepts:

- Stereopsis helps detect many three-dimensional abnormalities, such as diabetic macular edema, retinal neovascularization, exudative age-related macular degeneration (AMD), and glaucomatous cupping.
- A number of teleophthalmology systems have re-introduced stereopsis as part of the digital examination.
- Several methods are available to view digital stereo images, the simplest of which include (1) a side-by-side display that uses a specially-designed viewer, (2) analglyphs using glasses with an exact color match to the images, and (3) LCD shutter glasses.
- Stereoviewing software is available commercially as part of complete fundus camera systems.
- The necessity of stereopsis in teleophthalmology is still a contentious issue.

4.1 Introduction

Teleophthalmology attempts to recreate the clinical encounter, but at a distance. Stereopsis is an important aspect of the clinical encounter, as it helps to detect many three-dimensional abnormalities, such as diabetic macular edema, retinal neovascularization, exudative age-related macular degeneration (AMD), and glaucomatous cupping.

The concept of distant diagnosis in ophthalmology, or *teleophthalmology*, has been indirectly validated by large scale clinical trials [1–6] for its ability to track and record diabetic retinopathy, AMD, and glaucoma. The detection of three-dimensional pathology in these diseases is critical, and the incorporation of stereopsis is one technique by which the ability to diagnose disease is maximized.

Early teleophthalmology systems [7–14] utilized film to photograph the retina. Many of these early systems used a Polaroid camera coupled to a non-mydriatic fundus camera, making incorporation of stereo more difficult [7, 8, 10, 11, 14]. Today a number of teleophthalmology systems have re-introduced stereopsis as part of the digital examination.

Because a clinical examination provides binocular information via the slit-lamp and indirect ophthalmoscope, there are advantages to incorporating stereopsis into teleophthalmology systems. This is not without controversy, however, as many teleophthalmology groups believe that the advantages of stereopsis are outweighed by the difficulties inherent in capturing stereoscopic photographs. These groups have successfully developed monoscopic teleophthalmology systems [15–17], whereas other groups [18–20] continue to feel that stereopsis should be incorporated. The purpose of this chapter is to review the basics of stereoscopic photography, describe current stereoscopic teleophthalmology systems that have been described in the literature, and review issues regarding the incorporation of steropsis into teleophthalmology.

4.2 Methods of Stereoscopic Image Capture

In the following subsections we will discuss various techniques for capturing stereoscopic images.

4.2.1 Non-Simultaneous Technique

A stereophotograph has two images, one for each eye, that when viewed together provide three-dimensional information about the subject. The most common method of acquiring a stereophotograph is non-simultaneous capture via a corneal-induced parallax [21]. To create this, a photographer carefully lines up the fundus camera at one edge of the pupil, captures the first image of the stereopair, and then quickly moves the camera to the other edge of the pupil in order to capture the second image. Detailed and careful instruction to the patient is required to prevent refixation between images, which can result in a stereopair with variable three-dimensional information; in other words, patient refixation can alter the stereobase of the photographs, which is the main disadvantage of non-simultaneous techniques – variable stereobase.

Because most experienced photographers are able to obtain consistent, high quality results, in teleophthalmology applications, the skill level of the photographer becomes the limiting factor for consistent stereopsis. To minimize this effect, a retinal camera should maximize a photographer's ability to capture high quality retinal photographs, while minimizing photographic difficulty. Maberley et al. [22] showed that a non-mydriatic camera is easy to operate, irrespective of the experience of the operator. When combined with stereoscopic image capture, a non-mydriatic camera may be a very efficient solution.

To improve the quality variables inherent in manually acquired stereo photographs, *image splitters* have been developed. Mounted over the front barrel of a fundus camera, these devices allow capture of a stereo-image by movement of a glass plate. The glass plate works by optically shifting the viewpoint from which each image is captured, thereby providing the required image disparity needed for stereopsis. Because only the plate moves, the photographer need only line up the camera in one position, and then capture two non-simultaneous images.

The Allen stereo-separator is one example of an image-splitting device. The automated retinal imaging system (ARIS, Visual Pathways, Prescott, AZ) is yet another improvement on non-simultaneous stereoscopic imaging systems. Using a constant 2 mm stereobase, image shift is automated and occurs in approximately 65 ms. This compares with manually acquired photographs, which are temporally spaced two to three seconds apart. By providing autofocus and eye-tracking technology, the ARIS system efficiently and consistently captures quality stereophotographs.

4.2.2 Simultaneous Capture

Cameras that capture both images of a stereopair simultaneously have the advantage of a fixed stereo base. These cameras, such as the Nidek 3-Dx, typically use a separation of 3 mm (measured in the pupillary plane) to obtain simultaneous image pairs. Offered as both a standard fundus and non-mydriatic camera, it has the advantage of reproducibility. Nidek 3-Dx stereophotographs have shown efficacy for optic nerve head photography [23] and detection of clinically significant macular edema (CSME) [24].

4.3 Stereophotograph Viewing

Both film and digital methods are available for viewing film stereophotographs [25]. Slides can be placed side-by-side in 2×2 mounts and then viewed using either a Larson or Donaldson viewer. These viewers incorporate +5 diopter lenses as simple magnifiers, and are easy and straightforward to use. Some include built-in adjustability for viewers with different interpupillary distances.

More time-consuming methods are also available, such as the realist stereo slide mount, where photographs are meticulously placed to match the interpupillary distance of the viewer. Similarly, the View-Master disc is an option still in use for some ophthamic textbooks, but is not a practical one for clinical practice.

4.3.1 Digital

The following subsections cover a variety of methods for viewing stereo digital images.

4.3.1.1 Mirrored and Prismatic Viewers

Similar to film, there are a variety of methods to view stereo digital images. The simplest method is side-by-side display, in which two stereo images are displayed side-by-side on a monitor and then viewed using a specially designed viewer. These viewers use either a mirror or a prism to present the appropriate image to each eye. Images can also be displayed as over-under images, and then viewed with an appropriate mirror configuration to produce a stereoimage. Advantages of this technique are that there is no loss in color quality, image brightness, or image *ghosting*, wherein the information in one image is viewed by the other eye, thus decreasing the perceived stereoscopic information.

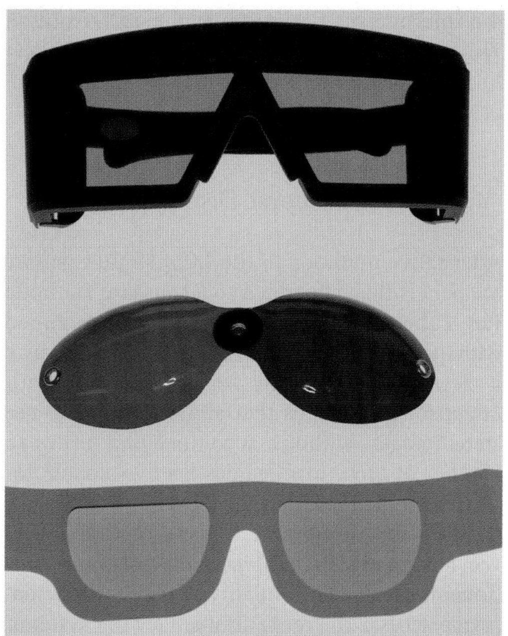

Fig. 4.1. Three different viewing systems for stereo photographs. From top to bottom, LCD shutter glasses, (StereoGraphics, Inc.) red-green anaglyph viewers, and polarized-lens glasses. LCD shutter glasses and anaglyph viewers can both be used for viewing digital stereo, whereas polarized lenses are used primarily for viewing film stereo photographs

4.3.1.2 Anaglyphs

Anaglyphs are stereoimages that present monochromatic images to each eye, with different colors used for each image. The most commonly used colors are red and green. Stereoimages are viewed using shutter glasses (Fig. 4.1) that utilize an exact color match to those used to create the image. This format has several disadvantages: (1) full-color images cannot be viewed with this technique, (2) viewers with color blindness may have difficulty appreciating the stereo effect, and (3) there may be ghosting due to inaccurate color matching. Instructions on how to create anaglyphs have been published on the Internet.

4.3.1.3 LCD Shutter Glasses

The most common method for stereo digital review are LCD shutter glasses (Fig. 4.1). This method requires a monitor with a high refresh rate, which enables the computer alternately to display the left and right images in rapid succession. To do this, the glasses are synchronized to the monitor, so that when the LCD shutter is activated before one eye – and therefore occluding it – the other eye is able to see its corresponding image. In other words, the left eye sees only the left image, and the right eye only the right image. Although the high refresh rate allows high-quality stereo to be viewed through the glasses, there is some cross-talk, or ghosting, that can degrade the stereo effect. However, by using phosphors with a fast decay rate, some manufacturers have developed displays that overcome this deficiency. With a faster decay rate, each image remains on the screen for a shorter amount of time, thereby decreasing the ghosting of each image. A limitation is that there may be a reduction in the amount of light that reaches the observer due to the intermittent occlusion of the LCD shutter. This may be a significant problem when viewing images that are captured with a shorter exposure or with a less intense flash.

4.3.1.4 Stereoscopic Displays

Alternative methods to the LCD shutter glasses are panels that can attach to a standard Cathode Ray Tube (CRT) computer monitor; combined with passive polarized eyewear, it can produce a viewable stereoimage. Also available are microlens array screens that allow a viewer to see stereoimages without accompanying eyewear. Neither of these formats has been evaluated for its teleophthalmology application.

The most important aspects of digital stereoviewing are the hardware and software components that facilitate quality display and efficient image access. The more simple viewing systems, such as the digital 2×2 mount, rely more on the viewer used than the computer hardware. The LCD shutter system requires a high-resolution CRT monitor that is capable of (1) refresh rates in excess of 100 Hz, (2) a high-end video card that can process two large digital image files quickly, and (3) a processor fast enough to integrate the two. However, there are commercial products that could work for teleophthalmology that perform at refresh rates of 70Hz (e.g., VRex).

Because computer processing speeds are constantly changing, the goal of a digital viewing system is to match hardware components so that the viewing of digital images is as easy as picking up two slide film photographs and placing them under a viewer. Stereoviewing software is available commercially as part of complete fundus camera systems, although sometimes, proprietary custom-designed software is used. Because stereoscopic viewing software specific to an ophthalmology application is not easily available – unless it is purchased as part of a commercial system – it is one of the more difficult aspects of creating a system independently.

4.4 Image Quality

The quality of any photograph depends on two variables: the camera and the film. In comparison between film and digital formats, film has been estimated to have a resolution equivalent of up to 11 megapixels. This estimate is based on the detail that 100 ISO, 35 mm film can provide before one is able to resolve the grain of the film. Considerable research has been done that compares digital photography to film. When evaluating the benefits of each, it is imperative to consider the fundus camera, photographic protocol, and the resolution of the digital back.

4.5 Stereoscopic Teleophthalmology Systems

The following subsections discusses teleophthalmology systems at various universities and organizations.

4.5.1 University of Alberta

This group is involved in the application of teleophthalmology to diabetic retinopathy, age-related macular degeneration, glaucoma, and hereditary retinal disorders [20, 26–28]. It works by capturing non-simultaneous digital images (six megapixel) of the disc and macula, while non-stereoscopic images are captured of the peripheral retina.

Evaluative studies [27, 20, 28] of this system have shown good correlation between stereo digital and stereo film for identifying most features of diabetic retinopathy. In particular, the identification of clinically significant macular edema (CSME) with this teleophthalmology system was found to correlate well with contact lens biomicroscopy (sensitivity 90.6%, specificity 90.4%, $\kappa=0.812$) [27]. This finding is significant, because it indicates that a stereoscopic teleophthalmology examination could closely approximate what is possible with a traditional clinical examination.

4.5.2 Joslin Vision Network

The Joslin Vision Network teleophthalmology system, which captures digital 0.3 megapixel stereoscopic photos without pupillary dilation using a Topcon TRC NW – 5S non-mydriatic camera, was first described in 2001 [18]. The Joslin group reported good image quality, and graded an equivalent number of eyes (1, 0.9%) ungradeable with both stereo digital and standard film photography. What is significant is that other studies utilizing non-mydriatic capture of fundus photographs have shown higher proportions of ungradeable images [29, 30]. Although the overall level of diabetic retinopathy correlated well with film for grouped, stratified levels of diabetic retinopathy ($0.6 < \kappa < 0.78$), six times as many eyes were ungradeable for retinal thickening when compared to film. It is possible that this was due to the difficulty in obtaining appropriate stereo separation through an undilated pupil.

4.5.3 Inoveon 3DT System

The Inoveon 3DT teleophthalmology system, which was first described in Inoveon's 2002 validation paper [19], compared digital stereo (three megapixel) to an identical protocol using standard stereoscopic film photography. The system was created to identify a referral threshold for one of three endpoints: (1) level 53 or greater, (2) macular edema, or (3) ungradeable images. Stereo digital identified 98.2% of patients (55/56) who had a threshold endpoint specified by standard film photography, although more patients were referred with stereo digital because of either ungradeable images, or over-reading of macular edema. The Inoveon group demonstrated that the sensitivity and specificity of a stereoscopic, digital, teleophthalmology imaging system can approximate Early Treatment Diabetic Retinopathy Study (ETDRS) grading of standard film for the identification of a defined threshold of disease.

Table 4.1. Comparison of key features of three stereoscopic teleophthalmology systems for evaluating diabetic retinopathy[a]

Teleophthalmology group	Fundus camera	Digital resolution (megapixels)	Mydriasis	Stereo viewing technique	Number of fields	Field size	Grading method
University of Alberta	Zeiss ff450i	6	Yes	LCD shutter glasses, SDI stereo viewer	7	30°	Modified ETDRS web site auto diagnosis
Joslin Vision Network	Topcon TRC NW-5S	0.3	No	LCD shutter glasses, proprietary software	3	45°	ETDRS
Inoveon 3DT System	Zeiss ff450	6	Yes	LCD shutter glasses, proprietary software	7	30°	ETDRS

[a] CSME = clinically significant macula edema, DR = diabetic retinopathy, NPDR = nonproliferative diabetic retinopathy

4.6 Additional Issues with Stereopsis in Teleophthalmology

4.6.1 Image Compression

4 Stereo digital photographs require twice the data storage of monoscopic photographs. Furthermore, because high-resolution cameras produce large files, some groups think that the storage requirements for stereoscopic systems are too great. New research [26] into image compression, however, indicates that the file size of high-resolution images is becoming less problematic for teleophthalmology systems.

4.6.2 Mydriasis

The need for mydriasis is dependent on several factors, the first of which is the type of fundus camera used. For instance, cameras such as the Zeiss ff450i require full dilation to capture high-quality photographs. Non-mydriatic cameras, however, are designed specifically to capture images without pupillary dilation. To do this, the user aligns the area of interest using an infrared camera, which decreases light-induced miosis. As a result, because both the pupil and stereobase are smaller, less three-dimensional information is obtained.

Several studies [29, 30] have indicated that the quality of images decreases when photographs are captured through undilated pupils. Because non-mydriatic cameras are so easy to use, even for the novice operator, the benefits of these cameras can be retained by dilating a subject prior to image capture.

4.7 Necessity of Stereopsis

The necessity of stereopsis in teleophthalmology is a contentious issue amongst teleophthalmology researchers that has not been resolved in the current literature [31]. Because stereopsis is such an important aspect of the clinical examination, incorporating it into the examination could perhaps reflect the underlying goal of a teleophthalmology system. With regard to diabetic retinopathy, systems that are designed solely to screen for the presence or absence of any level of diabetic retinopathy may function well without stereopsis.

One consideration, however, that may lead to more teleophthalmology groups adopting stereopsis may be improved cost-effectiveness: data from the ETDRS [32] showed that more patients would be referred if non-stereoscopic cues for the identification of CSME were used. Further research is needed to ascertain whether stereopsis is a necessity when developing a teleophthalmology system.

References

1. Age-Related Eye Disease Study Research Group (2001) The Age-Related Eye Disease Study system for classifying age-related macular degeneration from stereoscopic color fundus photographs: the Age-Related Eye Disease Study report 6. Am J Ophthalmol 132(5):668–81
2. DCCTR group (1993) The effect of intensive treatment of diabetes on the development and progression of long-term complications in insulin-dependent diabetes mellitus. N Engl J Med 329(14):977–986
3. DRSR group (1981) Diabetic retinopathy study report number 7: a modification of the Airlie House classification of diabetic retinopathy. Invest Ophth Vis Sci 21(1 Pt 2):210–226
4. ETDR study group (1991) Grading diabetic retinopathy from stereoscopic color fundus photographs: an extension of the modified Airlie House classification, ETDRS report number 10. Ophthalmology 98(5):786–806
5. Klein R, Klein B, Moss S, Davis M, DeMets D (1984) The Wisconsin epidemiologic study of diabetic retinopathy II: prevalence and risk of diabetic retinopathy when age at diagnosis is less than 30 years. Arch Ophthalmol 102(4):520–526
6. Klein R, Klein B, Moss S, Davis M, DeMets D (1984) The Wisconsin epidemiologic study of diabetic retinopathy III: prevalence and risk of diabetic retinopathy when age at diagnosis is 30 or more years. Arch Ophthalmol 102(4):527–532
7. Diamond JP, McKinnon M, Barry C, Geary D, McAllister IL, House P, Constable IJ (1998) Non-mydriatic fundus photography: a viable alternative to fundoscopy for identification of diabetic retinopathy in an Aboriginal population in rural Western Australia? Aust N Z J Ophthalmol 26(2):109–115
8. Harper CA, Livingston PM, Wood C, Jin C, Lee SJ, Keeffe JE, McCarty CA, Taylor HR (1998) Screening for diabetic retinopathy using a non-mydriatic

retinal camera in rural Victoria. Aust N Z J Ophthalmol 26(2):117–121
9. Higgs ER, Harney BA, Kelleher A, Reckless JP (1991) Detection of diabetic retinopathy in the community using a non-mydriatic camera. Diabet Med 8(6):551–555
10. Leese GP, Newton RW, Jung RT, Haining W, Ellingford A (1992) Screening for diabetic retinopathy in a widely spaced population using non-mydriatic fundus photography in a mobile unit. Diabet Med 9(5):459–462
11. Mohan R, Kohner EM, Aldington SJ, Nijhar I, Mohan V, Mather HM (1988) Evaluation of a non-mydriatic camera in Indian and European diabetic patients. Brit J Ophthalmol 72(11):841–845
12. Owens DR, Gibbins RL, Lewis PA, Wall S, Allen JC, Morton R (1998) Screening for diabetic retinopathy by general practitioners: ophthalmoscopy or retinal photography as 35 mm colour transparencies? Diabet Med 15(2):170–175
13. Penman AD, Saaddine JB, Hegazy M, Sous ES, Ali MA, Brechner RJ, Herman WH, Engelgau MM, Klein R (1998) Screening for diabetic retinopathy: the utility of nonmydriatic retinal photography in Egyptian adults. Diabet Med 15(9):783–787
14. Taylor R, Lovelock L, Tunbridge WM, Alberti KG, Brackenridge RG, Stephenson P, Young E (1990) Comparison of non-mydriatic retinal photography with ophthalmoscopy in 2159 patients: mobile retinal camera study. Br Med J 301:1243–1247
15. Boucher MC, Gresset JA, Angioi K, Olivier S (2003) Effectiveness and safety of screening for diabetic retinopathy with two nonmydriatic digital images compared with the seven standard stereoscopic photographic fields. Can J Ophthalmol 38(7):557–568
16. Hansen AB, Sander B, Larsen M, Kleener J, Borch-Johnsen K, Klein R, Lund-Andersen H (2004) Screening for diabetic retinopathy using a digital non-mydriatic camera compared with standard 35-mm stereo colour transparencies. Acta Ophthalmol Scand 82(6):656–665
17. Maberley D, Cruess AF, Barile G, Slakter J (2002) Digital photographic screening for diabetic retinopathy in the James Bay Cree. Ophthalmic Epidemiol 9(3):169–178
18. Bursell SE, Cavallerano JD, Cavallerano AA, Clermont AC, Birkmire-Peters D, Aiello LP, Aiello LM (2001) Stereo nonmydriatic digital-video color retinal imaging compared with Early Treatment Diabetic Retinopathy Study seven standard field 35-mm stereo color photos for determining level of diabetic retinopathy. Ophthalmology 108(3):572–585
19. Fransen S, Leonard-Martin T, Feuer W, Hildebrand P (2002) Clinical evaluation of patients with diabetic retinopathy: accuracy of the Inoveon diabetic retinopathy-3DT system. Ophthalmology 109(3):595–601
20. Tennant M, Greve M, Rudnisky C, Hillson T, Hinz B (2001) Identification of diabetic retinopathy by stereoscopic digital imaging via teleophthalmology: a comparison to slide film. Can J Ophthalmol 36(4):187–196
21. Wong D (1982) Textbook of ophthalmic photography. AL: Inter-Optics Publications, Birmingham, p 76
22. Maberley D, Morris A, Hay D, Chang A, Hall L, Mandava N (2004) A comparison of digital retinal image quality among photographers with different levels of training using a non-mydriatic fundus camera. Ophthalmic Epidemiol 11(3):191–197
23. Greenfield DS, Zacharia P, Schuman JS (1993) Comparison of Nidek 3Dx and Donaldson simultaneous stereoscopic disk photography. Am J Ophthalmol 116(6):741–747
24. Kiri A, Dyer DS, Bressler NM, Bressler SB, Schachat AP (1996) Detection of diabetic macular edema: Nidek 3Dx stereophotography compared with fundus biomicroscopy. Am J Ophthalmol 122(5):654–662
25. Saine PJ, Tyler ME (2002) Ophthalmic Photography: Retinal Photography, Angiography, and Electronic Imaging, 2nd edn. Butterworth-Heinemann, Boston, pp 97–136
26. Baker CF, Rudnisky CJ, Tennant MT, Sanghera P, Hinz BJ, De Leon AR, Greve MD (2004) JPEG compression of stereoscopic digital images for the diagnosis of diabetic retinopathy via teleophthalmology. Can J Ophthalmol 39(7):746–754
27. Rudnisky C, Hinz B, Tennant M, DeLeon A, Greve M (2002) High-resolution stereoscopic digital fundus photography versus contact lens biomicroscopy for the detection of clinically significant macular edema. Ophthalmology 109(2):267–274
28. Tennant M, Rudnisky C, Hinz B, MacDonald I, Greve M (2000) Teleophthalmology via stereoscopic digital imaging: a pilot project. Diabetes Technol Ther 2(4):583–587
29. Klein R, Klein BE, Neider MW, Hubbard LD, Meuer SM, Brothers RJ (1985) Diabetic retinopathy as detected using ophthalmoscopy, a nonmydriatic camera and a standard fundus camera. Ophthalmology 92(4):485–491
30. Perrier M, Boucher MC, Angioi K, Gresset JA, Olivier S (2003) Comparison of two, three and four 45° image fields obtained with the Topcon CRW6 nonmydriatic camera for screening for diabetic retinopathy. Can J Ophthalmol 38(7):569–574
31. Anonymous (2003) Current state and future direction of teleophthalmology in Canada: first Canadian ophthalmic telemedicine symposium. Can J Ophthalmol 38(5):349–351
32. Bresnick G, Mukamel D, Dickinson J, Cole D (2000) A screening approach to the surveillance of patients with diabetes for the presence of vision-threatening retinopathy. Ophthalmology 107(1):19–24

Chapter 5

Design Considerations for a Low-Cost Sustainable Ocular Telehealth Program

5

Jorge Cuadros

This chapter addresses the following

Key Concepts:

- As the field of ocular telehealth programs evolves, the positive and negative experiences from hundreds of demonstration ocular telehealth programs have led to the formation of guiding principles for future programs and institutional services.
- General principles are necessary to guide the development of economically feasible, effective, and sustainable telehealth programs.
- Areas that need to be addressed include:

1. Identifying specific needs
2. Interoperability and security
3. Outcomes measurements
4. Recognizing organizational and human factors
5. Adaptability and extensibility
6. Maximizing usability

5.1 Introduction

Hundreds of ocular telehealth programs have been developed since the inception of telemedicine in the 1960s, yet relatively few still exist. Programs in use today are based on years of demonstration projects and thoughtful work by knowledgeable task forces that have made it possible to bring remote eye care to every continent in the world. While governments, educational institutions, and health care organizations world-wide have made considerable investments in ocular telehealth programs, few projects have evolved into permanent services and many have disappeared altogether after the initial funding period.

As the field evolves from demonstration projects and feasibility studies to firmly established high throughput institutional services based on positive and negative experiences of existing programs, guiding principles for future ocular telehealth programs have been formed. Whether programs are created internally, shared with other organizations, or purchased from vendors, program directors, policy makers, educators, and clinicians should be aware of design considerations that will help them develop and deploy ocular telehealth programs that have lasting value.

This chapter provides an overview of some lessons learned and general principles for the development and implementation of economically feasible, effective, and sustainable ocular telehealth programs. We will not review accreditation, detailed technical standards, or cost-benefit analyses, since these subjects are covered in other chapters.

5.2 Recommendations for Telehealth Development

In June 2001, a group of telemedicine experts from nine countries presented a series of recommendations on the G-8 Global Healthcare Applications Sub-Project 4: International Concerted Action on Collaboration in Telemedicine [1]. Their recommendations for the global development of telemedicine centered on four main points: (1) developing process models that iden-

5

tify specific needs, (2) adopting interoperability and security standards, 3) creating outcomes measurements that target acceptability, distribution, and competence, and (4) identifying and allocating leadership, funding, incentives, and training that recognizes organizational and human factors.

Several other groups have echoed these points, while adding other important considerations. For instance, when the European Health Telematics Association (EHTA) convened in Geneva to present its work on development of telemedicine in Europe [2], it produced a list of key issues for interoperability in telehealth that emphasized human–human interaction, user needs, transcultural management, education and training (skills), and organizational development. Another key contribution, made by the Australian National Telehealth Committee (ANTC), is the concept that health care innovations and technological components evolve quickly, but that standards can take too long to implement. This point was distilled into the concepts of adaptability and extensibility, i.e., that the fundamental design of the system should ensure the ability to add new features without disturbing its existing structure.

A final recommendation comes from the study of networks and the connectivity of nodes within networks, with a focus on increasing the accessibility of a system greatly, which in turn, increases its use. In other words, usability can be maximized if barriers to access and use are minimized.

The following sections describe strategies for following the above-mentioned design considerations. Our group, the Optometric Eye Center at the University of California, Berkeley, has attempted to incorporate these six design considerations into EyePACS, our ocular telehealth program [3].

5.3 Identify Specific Needs

The use of information technology should be driven by needs and not by technology. This is a lesson learned by ocular telehealth groups that have invested in systems for the sake of modernization without a clear plan for using them. In contrast, the programs presented in this book are examples of successful programs that have focused on specific needs. These are programs that have a well-defined process model that justifies the use of telehealth. At the University of California, Berkeley Optometric Eye Center, we have identified specific needs during the pilot phase of the EyePACS program, which was deployed for the following specific tasks:

1. Referrals to ophthalmic specialists replaced the traditional method of faxing referral letters; at the same time, curbside consultations were provided for cases that did not require referral.
2. Educational courses integrated EyePACS into their curriculum for digital grand rounds, clinical assessment of interns, and for glaucoma treatment certification.
3. Using digital case presentations of glaucoma patients that were facilitated by the use of EyePACS, Web-based detection of glaucoma was studied through collaboration with ten glaucoma specialists scattered throughout the United States.
4. EyePACS has been used effectively for diabetic retinopathy screening and for training primary care physicians to detect sight-threatening retinopathy in their own patients.

5.4 Interoperability and Security

Electronic medical records, image archival systems, diagnostic instruments, and laboratory orders – in addition to telehealth programs – are directly affected by health information standards. Therefore, eye care clinicians should be aware of regulations in health care data occurring around the world.

Three relevant regulations are the US Health Insurance Portability and Accountability Act (HIPPA), Europe's EC 95/46 Directive, and Japan's HPB 517. In synthesizing these sources, we find that although there are some specific differences, there are a core set of security and privacy features. This is evident in each set of rules, which specify that protected health information is any information about health conditions, treatments, or payments that identifies an individual. The rules require that health care providers communicate the minimum necessary amount of protected health information, that patients have access to their own protected health information and can make corrections, and that patients can withhold permission to use information. The rules apply mostly to electronically submitted claims, but can encompass all clinical communication, including paper records. For research and archival purposes, data may be *sanitized*, i.e., data fields that include identifying patient information are removed before transmittal. However, information that is de-identified is not protected health information, and can be freely used and disclosed.

5.4.1 Health Information Standards

Other health information standards for data transmission allow eye care clinicians to (1) easily exchange information with other clinicians, including those in other specialties, (2) adapt new applications to existing systems without undue effort and expense, and (3) electronically exchange information with other health care and administrative organizations. An overview of key standards and related organizations follow.

5.4.1.1 HL7

HL7 is one of the six American National Standards Institute(ANSI)-accredited standards development organizations designated by HIPPA that is also part of an international effort called Integrating the Healthcare Enterprise (IHE). HL7 develops specifications, the most widely used of which is a messaging standard that enables disparate health care applications to exchange key sets of clinical and administrative data [4]. Most standards development organizations produce standards (sometimes called *specifications* or *protocols*) for a particular health care domain, such as pharmacy, medical devices, imaging, or insurance (claims processing) transactions. HL7's domain is clinical and administrative data.

5.4.1.2 CDA and VisionML

The CDA (Clinical Document Architecture), which is part of HL7's Reference Information Model (RIM), specifies the data objects and relationships between objects involved in health care communication. By incorporating this data structure in an ocular telehealth system, programs can greatly facilitate interoperability of clinical data and speed up their development. The CDA Standard, which has been published as an ANSI-approved standard, brings the health care industry closer to a standardized electronic medical record. By leveraging the use of Extensible Markup Language (XML), the HL7 Reference Information Model, and coded vocabularies, the CDA makes documents both machine- and human-readable, so that they are easily parsed and processed electronically, and also easily retrieved and used by the people who need them. CDA documents can be displayed using XML-aware web browsers or wireless applications, such as mobile phones or other hand-held devices.

VisionML is a proposed XML standard whose proponents are optometrists and optical vendors world-wide. It is used for exchanging data among optometric and optical business entities [5].

5.4.1.3 DICOM

The Digital Imaging and Communications in Medicine (DICOM) standard was created by the National Electrical Manufacturers Association (NEMA) to aid the distribution and viewing of medical images. As an international organization, it has chartered an ophthalmic standards committee (Work Group 9) for the purpose of developing a common format for data output from diagnostic instruments. Representatives of the major vendors of ophthalmic instruments have supported this effort in order to allow data from applications such as visual field analyzers, digital imaging devices, and electronic medical records to share a common user interface [6]. Consider DICOM compliance when procuring diagnostic instruments such as nerve head analyzers, visual field analyzers, and digital imaging devices.

5

5.4.1.4 De Facto

Interoperability is also aided by de facto standards – standards that arise simply because a majority of users adopt them. A very prominent standard for information technology at this time is the Internet web browser. Users can access the vast majority of shared documents now via the Internet because of this dominant standard. A computer program that delivers its results into a web browser can interact with users without regard to location or computer operating system. Similarly, in health care the problem-oriented exam record is a salient example of a widely accepted de facto standard, since it is the most common way that clinicians communicate with each other about patients.

Programs that incorporate health care data standards, such as HL7, DICOM, and de facto, may be more useful to clinicians in the long term.

5.4.2 Health Information Security

The security of any information system is comprised of three essential components: confidentiality, integrity, and availability [7]. For it to be secure, information must be (1) inaccessible to those who are not authorized to access it (confidentiality), (2) protected from destruction and/or unauthorized alteration of any kind (integrity), and (3) readily available to those authorized to access it (availability).

Electronic information and communication systems have evolved more rapidly than the mechanisms to effectively protect the confidentiality and integrity of the information they convey. Computer-related security incidents reported to the Computer Emergency Readiness Team (CERT) Coordination Center at Carnegie-Mellon University have more than doubled every year since 1998, as have the annual number of reported security vulnerabilities [8]. Increasing frequency of Internet fraud, identity theft, and attacks upon the network infrastructure and confidential data of governmental and private organizations has stimulated public awareness of the need for improvements in the protection of personal information provided to their employers, schools, and places of business.

The Health Insurance Portability and Accountability Act (HIPPA) of 1996 [9] and the Family Educational Rights and Privacy Act (FERPA) of 1974 [10] are two examples of US legislation that explicitly define the ongoing responsibilities of health care administrators to protect the personal information of individuals to whom they provide clinical and educational services. This protection extends beyond that related to the invasion of privacy and malicious attacks against organizations and individuals. Information security also includes protection from the inadvertent destruction or corruption of information due to failures of hardware or software, losses due to carelessness, ignorance, or accident on the part of authorized users, and those resulting from natural disasters such as fire, flood, earthquake and unexpected surges or loss of electrical power.

5.4.2.1 Technological Neutrality

Any recommendations or guidelines concerning technology must provide for the wide variety of technological infrastructure employed among the different clinical settings. Different proprietary computing platforms (e.g., such as those based upon Microsoft, Macintosh, UNIX, Linux, etc., operating systems) all vary in the prevalence and nature of their security vulnerabilities. General guidelines for information security must allow for such differences.

5.4.2.2. Differences of Administrative Structure

Clinical settings also differ widely in their organizational structures. This results in a wide array of different opportunities and constraints within which the administrators of different institutions can operate. While a setting that is part of a larger organization might benefit from greater technological infrastructure and support staff, it is also likely to have tighter constraints and less of a voice in determining exactly how those resources are configured and deployed. A more independent setting may be more restricted in its technological resources but have more flexibility and control over them. Security guidelines related to administrative policies and their enforcement must take into account such differences in administrative structure.

5.5 Other Considerations

In the following subsections we will discuss issues to be considered in order to optimize the probability of positive outcomes with oculartele health programs.

5.5.1 Outcomes

Just as with other medical interventions, telehealth requires validation to ensure that desired outcomes are being achieved. In addition to the many studies that have supported the clinical viability of ocular telehealth, each program director should measure the performance of their particular program. The acceptability of the system by users and administration should be assessed. How well the program covers the target users and services should be measured. Continuous assessment of the competence of participants via accreditation and certification will ensure that an acceptable level of quality is met.

5.5.2 Recognize Organizational and Human Factors

Sim and Miller [11] created a list of barriers and potential solutions for continued use of information systems in health care that are quite applicable to developing successful telehealth and distance education. Topics to consider include:

- Uncertain financial benefits: systems must generate real benefits for the users.
- Excessive time commitment by clinicians: clinicians must be able to use systems with no additional time required to see patients or teach students.
- Complex technology and user interfaces: learning time must be minimal as new users are added to the system.
- Difficult complementary changes and inadequate support: clinicians and teachers need administrative support to incorporate non-technical organizational changes and new programs in to their practice.
- Clinician attitudes: proponents of the programs within the organization, as well as positive "can-do" attitudes, will greatly influence the use of programs, and are essential for solving system-related usability problems.

The above list underscores that the success of a program greatly depends on non-technical factors, and that identifying leaders and champions, allocating resources, and obtaining adequate funding, all play key roles.

5.5.3 Adaptability and Extensibility

These words "adaptability" and "extensibility" refer to (1) the ability of a system to be extended into previously undefined applications, and (2) how easily programs can be adapted to unforeseen uses. The rapid evolution of information technology makes it impossible to assure that any approach to electronic data that is effective today will remain effective over time. Elaborate and costly programs have quickly become obsolete, because they were not adapted to changes.

A system that accommodates change as new procedures, protocols, and technology arise will have a longer useful life. Specifically, by understanding a system's metadata, and the underlying, unchanging structure and hierarchies of health information, it is possible to design flexible data models that can accommodate change without altering the core structure. Medical informatics experts have been actively discovering this ontology and conceptual framework for several decades in efforts such as systematized nomenclature for medicine (SNOMED) CT [12] and Unified Medical Language System (UMLS) [13]. These frameworks should be incorporated wherever possible in the design of new programs.

5

5.5.4 Minimize Barriers to Access and Use

Users of clinical information systems typically have low thresholds for abandoning new health information technologies. New applications are more likely to be adopted if they (1) function with existing tools and applications, such as word processors, e-mail and web browsers, (2) conform to existing tasks, such as recording patient information or generating patient reports, and (3) require only a few steps to complete a given task.

With these criteria in mind, systems should be made to function on all common platforms and browsers, to use familiar interface formats, and to be accessible with minimal navigation.

The cost of using a system is another variable that often affects a system's accessibility. Current proprietary systems can be too costly or impose unacceptable usage fees in developing countries and community clinics. Open source software is a free and sometimes viable alternative to costly proprietary systems. The term *open source* is defined by the Open Source Initiative (OSI) [14] as the availability of the computer program code, which can be viewed, redistributed, and modified by other programmers who may wish to set up similar applications, or to develop the program for diverse applications. Open source means freedom to download the software, use it, modify it and even distribute it (under the terms of the general public license).

If open source is not possible, another approach is to provide open access to programs. This would mean that access is free, but that the program code can not be modified by users. This option is not as optimal as open source, however, because it lacks the essence that allows open source programs to evolve through changes from users.

5.6 Conclusion

It is important to view telehealth as a program that is evolving within the larger context of medical informatics, so that programs can be truly integrated into practices, and are not simply developed as interesting but isolated demonstration projects. As programs and methods are integrated into health care, and they gain wide acceptance in day-to-day work, then telehealth care will simply become part of health care, in the same way that other innovations have been incorporated into daily medical practice. Sustainability of ocular telehealth progrms is not as much a guiding principle as it is a reward for applying the principles of interoperability, adaptability, accessibility, and security.

References

1. Lacroix A, Lareng L, Padeken D, Nerlich D, Bracale M, Ogushi Y, Okada Y, Orlov O, McGee J, Wootton R, Sanders J, Doarn C, Prerost S, Mc Donald I (2002) International concerted action on collaboration in telemedicine: final report and recommendations of the G-8 Global Healthcare Applications Project-4. http://www.mi.med.u-tokai.ac.jp/g7sp4/final.RTF. Cited 4 Oct 2005
2. Richardson R, Schug S, Bywater M, Williams D (2002) Position paper for the development of e-health Europe: thematic working group 2 "e-Health and Telemedicine" of the European Health Telematics Association. www.medgraphics.cam.ac.uk/Downloads/EHE_0003.PDF. Cited 4 Oct 2005
3. Cuadros J, Sim I (2004) EyePACS: An open source clinical communication system for eye care. Medinfo, pp 207–211
4. Health Level 7 (2005) Vision Data Standards Council. www.hl7.org/about/ 5. Cited 4 Oct 2005
6. American Academy of Ophthalmology Information Statement (2002) www.peterscherer-edv.com/standards/aao2.htm. Cited 4 Oct 2005
7. Director of Central Intelligence Directive (1999) Protecting sensitive compartmental information within information systems: Director of Central Intelligence Directive 6/3, 5 June. Federation of American Scientists, Washington, DC
8. CERT/CC Statistics (1988–2003) CERT-Coordination Center, Software Engineering Institute, Carnegie-Mellon University. www.cert.org/stats/cert_stats.html#incidents. Cited 4 Oct 2005
9. Office of the Secretary, Federal Register (2003) Health insurance reform: security standards; final rule. Department of Health and Human Services, Part II 68(34):8334–8381
10. Department of Education (2000) Family educational rights and privacy; final rule. Department of Education. Federal Register, Part V 65(130):41852–41863

11. Miller RH, Sim I (2004) Physicians' use of electronic medical records: barriers and solutions. Health Aff (Millwood) 23(2):116–126
12. SNOMED International.(2005) www.snomed.org/snomedct/index.html. Cited 4 Oct 2005
13. Unified Medical Language System (2005) National Library of Medicine. www.nlm.nih.gov/research/umls/umlsmain.html. Cited 4 Oct 2005
14. Open Source Initiative (2005) www.opensource.org. Cited 4 Oct 2005

Chapter 6

Information Technology in Ophthalmology and Medicine: Patient Education Kiosks

6

Leonard Goldschmidt

We acknowledge the generous support of the California Telemedicine and eHealth Center. Opinions expressed in this paper are not necessarily those of the Department of Veterans Affairs.

This chapter addresses the following

Key Concepts:

- Information technology used in patient education can work together with teleconsultation to lead to healthier and better informed patients who require less costly medical interventions.
- The overall aim of patient education is to allow patients to take control of their health, and to increase their compliance with recommended guidelines that are designed to improve health.
- Efforts have been made to provide easy-to-access and validated health information for patients
- A patient education and service kiosk was set up to provide a range of health information that was written in English and Spanish.
- Most survey respondents found the patient information useful, and may be more likely to follow health care providers' advice as a result.

6.1 Introduction

Most physicians are taught to be proactive in pursing the goal of a healthy patient. Eye care professionals, too, believe strongly that patients should be given the information they'll need to improve the longevity and quality of their vision. Yet in the western world, with a focus on managed health care, cost containment, and efficiency, such educational interventions and advice may not play the more prominent role that many eye professionals would assign to them.

Within the past decade, information technology (IT) has played a prominent role in facilitating such educational goals. A dizzying array of health-related sites is maintained on the World-Wide Web; originating from an amazing variety of individuals and organizations, thye represent widely diverse quality and approaches [1]. Those patients who are able to utilize this resource may potentially benefit, but only if the information they select is accurate and beneficial [2]. This means that information on the Internet is both factual and mythical, yet patients may find both types of information compelling.

Rational and well-conceived investments in patient education can lead to healthier and better informed patients who require less costly medical interventions [3–7]; additionally, such patients are more likely to follow their health care providers' instructions [8–10]. Concomitantly, people are often stratified between those who have little or no access to health-related information, and those who have easy, extensive information via the Internet [11, 12].

This chapter reviews efforts to equalize this disparity by providing easy-to-access and validated health information. We attempt to measure peoples' responses to our intervention, as well as to increase the odds of improving selected health outcomes. As other leaders of the Internet revolution have acknowledged "if the Internet is to be successful in improving the delivery of health care, it must not be reserved only for academic institutions: the process must begin in the doctor's office" [13]. The effort we report on here builds on earlier work limited to eye education [8, 9], while retaining the goal of creating an easy to use, health information resource for patients: a bilingual, touch-screen, information and education kiosk located in a convenient, accessible area of the waiting room. However, while the kiosk location is prominent and public [14], at the same time, it is designed to provide patient privacy during use (for instance, spoken content may be muted).

An important innovation of the touch-screen health education kiosk is the ability for the patient – after viewing multimedia, validated content – to print redeemable vouchers for appropriate clinical care. This care may include diabetic eye and foot examinations, as well as influenza and pneumonia shots, and mental health appointments. In addition to allowing patients to take control of their health, the overall aim of the kiosk is to increase compliance with personally recommended guidelines that are designed to improve health.

6.2 High-Tech Patient Education in the Patient Waiting Area

The patient education resource is a point-of-care (clinic waiting room) touch-screen kiosk that has been designed and validated as a user friendly interface between the patient and validated health information (Fig. 6.1). Large radio buttons on the touch screen provide the primary user input tool, and both visual and auditory output is incorporated in the content, unless muted by the patient (an on-line keyboard is present at web site locations supporting searches or text notation).

6.2.1 How It Works

A dedicated printer provides a hard copy (take home) version of patient-selected information. People select their preferred language (Spanish or English) and use the buttons to navigate preselected (licensed and validated) multimedia information on the kiosk's hard drive, or they can choose to view Internet medical web sites (Fig. 6.2). Currently available licensed material, which is updated quarterly, covers the following: diabetes, cancer, disabilities, hypertension, cholesterol, back pain, heart disease, traveler's tips for staying healthy, a complete compendium of medications, herbal medications and drug interactions, as well as an electronic library of illnesses and conditions that are explained at an elementary school educational level.

6.2.2 Modules

The modules on diabetes are not restricted to retinopathy, but also provide an overview of many aspects of the disease, including meal planning, type II diabetes and an explanation of digital retinal imaging, etc. In addition, approximately 20 selected English and Spanish language health-related web sites are accessible through the touch-screen kiosk, at high broadband speed, in a seamless touch-screen manner. Sites include those providing information on acquired immune deficiency syndrome, heart and lung disease, cancer, urologic conditions, several mental health web sites, as well as several general health web sites and the National Library of Medicine site. Information content can be updated through the wide area network and changed easily by the kiosk administrator. In addition to patient education, medication refill is an important function of the kiosk at our organization.

6.2.3 Usage

Patient use of the kiosk is voluntary and initiated either at the recommendation of a health care provider, clinic volunteer, or by the patient who notices the kiosk in the waiting areas of the California county hospitals or Department of Veterans Affairs clinics where they are installed. Our subject population is thus self-selected. Evaluation of kiosk usage is ongoing and largely automatic, built into the systems integration

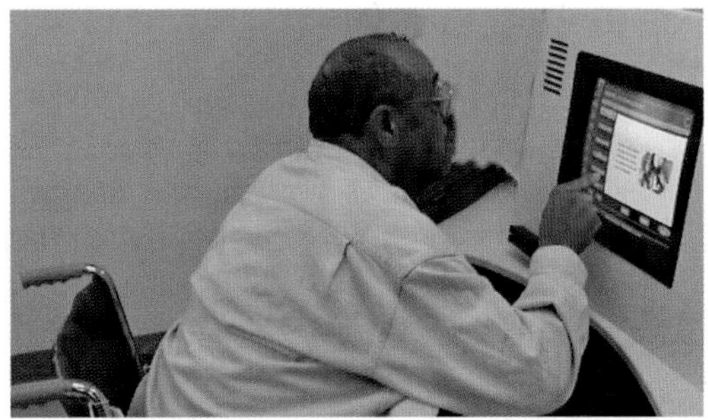

Fig. 6.1. A patient using the patient education and service kiosk (reprinted with permission)

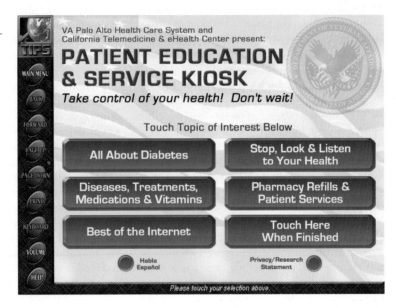

Fig. 6.2. Introductory screen image from the patient education and service kiosk

and touch-screen recording software. As of the most recent published report [15], 38,868 user sessions have been recorded over the 2.5 years that the original three kiosks have been in place. Two kiosks have been active for the entire period and one was installed a year after the original devices. To date, 2,878 users participated in the on-line survey questionnaire (representing 7.4% of all user sessions). During 2004, approximately 30 similar units have been installed in our health care system, which ranges from Reno, NV to Honolulu, HI. Similar kiosks have also been installed at Indian Health Service facilities in Arizona and the Kaiser Permanente Health Care System in Northern California.

The summarized results are from three different hospital or clinic locations, and each device can provide vouchers redeemable for clinical services [15]. The kiosk software records the touches of users and provides information on the number of individuals initiating a session and the number of locations accessed within the program. In accordance with our institutional review board protocol, respondents did not have to answer all questions if they did not wish to, however users averaged 1,873 responses for each question on our survey. Data from the survey shows that:

- Seventy-three percent of kiosk users were doing so for the first time.
- Seventy percent were using the kiosk at their own volition, rather than at the recommendation of their doctors or staff.

Patient reactions to the kiosks were positive:

- Eighty-four percent of respondents thought that the kiosk was generally well located.
- Eighty-two to eighty-four percent (repeat internal validation questions) said the instructions for the kiosk were easy, or somewhat easy, to follow.
- Ninety percent of respondents stated that the information on diabetes was helpful to them.
- Sixty-eight percent of respondents found some or all of the information they were looking for on the kiosk.
- Eighty-five percent said they would use the kiosk in the future.
- Seventy-one percent of people said that the information on the kiosk was helpful in understanding their health.
- Eighty-seven percent of people said the clinic had more to offer because of the patient education kiosk.
- Eighty-two percent said it was very likely (56%) or somewhat likely (27%) that what they learned at the kiosk would help them follow a health provider's advice.

Most importantly, in the year following the introduction of the kiosk intervention, a 14% increase was recorded (2002/03 influenza season) in the number of patients receiving influenza vaccinations within the VA Palo Alto Health Care System, compared to the prior year (2001/02 influenza season) [15]. This increase was sustained in the 2003/04 influenza season.

Since patients can use different sites, at times, for different clinical services, and are not necessarily inclined to print vouchers for eligible services, a direct cause and effect cannot be determined between the kiosk education and the observed increase in influenza immunizations. Future plans call for having a paid assistant or volunteer at selected kiosks to better assess the efficacy of the tool in affecting clinical outcomes.

6.3 Summary

We have created a patient education and service kiosk that provides a range of health content both in English or Spanish. The kiosk presents validated information on diabetes, cancer, disabilities, hypertension, cholesterol, back pain, heart disease, and traveler's tips for staying healthy. The content has been developed using tested principles of health education and is based especially on data showing that patient control of certain health variables can affect the clinical outcome of disease [16, 17], particularly diabetes. Kiosks also offer patients an opportunity to better utilize free time around or between appointments by acquiring useful health information.

Databases of diseases, medications, and herbal supplements have been licensed and are available. Most patients found the kiosk easy to use and are likely to use it again. By allowing patients to print out and take home accurate detailed information for later review, retention and utilization of important health-related information is promoted. In addition, the printed information can be shared with family and friends, increasing the likelihood that patient caregivers have accurate information for supporting the patient.

Most survey respondents found the information useful and feel the clinic has more to offer because of the kiosk. The kiosk provides physicians, allied health professionals, and hospitals the opportunity to provide their patients with the maximum amount of information during each clinic visit and to ensure that the information is relevant to the patients' needs and interests. Most significantly, patients felt they would be more likely to follow health care providers advice because of the kiosk (>82%), and there was a recorded 14–16% increase in the number of influenza shots dispensed after the introduction of the kiosk, although there may well be other unknown factors that influenced this finding.

In conclusion, the kiosk has the potential to make every encounter with patients an opportunity to favorably influence clinical outcomes, and to enable people to have more control over their health.

References

1. Silbert WM, Lundbert GD, Musacchio RA (1997) Assessing, controlling, and assuring the quality of medical information on the Internet. JAMA 277:1244–1245
2. Brown M (1998) The HealthMed retrievers: profiles of consumers using online health and medical information. Cyber dialogue, New York, NY
3. Brown SJ, Lieberman DA, Gemeny BA, Fan YC, Wilson DM, Pasta DJ (1999) Educational video game for juvenile diabetes: results of a controlled trial. Med Inform 22:77–89
4. Robinson, TN, Patrick K, Eng,T, Gustafson D (1998) Science panel on interactive communication and health: an evidence-based approach to interactive health communication. JAMA 280(14):1264–1267
5. Johnson KB, Ravert RD, Everton A, Wang DJ (1998) Hopkins Teen Central; a preliminary assessment of an Internet-based support system for children with cystic fibrosis. In: American Medical Informatics Association Spring Congress Abstract Book, Philadelphia, PA, p 61
6. Banzer E, Florance V (1998) Kiosk access to AIDS information in public settings. In: American Medical Informatics Association Spring Congress Abstract Book, Philadelphia, PA, p 49
7. Asare AL, Pfalz C, Patrick TB, Caldwell CW (1998) Enhancing the education and counseling process for patients undergoing genetic testing by providing Internet accessible information. In: American Medical Informatics Association Spring Congress Abstract Book, Philadelphia, PA, p 62
8. Goldschmidt L, Goodrich GL (2000) Multimedia patient education in the office. Ophthalmol Clin North Am 13(2):239–247
9. Goldschmidt L, Goodrich GL (2003) Patient education and service kiosk: health education at the point-of-care. Int J Health Care Eng 11(5):321
10. Goldschmidt LP, Goodrich G, Patton R, Shyshka J (1998) Computer enhanced patient care: effectively delivering medical information to the patient. In: American Medical Informatics Association Spring Congress Abstract Book, Philadelphia, PA, p 91
11. Fersuson T (1998) Digital doctoring: opportunities and challenges in electronic patient–physician communication. JAMA 280:1361–1362
12. Simonsis K (1999) A focus group to evaluate proposed communication vehicles being developed in support of VA eligibility reform. VHA Health Administration Services, Washington, DC
13. Fotsch E (2000) The effect of the World-Wide Web on you and your patients. Ophthalmol Clin North Am 13(2):261–270
14. Strecher VJ (1998) Michigan interactive health kiosk demonstration project, annual report. University of Michigan School of Public Health, Ann Arbor, MI
15. Goldschmidt LP, Goodrich GL (2004) Development and evaluation of a point-of-care interactive patient education kiosk. J Telemed Telecare 10(1):32–32
16. UK Prospective Diabetes Study (UKPDS) Group (1998) Intensive blood-glucose control with sulphonylureas or insulin compared with conventional treatment and risk of complications in patients with type 2 diabetes (UKPDS 33). Lancet 352:837–853
17. UK Prospective Diabetes Study (UKPDS) Group (1998) Tight blood pressure control and risk of macrovascular and microvascular complications in type 2 diabetes (UKPDS 38). Br Med J 317:703–713

Chapter 7

Online Retinal Image Database and Analysis System With JPEG 2000 Metadata Embedding

Opas Chutatape

7

This chapter addresses the following

Key Concepts:

- Because it offers efficiency and flexibility in accommodating a wide range of information, there are many advantages to using JPEG 2000 in medical imaging in telemedicine.
- With its operating concept, design, and structure, the goal of the Web-based fundus image database system (WFIDS) is to be a platform for wide-scale research work.
- The structure and mechanisms of the Extensible Markup Language (XML) document is designed for embedding data in JPEG 2000.
- Because existing Web browsers do not natively support JP 2000, a plug-in has been developed to view JP2 images on the web page.
- There are security issues surrounding the metadata, and various approaches to implement security.

7.1 Introduction

Substantial work has been done at multiple sites documenting and speculating on the potential social and economic benefits that telemedicine can bring. However, until satisfactory transmission of clinical information is satisfactory, society will not be able to benefit from implementing telemedicine. To have "satisfactory transmission" means that the information is of adequate quantity and of sufficient quality to allow for diagnostic accuracy. Convenience, an acceptable time between data acquisition and analysis, and the cost-effectiveness of each transmission modality must also be addressed as potentially disrupting the clinical practice of both the primary and secondary site physicians.

Detecting and grading of diabetic retinopathy by means of digital retinal images sent via the Internet have been attempted, and the diagnostic results have been assessed by a number of ophthalmologists. An evaluation [1] was reported, based on non-stereo digital images obtained from a CR5-45NM Canon non-mydriatic fundus camera equipped with a video camera (Sony DX950). Four JPEG images covering various regions of the single eye and with a compression ratio of 1:3 were transmitted via the Internet. The results showed that the presence or absence of diabetic retinopathy could be correctly assessed by inspection of the test images. In most cases, good agreement was found between the gradation made from the images and the gradation made by direct examination of the eyes. These findings are among several that suggest that the technique is suitable for diabetic retinopathy screening.

The development of an automated retinal imaging system has been an ongoing research activity at Nanyang Technological University, Singapore, for many years. It has initiated new techniques in retinal image analysis for the detection of landmarks, abnormalities and their classification, and three-dimensional visualization [2–7]. These techniques have potential use as diagnostic tools for non-proliferative diabetic retinopathy (NPDR) and glaucoma. For landmark detection, various algorithms are being created for detection and tracking of blood vessels, optic disc localization, and boundary estimation. In the detection of abnormalities, particular attempts are being made to detect and classify bright lesions (i.e., exudates and cotton wool spots) and dark lesions (which are limited to hemorrhages and microaneurysms). Three-dimensional optic disc surface reconstruction and parameter estimation from ordinary stereo retinal images is another promising research activity for studying and detecting glaucoma with cost-effective tools. An attempt to set up an online system has led to the Web-based fundus image database system (WFIDS), which has many features suitable for small clinics. This system, when fully integrated with other diagnostic software tools, can be used as a model of an independent telemedicine system that can be extended to other patients' healthcare requirements.

In typical telemedicine applications that mostly involve interactive communication, the speed of medical data transmission must be real-time, while maintaining a high quality of data at the same time. In e-health, which relies on the Internet, the speed is largely dependent on the traffic conditions of the heterogeneous networks involved. Both applications unavoidably must have a small data size to increase transmission speed, and at the same time, keep sufficient information and implement a flexible data format to accommodate a wide range of applications. Among the many image formats available, JPEG 2000 was tested [8, 9] and shown to offer a number of suitable features that are useful for medical applications, such as progressive transmission, region of interest (ROI) coding, and metadata embedding. The metadata allows a good deal of flexibility to accommodate a wide range of medical and non-medical data integration.

7.2 Web-Based Fundus Image Database System (WFIDS)

In the following subsections we will provide an overview of the operation and database system of the Web-based fundus image.

7.2.1 Operation Overview

Our research group at Nanyang Technological University has embarked on the Web-based fundus image database system for different users that are hypothesized into seven categories: administrator, photographer, doctor, patient, public, researcher, and Web master, (Fig. 7.1). Researchers can use this system for on-line research collaboration, while the public can access it through information and education on health care. Interaction with the server is bi-directional in that users can retrieve and input various data to the server. Two groups of interactions between users may be handled: Administrator–Doctor–Patient interactions and Photographer–Doctor–Researcher interactions.

7.2.1.1 Process Flow

In addition to research collaboration and public information, WFIDS simulates the process flow that a patient will normally go through when visiting an eye clinic. A patient initially fills in a form and passes it to the administrator. The administrator then registers the patient to WFIDS and creates a username for the patient for login purposes. The administrator has the privilege to register a new user, be it a doctor, patient, researcher, photographer, or another administrator. The patient is then assigned to a doctor to undergo an initial eye checkup. The patient may be required to have a photograph of the retina taken, due to eye diseases or other diseases related to retinal appearance. The patient proceeds to the eye photography room for an eye imaging session. The photographer then takes the fundus image of the patient, logs in to WFIDS, goes to the upload page, enters the patient's registration ID, and uploads the image to the server. Since the fundus camera is connected to a front-end personal computer through a USB port, the image is immediately available in digital format and ready for uploading. At this point in time, the image is readily available to everyone with viewing privileges, regardless of location.

When a doctor enters the web site, notification of the new patient image is automatic. The doctor then views the new image, and gives a

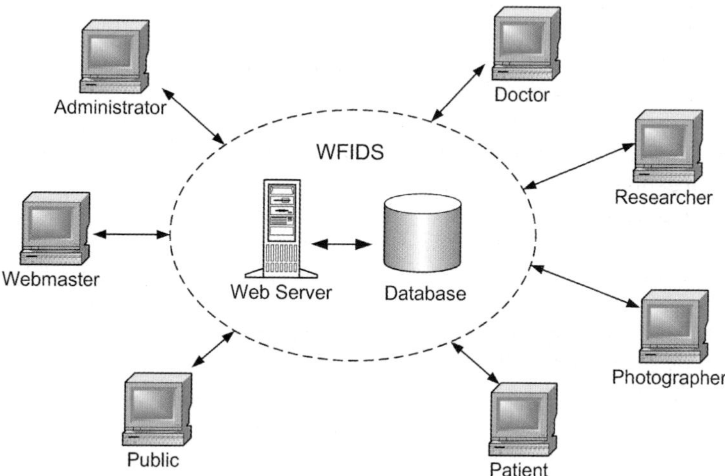

Fig. 7.1. Structure and users of Web-based fundus image database system (WFIDS)

diagnosis and recommendation. The doctor can use the image processing software tools provided to help identify certain abnormalities in the retina. All fundus images and diagnoses are stored in the database, hence doctors are able to keep track of patient history. Each patient is given a username and password to login to the WFIDS. Given controlled access, patients are able to update their profiles, view their eye images and their diagnoses. Furthermore, there is an integrated mailing system where a party can send a message to someone elsewhere in the system. In this way, patients are able to send questions from their homes to their doctors. An appointment can also be made using this internal mailing system. Researchers and the general public are also given access to WFIDS. In WFIDS, they are able to look for information pertaining to eye care, read any available journals or publications, access public web links, etc.

7.2.1.2 NetMeeting

In addition to the internal mailing and appointment system, NetMeeting is available on system as a basic means of synchronous communication. IP addresses are logged by the system as a user logs in, so any user will be able to contact anyone who is concurrently accessing the web site. With the availability of the internal mailing system, appointment system in the WFIDS, and Netmeeting, interaction among medical personnel and patients can be made more natural.

7.2.2 Database System Overview

The functional block diagram (Fig. 7.2).of the WFIDS system can be divided into three layers They are:

1. Presentation layer: This layer uses active server pages (ASP 2.0) technology supported by VBScript and JavaScript languages for the server and client scripting respectively, in order to provide a Hypertext Markup Language (HTML) presentation to the client.
2. Business logic layer: This layer also uses ASP technology. It provides some data processing before it is passed over to the presentation layer for display. The presentation and business logic layers reside in Internet Information Services (IIS 5.0), which runs on the Windows NT 4.0 Server.
3. Database layer: Structured Query Language (SQL) Server 7.0 is used as the database. Stored procedures offered in the SQL Server are also used for data retrieval and update. An Open DataBase Connectivity (ODBC) connection is used between the Active X Data Objects DataBase and the SQL Server.

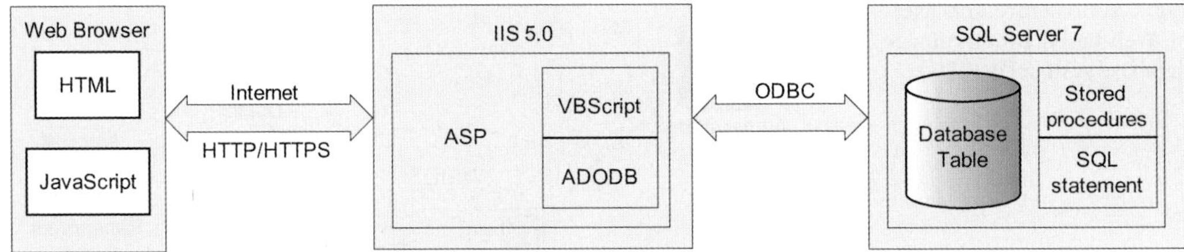

Fig. 7.2. Overview of Web-based fundus image database system (WFIDS)

7

7.3 Web Page Flow Design

The design of web page flow is based on *use case* representation, i.e., a representation of a typical sequence of actions that an "actor" performs in order to complete a given task. The flow of the ASP pages is branched out by the role of the user who logs in to the system (Fig. 7.3). Since many functions are common to many users, these common functions are reused and the same ASP pages are called.

7.4 JPEG 2000 Implementation and Data Embedding

Among the various JPEG 2000 functionalities implemented in WFIDS, the one described here is the embedding of diagnostic and other information into the fundus image JPEG 2000 file, so that the image can be integrated with its relevant data and transported as a single entity. Although the DICOM standard is a well known alternative, and it already has transfer syntax for JPEG 2000 image compression, various non-pixel data attributes in the DICOM can be fulfilled by the basic JPEG 2000 file format together with its embedded data. Furthermore, web browsers do not natively support DICOM images or JPEG 2000. Hence it is neither necessary nor an efficient approach to use DICOM when considering it from a transmission efficiency and utility point of view.

7.4.1 Structure of the JPEG 2000 File Format [10, 11]

The basic and minimal JPEG 2000 file format is called JP2. A JP2 file contains a sequence of boxes. Each box encapsulates one element of the file, such as a code stream or a group of metadata fields. A box can also encapsulate other boxes as part of its data, and such a box is called a super box. Each box contains header and contents fields. The box header starts with a four bytes length field (L) followed by a four bytes *box type* field (T), and eight bytes *extended length* field (XL) if required. The fields are encoded in big-endian unsigned integers, which means that the value must be transformed into little-endian format, the format used in Intel-processor based personal computers. Any application needs to properly parse the file with:

- The signature application and application profile boxes, allowing the file to be recognized as being a part of a JPEG 2000 family
- The header box containing the standard image header information, such as image size, resolution, bit depth, and color space
- The contiguous code stream box, containing the JPEG 2000 compressed image data.
- Metadata boxes, allowing vendor-specific and non-image data to be embedded within the file

The JP2 file format structure is illustrated in Fig. 7.4.

7.4.2 Mechanisms

The JPEG 2000 file format provides two mechanisms for embedding user-defined metadata into a file: an XML box, or a Universal Unique Identifier (UUID). As XML is designed to provide a software–hardware independent, and an easy way of sharing data on the Internet, it is considered more suitable to this application.

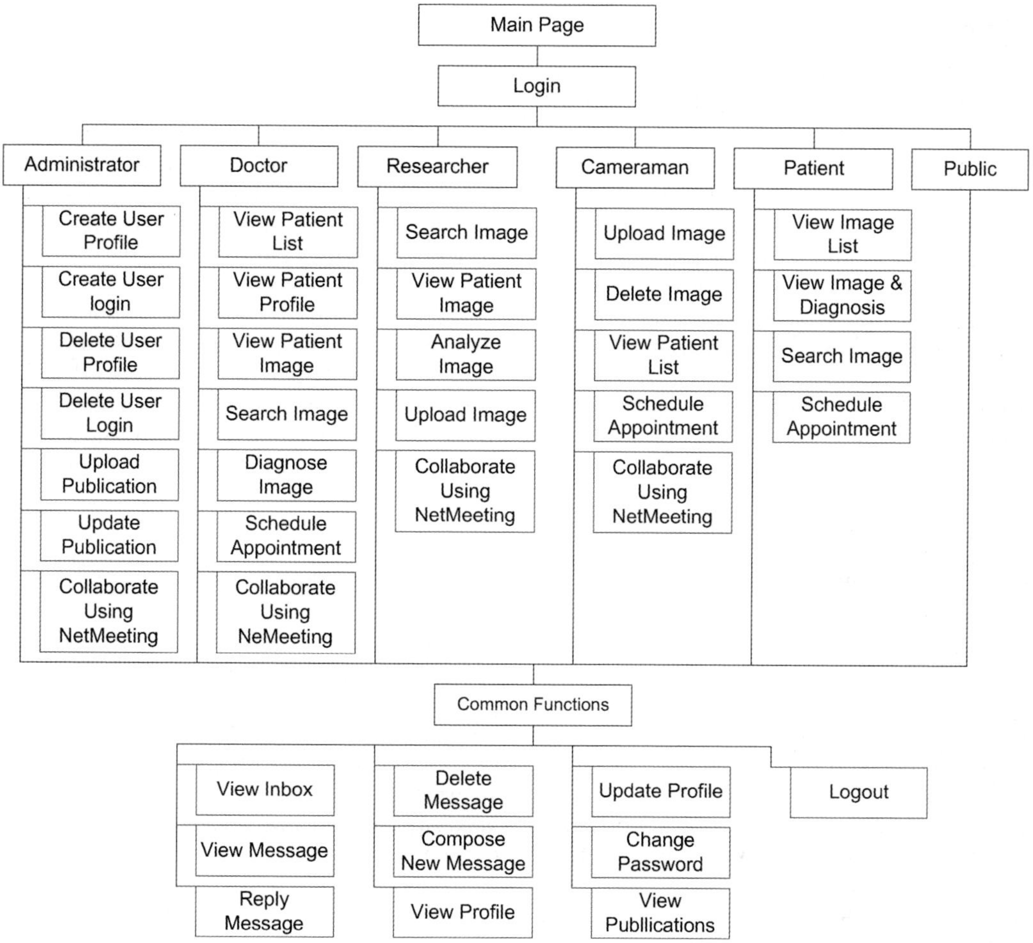

Main Page
Login

- Administrator
  - Create User Profile
  - Create User login
  - Delete User Profile
  - Delete User Login
  - Upload Publication
  - Update Publication
  - Collaborate Using NetMeeting
- Doctor
  - View Patient List
  - View Patient Profile
  - View Patient Image
  - Search Image
  - Diagnose Image
  - Schedule Appointment
  - Collaborate Using NeMeeting
- Researcher
  - Search Image
  - View Patient Image
  - Analyze Image
  - Upload Image
  - Collaborate Using NetMeeting
- Cameraman
  - Upload Image
  - Delete Image
  - View Patient List
  - Schedule Appointment
  - Collaborate Using NetMeeting
- Patient
  - View Image List
  - View Image & Diagnosis
  - Search Image
  - Schedule Appointment
- Public

Common Functions

- View Inbox
- View Message
- Reply Message
- Delete Message
- Compose New Message
- View Profile
- Update Profile
- Change Password
- View Publlications
- Logout

Fig. 7.3. Flow structure of Web page

Defining the building blocks of an XML document is further implemented through the XML schema, which is considered more advantageous than the alternative Document Type Definition (DTD). The Microsoft XML Core services (MSXML) 4.0 Software Development Kit was used in the WFIDS work discussed in this chapter.

7.5 Software Design and Implementation

In the following subsections we will discuss the JP2 Metadata classes for accessing, storing, and handling JP2 files.

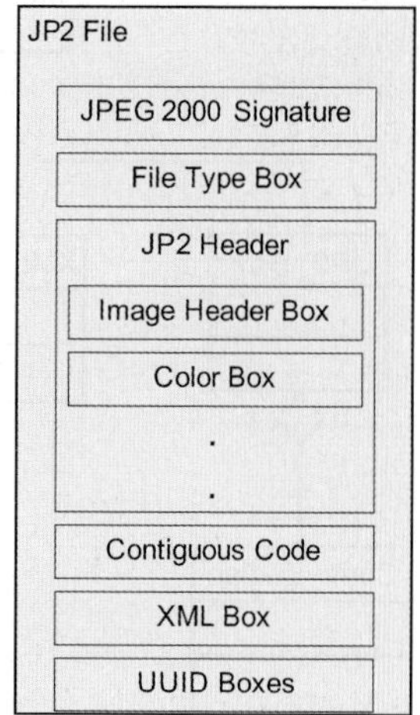

Fig. 7.4. Structure of JP2 file format

7

7.5.1 JP2 Metadata Classes

JP2 Metadata, an embedding library that contains various functions to handle the JP2 files and embed the metadata, was developed for WFIDS. This library can be divided into three main classes according to functionality. The first class is designed to read, write, and verify JP2 files. The second class is designed for reading and storing individual boxes into appropriate JP2 files. The last class is for handling XML metadata. The relationships between all of these classes are shown in the overall class relationship diagram (Fig. 7.5), using Unified Modeling Language (UML) specifications [12].

7.5.2 Accessing: JP2_Meta Class

JP2_Meta class was written for accessing JP2 files. It also acts as the main class and interface for the JP2 metadata library. To access a JP2 file, file I/O and memory I/O classes are required. The three generic classes for I/O access (CxFile, CxIOFile, and CxMemFile) are taken from the CxImage Library [13].

7.5.3 Storing: JP2_Box Class

The JP2_Box class was written for accessing and storing the data for a box in the JP2 file. When reading a JP2 file, the file needs to be loaded to the memory box by box, using the JP2_Box class. Because the number of boxes can vary, it is more appropriate to use a list instead of an array. Writing a JP2 file simply means writing the entire list of JP2-Box objects into a JP2 file.

The box length and box type in the JP2 file are stored in big-endian format, while the personal computer system uses little-endian format. Hence there is a need to convert from one format to another when reading from or writing to a JP2 file. Class Conv_Endian was written to perform this conversion.

7.5.4 Handling: XML_Metadata

The XML_Metadata class contains a wide range of functions related to XML and XML schema, including loading and saving XML documents, setting and getting data from the XML document, and verifying the XML document against an XML schema. It makes use of MSXML 4.0 SDK, which provides functions for the XML

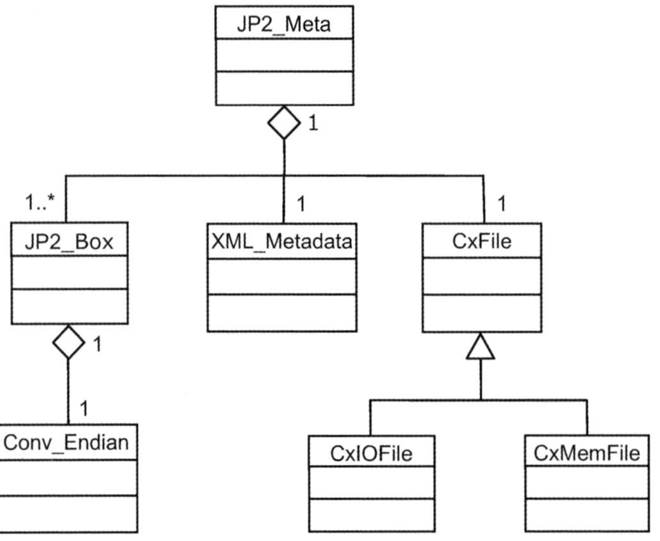

Fig. 7.5. Diagram of overall class relationship

parser, XML Document Object Model [14, 15], and XML schema.

Interfacing with MSXML is accomplished using smart pointer classes, for which the MSXML headers and libraries were imported by inserting the following two statements at the beginning of the codes: (1) #import <msxml4.dll>, and (2) using namespace MSXML2. The first statement instructs Visual C++ to generate the type library information contained in the *msxml4.dll* library. As a result, two header files, *msxml4.tlh* and *msxml4.tli*, are created. These files contain the required type library information, with interfaces also wrapped in smart pointer classes.

The second statement imports the namespace to the project, so that the Document Object Model Application Program Interfaces can reference them without explicitly specifying their namespace [15].

7.6 Implementation

In the following subsections we will discuss implementing the XML document and JP2 images on the Web page.

7.6.1 XML Document

The structure of our XML document (Fig. 7.6), which was designed to store the diagnosis data, has a root element **BMERC (Biomedical Engineering Research Center)** that is used to identify the XML metadata required for the application. A temporary Uniform Resource Identifier (URI) of jp2meta.xsd assigned to the namespace is supposed to be replaced with the permanent Uniform Resource Locator (URL) of WFIDS afterward.

The data represented in the XML document is categorized into five main categories: personal information, medical information, image information, diagnostic information, and clinical information. The modeled information that is provided is considered to be sufficient for the application. The XML document structure can be changed to accommodate additional information, as required.

```
<?xml version="1.0" ?>
<BMERC xmlns="jp2meta.xsd">
  <PERSONNEL_INFO>
    <PATIENT_ID/>
    <FIRST_NAME/>
     <LAST_NAME/>
    <GENDER/>
    <DATE_OF_BIRTH/>
    <BLOOD_TYPE/>
    <HEIGHT/>
    <WEIGHT/>
  </PERSONNEL_INFO>
  <HEALTH_INFO>
    <BLOOD GLUCOSE LEVEL/>
    <BLOOD_PRESSURE/>
    <CHOLESTEROL_LEVEL/>
    <HEART_PROBLEM/>
    <DRUG_ALLERGY/>
    <OTHER_PROBLEMS/>
    <DOCTOR_COMMENT/>
  </HEALTH_INFO>
  <IMAGE_INFO>
    <DATE_TAKEN/>
    <TAKEN_BY/>
  </IMAGE_INFO>
  <DIAGNOSTIC_INFO>
    <DATE_DIAGNOSED/>
    <DIAGNOSED_BY/>
    <NDR/>
    <NPDR_CLASS/>
    <PDR_CLASS/>
    <HEMORRHAGE_PRESENCE/>
    <OPTIC_DISC_CONDITIONS/>
    <BLOOD_VESSEL_PATTERN/>
    <DOCTOR_COMMENT/>
  </DIAGNOSTIC_INFO>
  <CLINIC_INFO>
    <CLINIC_NAME/>
    <CLINIC_PHONE/>
    <CLINIC_EMAIL/>
    <CLINIC_ADDRESS/>
  </CLINIC_INFO>
</BMERC>
```

Fig. 7.6. Structure of our XML document designed for embedding of data was used to store the diagnosis data

7.6.2 Viewing JP2 Images on the Web Page

The current popular web browsers, Internet Explorer and Netscape, do not have built-in support for JPEG 2000 images, unlike other more established image coding formats like JPEG, Bitmap (BMP) and GIF. Therefore, the <img> tag in HTML cannot be used for displaying JPEG 2000 images. An ActiveX object or browser plug-in is required to view JP2 images. There are a few browser plug-ins available for download free of charge [16, 17]. A browser plug-in to view JP2 images was also developed and implemented in WFIDS.

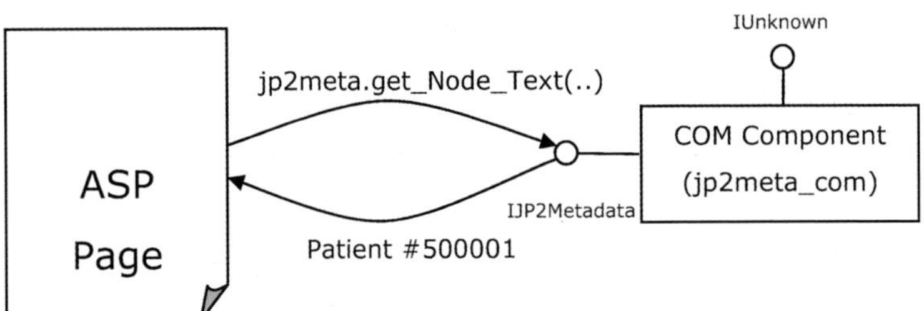

Fig. 7.7. Lollipop diagram illustrating the interface between active server pages (ASP) Web page and the COM component, jp2meta_com.

7.6.2.1 Porting the Data Embedding Function to Web

In order to port the data embedding functions written as a C++ Class to the ASP web page, a component object model (COM) component was written. The function of embedding XML metadata into a JP2 file was ported to a COM component so that the code can be re-used when implementing the function to the ASP web page. The lollipop diagram (Fig. 7.7) illustrates the interface between the ASP Web page and the COM component, jp2meta_com.

7.6.2.2 Interface for COM Component

The interface for the COM component, IJP2Metadata, was created by adding CJP2Metadata Class to the jp2meta_com project file. The Class CJP2Metadata (Table 7.1) provides only the essential functions of the JP2 Metadata Library.

A physician can annotate the JP2 image (Fig. 7.8) with metadata embedded at the right side to indicate the diagnosis, whereas the left image is the original one and cannot be changed. After the diagnostic annotation has been done, the doctor can then save the image.

Table 7.1. Description of class CJP2 metadata

Class CJP2Metadata	
Class Member Objects	**Description of Member Objects**
jp2meta	A J P2_Metadata object. Contain JP2 Metadata Library.
Class Methods:	Description of Member Objects:
validate_JP2_file()	File stream validate function to validate the JP2 file specified.
validate_JP2_mem()	Memory stream validate function to validate the memory buffer specified.
load_JP2_file()	File stream load function to load from the JP2 file specified.
load_JP2_mem()	Memory stream load function to load from the memory buffer specified.
write_JP2_file()	File stream write function to write to the JP2 file specified.
write_JP2_mem()	Memory stream write function to write to the memory buffer specified.
get_Node_Text()	Select a single node using XPath syntax and get the text of the current node selected.
set_Node_Text()	Select a single node using XPath syntax and set the text of lhe current node selected.
validate_XML()	Validate XML data to check whether it is the format specified by XML schema loaded.
load_XSD_file()	Load XSD file from file specified.

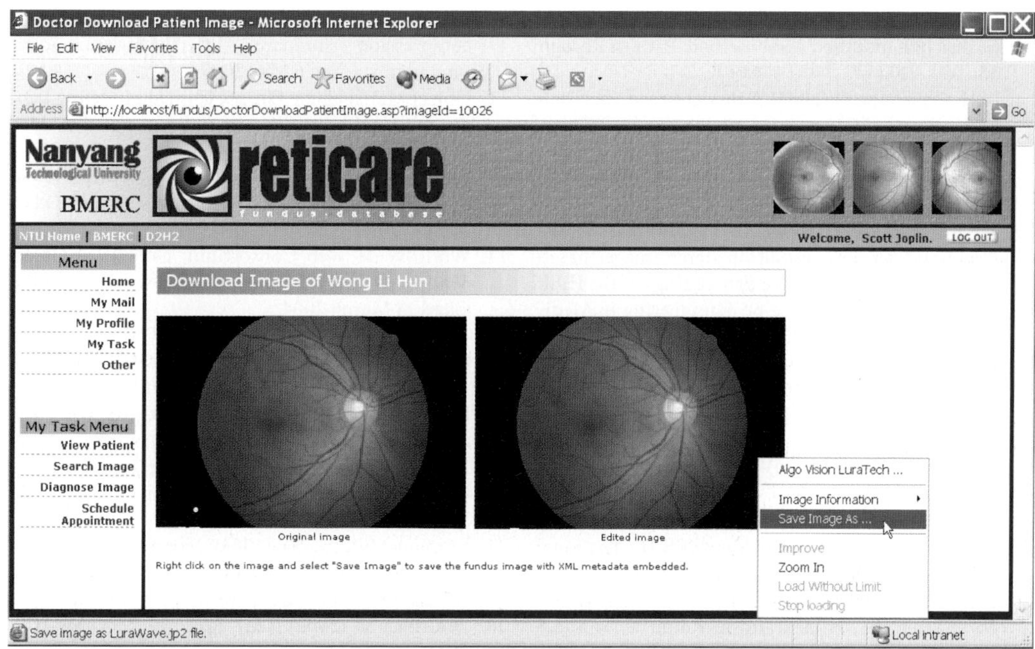

Fig. 7.8. Downloading of JP2 image with metadata embedded

7.7 Discussion and Conclusion

Throughout this chapter, we have been describing the implementation of the JPEG 2000 standard in WFIDS, which involved the writing of a software library (the JP2 Metadata library) to embed diagnostic metadata into the fundus image coded in JP2 format. The embedded data is stored in XML format and validated using XML schema. The library is then ported into a COM component and used to embed data from the database to the JPEG 2000 images.

The use of JPEG 2000 metadata for medical imaging should be justifiable in cases where the rigid non-pixel data formats used in DICOM are not required. The use of XML metadata is more natural and easily extensible. For the security of metadata, XML security standards such as XML encryption [18, 19] to encrypt the data, and XML signature [18, 20] to digitally sign the data for the purpose of preventing unauthorized changes, should be considered. The XML Security Library [21] can be used to implement this feature.

JPSEC, Part 8 of the JPEG 2000 standard [22], which is currently being worked on by the JPEG committee, may provide a better solution for solving both problems. The committee is proposing to standardize tools and solutions in terms of specifications in order to ensure the security of transactions, and the protection of contents (IPR) and technologies (intellectual property), while also enabling applications to generate, consume, and exchange JPEG 2000 Secured bitstreams.

References

1. Gomez-Ulla F, Fernandez MI, Gonzalez F, Rey P, Rodriguez M, Rodriguez-Cid MJ, Casanueva FF, Tome MA, Garcia-Tobio J, Gude F (2002) Digital retinal images and teleophthalmology for detecting and grading diabetic retinopathy. Diabetes Care 25(8):1384–1389
2. Gang L, Chutatape O, Krishnan SM (2002) Detection and measurement of retinal vessels in fundus images using amplitude modified second-order gaussian filter. IEEE Trans Biomed Eng 49(2):168–172

3. Li H, Chutatape O (2003) Boundary detection of optic disk by a modified ASM method. Pattern Recogn 36:2093–2104
4. Li H, Chutatape O (2003) A model-based approach for automated feature extraction in fundus images. In: Proceedings of the 9th IEEE International Conference on Computer Vision (ICCV 2003), Nice, France, pp 394–399
5. Xu J, Chutatape O (2004) 3-D Optic disk reconstruction from low-resolution stereo images based on sub-pixel matching. In: Proceedings of the IEEE International Conference on Engineering in Medicine and Biology (EMBS 2004)
6. Dandapat S, Xu J, Chutatape O, Krishnan, SM (2004) Wavelet transform domain data embedding in a medical image. In: Proceedings of the IEEE International Conference on Engineering in Medicine and Biology (EMBS 2004)
7. Dandapat S, Chutatape O, Krishnan SM (2004) Perceptual model based data embedding in medical images. In: Proceedings of the IEEE International Conference on Image Processing (JCJP 2004)
8. Foos DH, Muka E, Slone RM, Erickson BJ, Flynn MJ, Clunie DA, Hildebrand L, Kohm K, Young S (2000) JPEG 2000 compression of medical imagery. In: Blaine G, Siegel E (eds) Proceedings of SPIE vol 3980, PACS Design and Evaluation: Engineering and Clinical Issues, pp 85–96
9. Foos DH, Muka E, Slone RM, Erickson BJ, Flynn MJ, Clunie DA, Hildebrand L, Kolm K, Young S (2000) JPEG 2000 compression of medical imagery. In: Blaine G, Siegel E (ed) Proc. of SPIE Vol. 3980, PACS Design and Evaluation: Engineering and Clinical Issues
10. Houchin JS, Singer DW (2002) File format technology in JPEG 2000 enables flexible use of still and motion sequences. Signal Process Image Commun 17(1):131–144
11. Adams MD (2002) The JPEG-2000 still image compression standard. http://www.ece.uvic.ca/~mdadams. Cited 6 May 2005
12. Object Management Group, Unified Modeling Language (UML) http://www.uml.org. Cited 6 May 2005
13. Pizzolato D (2003) CxImage v 5.8. http://www.codeproject.com/bitmap/cximage.asp. Cited 23 Feb 2004
14. World-Wide Web Consortium, Document Object Model (DOM) (2004) http://www.w3.org/DOM. Cited 14 March 2004
15. Microsoft Developer Network, DOM Developer's Guide of Microsoft XML Core Services (2003) http://msdn.microsoft.com/library/default.asp?url=/library/en-us/xmlsdk/htm/xml_mth_sz_01k5.asp. Cited1 Oct 2003
16. LuraWave, LuraWave JP2 Browser Plug-in (2003) http://www.algovision-luratech.com. Cited 1 Oct 2003
17. Morgan-Multimedia (2003) Morgon JP2 Browser Plug-in. http://www.morgan-multimedia.com/JPEG2000. Cited 1 Oct 2003
18. Dournaee B (2002) XML Security. McGraw-Hill/Osborne, New York
19. W3C, XML Encryption Working Group (2004) http://www.w3c.org/Encryption/2001/. Cited 10 Feb 2004
20. W3C, XML Signature Working Group (2004) http://www.w3c.org/Signature/. Cited 10 Feb 2004
21. Sanin A, XML Security Library (2004) http://www.aleksey.com/xmlsec/. Cited 10 Feb 2004
22. JPEG, JPEG 2000 Security (Part 8) (2004) http://www.jpeg.org/jpeg2000/j2kpart8. Cited 10 Feb 2004

Chapter 8

Telemedicine and Law

8

Neera Bhatia

This chapter addresses the following

Key Concepts:

- When a doctor provides an evaluation of a patient's condition, upon which a patient relies, a *duty of care* exists, even if the doctor–patient relationship is not face-to-face.
- Telemedicine has revolutioned changes in the way health care is delivered, but the legal and ethical implications of this mode of medical delivery have not progressed as rapidly.
- Telemedicine raises questions about potential threats to patient confidentiality and the resolution of medical negligence cases.
- Most professional associations and regulatory authorities have yet to devise guidelines and standards that establish and resolve telemedical negligence claims.
- It is important that patients be educated about informed consent – a fundamental aspect of medical law and ethics – so that they understand the potential risks associated with telemedicine and how it differs from traditional medical intervention.
- It is difficult to predict how the law will resolve these legal and ethical issues, although it should become clearer as precedents are set.

8.1 Introduction

Traditionally, a patient–doctor relationship was formed face-to-face in the doctor's examination room or through home visits. This long-standing practice was somewhat obscured by the introduction of the telephone by Alexander Graham Bell in 1876; doctors were often the first to use the telephone as they saw the potential of technology to assist them in their profession. By way of example, in the case of *Bienz vs Central Suffolk Hospital* [1], it was held that a telephone conversation in which a doctor provided medical advice that a patient relied on still constituted a patient–doctor relationship even though the interaction was not conducted face-to-face. Furthermore, as long the doctor provided some level of evaluation of the patient's condition, and the patient relied on this evaluation, a relationship is formed and a duty exists. This is one of the earliest examples of telemedicine in its simplest form. An early illustration of telemedicine in practice can be dated back to the early 1920s in Norway in Haukeland hospital, where ships at sea could obtain help and advice from doctors in the hospital via radio in cases where there had been accidents or illness while at sea.

The 1990s saw a great boom in the development and progression of technology, when multimedia systems and telecommunications businesses actively sought to produce and share more compact technology data across several networks, using significantly fast communication channels.

Today, the European Commission (EC) has defined telemedicine as "the investigation, monitoring and management of patients and the education of patients and staff using systems which allow ready access to expert advice and patient information, no matter where the patient or relevant information is located" [2].

8.2 The Legal Implications of Telemedicine

Although the evolution of telemedicine has been productive, and it has essentially generated major and often revolutionary changes in the way health care is delivered, the legal and regulatory sphere concerning telemedicine and its legal and ethical implications has not progressed as rapidly.

A number of issues have surfaced within medical law and its common application to everyday situations. prior to the introduction of telemedicine, the use of more technological methods of treatment that are often perplexing required lengthy consideration by judges and academics in medical law and ethics.

The medical canvas has become somewhat more clouded by the use of telemedicine. For instance, a key consideration is the resolution of medical negligence that can potentially arise through *Trans-Atlantic* surgical procedures. It also raises a substantial number of questions about potential threats to patient confidentiality.

8.2.1 Medical Negligence

Patient autonomy – the concept that individuals have personal sovereignty and the right to protect and control their bodies and property – is a fundamental concept in medical law. Because there is a natural imbalance in the doctor–patient relationship, the right to autonomy endeavors to limit the power of the doctor while protecting the patient from any unwarranted bodily intrusion, such as surgery without consent, or public disclosure of medical information.

8.2.1.1 Lack of Guidelines

Most professional associations or governing bodies have yet to devise strategic guidelines or a universal set of standards to follow should there be an unfortunate occurrence or medical blunder that involves the use of telemedicine. Regulatory authorities, too, have not devised or adjusted procedures in establishing and resolving medical negligence claims in accordance with the ever-evolving innovations in delivering healthcare in the 21st century.

The lack of guidelines in this area may possibly be due to the minimal number of cases of medical negligence in relation to invasive telemedical procedures, which would assist in creating fundamental legal principles and procedures to follow where telemedicine is used.

8.2.1.2 Establishing Boundaries and Liability

The dynamic nature of telemedicine has made it possible for doctors located in one country to perform intricate and often complex surgery on a patient in a completely different country. At the same time, a key aspect that is of growing concern is the need to create jurisdictional boundaries that establish liability within the emerging field of *telemedical negligence*.

Because of differing legal rules among its 52 states, the United States (US) has dealt with this issue. In *Prince vs Urban* [3], several telephone consultations between a patient from California and her Illinois-based doctor who provided repeat prescriptions was deemed as an insufficient basis to establish the Californian courts' jurisdiction over the doctor for purposes of making the doctor answerable to the patient's negligence claim [4].

The decision in this case would have been markedly different if the doctor had advertised her services in California, and if she had built a rapport with or directly treated other patillents. We do not yet know how the law will make decisions on such jurisdictional issues in other parts of the world, such as in England where legal rules do not vary from town to town; nor do we know the legal outcome in resolving medical negligence claims in a situation wherein a doctor is located in one country and the patient in another.

8.2.1.3 Patient-Provider Proof

In medical negligence cases, traditionally the onus is on the patient (the claimant) to prove that the doctor (the defendant) formed a relationship with that patient, much like the signing of a contract, and consequently, the doctor owes a duty of care toward that patient. The patient must then prove that the doctor breached this duty of care by failing to conform to the accepted standard of care, which directly caused or led to cause detriment to the patient.

Proving that a duty of care was owed may be difficult when a doctor and patient are in different parts of the world. Another challenge to prove: whether a telemedical meeting is sufficient to establish that a duty of care was owed, be it via teleconferencing, telephone, or e-mail. For example, a remote specialist who does not perform a hands-on examination, but rather uses high tech robotic machinery, could be regarded as delivering less than adequate care. Or if compressed digital images that are not reconstructed well causes the loss of valuable diagnostic information, it may be difficult for a doctor to make a diagnosis, which, in turn, could cause the patient further harm, or possibly even death.

8.2.1.4 Global Standard of Care

It would seem that in order to limit or control ambiguity when measuring the standard of care that is owed to patients receiving telemedicine care, would be to create a *global* standard of care that can be used to establish medical negligence or malpractice. It would also be markedly valuable for both legal and medical practitioners to have a uniform set of principles or rules that can be used to govern the way in which claims of medical negligence are handled.

8.2.2 Patient Privacy and Confidentiality

Because highly sensitive medical histories or diagnoses are easily accessible either visually or verbally through telemedicine, the opportunity exists to breach patient privacy and confidentiality. It may often not be possible to set controls or to establish safeguards for accessing such information, especially with the use of intranet systems and internal e-mail, potential computer viruses, or electricity failure, which could wipe out entire data bases with no back-up files.

Essentially, technology can only be a success when it is controlled by humans and human intelligence, and invariably humans make errors. Misdialed telephone numbers, faxes that are left unattended, or external interception of video or other transmission lines make it extremely easy for patient confidentiality to be breached. Because of this, it has been suggested that greater safeguards, and attention be placed on the potential exposure of patient medical information, by incorporating encryption or access codes to personal, often highly sensitive information.

8.3 Informed Consent

A fundamental aspect of medical law and ethics is informed consent, and the right of the patient to know and understand the risk involved in medical procedures or treatment. Although patients may generally welcome the use of telemedicine, which could potentially save their life or assist them in gaining medical treatment and advice from some of the world's most renowned medical professionals, it is important that patients understand the potential risks associated with telemedicine. These include those already discussed about privacy and confidentiality, and how telemedicine differs from traditional *hands-on* medical intervention. This could be addressed by inserting an additional clause in traditional consent forms that would provide patients with the option of accepting or declining telemedical procedures.

8.4 The Way Forward

The issues discussed and raised in this chapter are meant to serve as an introduction to the vast number of ambiguities, obscurities and complexities which saturate medical law, ethics and innovative technology. Although telemedicine has played a prominent and vital role in the development and advancement of medicine since the last millennium, it would seem that it is only now, in the 21st century, that its application and potential future development is being examined with greater scrutiny.

At the same time, the law has not progressed as rapidly as telemedicine technology. To fill the gap, a structured legal and ethical framework that meets the needs of providers and patients participating in telemedicine, and that reflects the use of technology on a daily basis, is needed to determine what are often life or death decisions.

Currently, it is difficult to determine or predict how the law will resolve legal and ethical telemedicine issues, such as medical negligence, although this is likely to become clearer as cases are tested and settled, and precedents are created. Because such a time is fast approaching, it would be wise for medical and legal practitioners to prepare for the numerous dilemmas and conundrums that are likely to arise.

References

1. Bienz vs Central Suffolk Hospital (1990) 557 New York, Supreme Court Division 139
2. Advanced Informatics in Medicine (AIM) (1990) Commission of the european communities; supplement application of telecommunications of health care telemedicine. AI 1685
3. Prince vs Urban (1996) 49 California Appeal 4th: 1056, 1066; 57 California report 2d 181 (Ct App, 4th appeal district, division 3)
4. Viegas S, Dunn K (1998) Telemedicine: practicing in the information age. Lippincott, Raven Publishers, Philadelphia, PA

Chapter 9

Cost-Effectiveness of Teleophthalmology in Diabetic Retinopathy Screening

9

I-van Ho, Nitin Verma

This chapter addresses the following

Key Concepts:

- Diabetic retinopathy represents a significant fiscal burden to public health.
- Economic limitations necessitate the detailed, cost-effective analysis of any diabetic screening program.
- The diabetic eye screening service provided by a teleophthalmic unit was compared with an ophthalmologist-based screening service, covering the Top End of the Northern Territory of Australia.
- The teleophthalmic diabetic eye screening program was shown to be more cost-efficient, with a payback period well within the estimated life span of the equipment.
- A sensitivity analysis revealed that capital cost fluctuations of up to 230% would not affect the cost-effectiveness of the program.
- The continuity, familiarity and acceptability of the screening program are likely to increase, which in turn will increase its efficiency.

9.1 Introduction

The restraints of economic limitations necessitate a detailed, cost-effective analysis of diabetic screening programs. This is particularly applicable to rural and remote areas of Australia, because distance and lack of medical and specialty services in these areas often result in delivery of services that are not cost-effective.

Diabetic retinopathy represents a significant public health burden that impacts the medical, functional, and psychological status of patients. Furthermore, ailments such as blindness that can result from diabetic retinopathy continue to create a significant economic burden on Australia. To address such fiscal concerns, the National Health and Medical Research Council (NHMRC) and the international medical community endorse regular screening for diabetic retinopathy, and prompt and appropriate treatment programs, when indicated.

9.2 Cost-Effectiveness and Cost-Benefits

A cost-effectiveness analysis can shed light on the range of benefits as well as the costs surrounding a decision that aggregates the effects over time. Using an approach called *discounting*, it is possible to arrive at a dollar-denominated *present value* that, in concept, is comparable with other governmental uses for scarce financial resources, including leaving them in the hands of taxpayers.

Reports from the United States (US) have shown that the detection and treatment of diabetic retinopathy is not only cost-effective, it is actually cost-saving from both governmental and societal perspectives. Indeed, it is estimated that the potential savings in the United States exceeds 600 million USD annually [1]. A detailed analysis of the cost-effectiveness of screening and treating diabetic retinopathy – with an estimated screening rate of 60% – showed that the overall cost-effectiveness is 3,190 USD per Quality Adjusted Life Years (QALY) [2]. Interestingly, the greatest cost-savings is for Type 1 diabetics, even though they survive longer and also have an increased incidence of proliferative retinopathy.

Laupacis and co-workers have suggested that health interventions costing less than 20,000 CAD per QALY are being adopted by certain societies [3]. The literature also supports well-implemented diabetic eye screening programs, because they are cost-effective for both health budgets and the public health. Of course, no tool is perfect, and cost-effectiveness analyses have limitations. For example, criticisms result (1) from the rudimentary techniques used to measure diverse benefits and costs in dollar terms, (2) equity concerns left unrecognized in the present value calculation, and (3) the fact that, to some, environmental concerns are allocated to ethics, rather than economics. Because of such criticisms, all cost-effectiveness analyses must be tempered with consideration for each individual, and health services should not be driven soley by economic considerations.

All efficient screening programs should be followed by effective and efficient treatment program. This is because we know, for instance, that prompt laser treatment for diabetic retinopathy prevents in excess of 90% of blindness from the disease.

9.3 Economic Definitions

In the following subsections we will discuss key terms used in cost-effectiveness analyses of teleophthalmology in diabetic retinopathy screening.

9.3.1 Payback

The payback method is the simplest measure to calculate. The payback method simply calculates how many periods/years into the future it takes for a capital project to generate net income to repay the initial investment (Fig. 9.1).

9.3.2 Net Present Value (NPV)

Net present value (NPV) is the *present value* of a future net benefit stream that reflects the time value of money. NPV considers all future cost-benefit flows over the life of the investment. The method yields one value that is easily interpreted. If the value is positive at a required rate of discount or interest, the project yields benefits that exceed its costs. If the value is negative, costs exceed benefits and therefore it is not fiscally prudent to invest or fund. Economists commonly use a discount rate of 4–5%, as it is the rate over inflation at which the government typically borrows funds [5].

9.3.3 Internal Rate of Return (IRR)

Decision makers are often more comfortable with value expressed in percentage terms rather than some other metric. The Internal Rate of Return (IRR) is a method that expresses value in terms of a percentage. Essentially, the IRR is the discount rate that makes the discounted value of future cost-benefit flows exactly equal the initial investment. In other words, it is the percentage return on investment above capital costs. In most economic circles, an IRR above 5% is sufficient for public sector investment and funding.

The IRR and NPV are, in effect, different ways of representing the future benefit of current investment. This is shown in Fig. 9.2.

The point where the graph intersects 0 AUD represents the equating of future benefit streams with current capital investments. The discount rate at this point represents the IRR. The discounted net cash flow corresponding to the arbitrary 5% discount rate represents the NPV.

9.4 Cost-Effectiveness of Diabetic Eye Screening Program in Australia

There are approximately 1300 diabetics in the rural and remote Top End of the Northern Territory in Australia, according to the authors' chart reviews and database collected from the community clinics and Territory Health Service (THS) chronic disease registers.

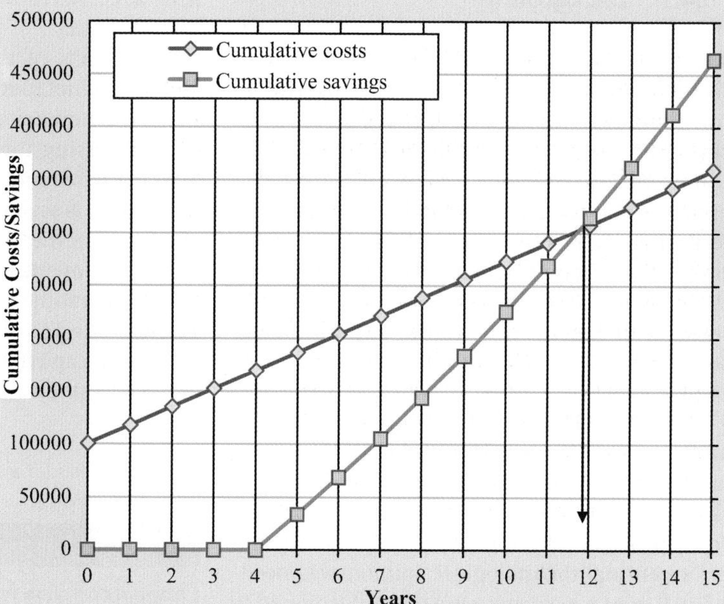

Fig. 9.1. Payback period in years

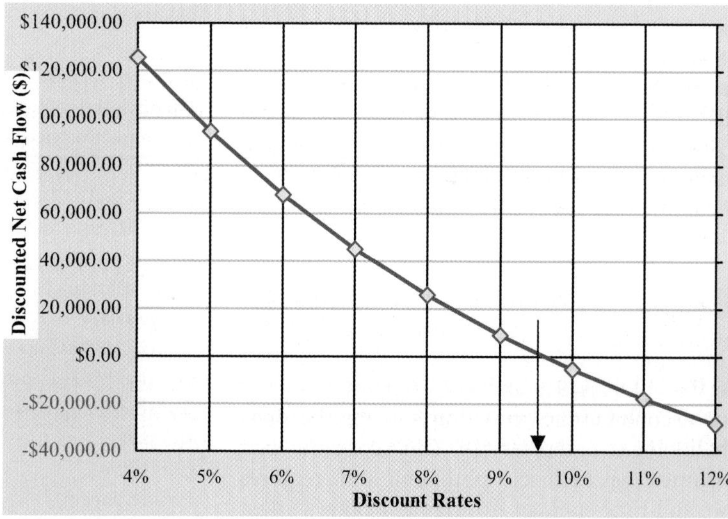

Fig. 9.2. Results of cost-effective analysis based on net present value (NPV) and internal rate of return (IRR) on investment

Capital and operating costs (Table 9.1) were used, and analyses were done comparing the existing Teleophthalmic Unit (TU) with the ophthalmologist-based screening service, as aspect of the Katherine Region, Rural Darwin and East Arnhem District.

The estimated results of cost-effectiveness analysis include the pay-back period, NPV at 5% discount rate, and IRR.A sensitivity analysis was included to test the sensitivity of the cost-effectiveness analysis (in terms of pay-back period, NPV and IRR) when capital cost escalates and efficiency improves.

9.4.1 Background

All diabetic patients had their corrected (and therefore, best) visual acuity recorded prior to mydriasis with tropicamide (1%) and phenylephrine (2.5) The teleophthalmic diabetic screening team took two 45° non-stereoscopic images of each eye: one macular centerd and one disc-centerd, The TOPCON TRC-NW5S digital non-mydriatic fundus camera fitted with a Sony DXC 950P 3-chip CCD-video camera was used in the imaging of the patients' fundi, and all images were archived on CD ROM in uncompressed bitmap format.

The CD ROMs were transported within one week to Royal Darwin Hospital (RDH) via courier services for analysis and grading by the resident ophthalmologist. Images were compressed to a JPEG 17:1 ratio format for e-mail to RDH if an urgent ophthalmological opinion was needed. All laser treatments were promptly offered to those with sight-threatening diabetic retinopathy by being transferred to the nearest regional hospital at the next scheduled eye clinic; urgent cases were transferred to RDH for immediate treatment. Patients with non-sight threatening diabetic retinopathy were scheduled for repeat eye examinations by the mobile teleophthalmic diabetic screening team within the NHMRC's recommended period.

9.4.2 Cost of Diabetic Eye Screening

Costs for providing a diabetic eye screening service (Tables 9.1 and 9.2) were determined for teleophthalmic screening and for the ophthalmologist-based service. This economic data assumes that each teleophthalmic unit requires two full-time staff, an Aboriginal health worker, and a nurse, who work closely with a full-time ophthalmologist in Darwin. It is with this staffing level that the program was implemented in the Top End.

All costs were determined from expenditures in the years 2000 and 2001, which include the complete cost for providing a diabetic eye screening service to all 32 rural and remote communities in the Top End. This economic data excludes the Darwin urban diabetic population, with a conservative estimate of an additional 2500 diabetics.

The results of the cost-effectiveness analysis (Table 9.3) includes screening 700 patients annually – the number of patients screened over the last year, using the mobile teleophthalmic diabetic eye screening service. The life of the capital investment is seven years, as advised by the manufacturers of the teleophthalmic equipment; minor replacements and maintenance are included under operating costs. In addition, sensitivity analysis was performed to estimate the effect of increasing capital costs on the cost-effectiveness of the teleophthalmic program (Table 9.4).

Table 9.1. Costs for a single unit teleophthalmic diabetic eye screening team

	AUD
Capital cost (non recurring)	
Fundus camera + portable computer	77,000
Review station computer	10,000
Color printer	600
Travel case	1,000
Total capital cost	88,600
Operational cost (yearly)	
Equipment service	1,000
Vehicle hire ($700/month)	8,400
Vehicle fuel (120 L @ $1.10/L)	1,320
Plane tickets + freight (for 2 persons)	10,510
Accommodations (for 2 persons)	3,200
Travel allowance (for 2 persons)	4,000
Nurse salary	45,000
Aboriginal health worker salary	32,000
Ophthalmic secretary salary	32,000
Ophthalmologist salary	150,000
Internet access	720
CD-ROMs	50
Printer paper	1,500
Printer cartridge	300
Medication	870
Courier services	425
Total operating cost	**291,295**

9.5 Discussion

Based on our three assessments, it is clear that teleophthalmic diabetic eye screening programs are effective, cost-effective methods of screening for diabetic retinopathy in the rural and remote regions of the Top End. Cost-effectiveness analysis with an internal rate of return (IRR) of 62.7% is extremely high, and is more than sufficient for public sector investment and funding. A payback period of two-and-a-half years is very attractive, and a positive net present value (NPV) of 111,121 AUD at 5% discount rate is attractive for public investment. A sensitivity analysis reveals that a capital cost fluctuation of up to 230% will not affect the cost-effectiveness. Increasing capital cost by 240% makes the NPV negative at 5%, and reduces the IRR to 3.7%. However, an IRR of 3.7% indicates that the investment is still marginally cost-effective at this level.

Table 9.2. Costs for ophthalmologist based diabetic eye screening service

	AUD
Capital cost (non-recurring)	
Lenses + ophthalmoscopes	6,000
Equipment case	500
Total capital cost	6,500
Operational cost (yearly)	
Ophthalmoscope battery	100
Vehicle hire ($700/month)	8,400
Vehicle fuel (120 L @ $1.10/L)	1,584
Plane tickets (1 person)	32,950
Accommodations (1 person)	4,700
Travel allowance (1 person)	3,465
Nurse co-coordinator salary	58,000
Ophthalmic secretary salary	32,000
Ophthalmologist salary	150,000
Community AHW salary	32,000
Medication	870
Total operating cost	**323,969**

Table 9.3. Cost-effectiveness analysis for teleophthalmic screening service

Cost-effective Analysis	
Pay-back period	2.5 years
NPV @ 5% (AUD)	111,121
IRR	62.66%

It is clear that teleophthalmic diabetic eye screening programs are cost-effective (Fig. 9.3), and that they suggest cost savings for future investment. At the same time, it can be seen that although there is minimal initial capital cost for the ophthalmologist-based screening, this method of screening for diabetic eye diseases in the Top End results in continual investment losses after two-and-a-half years. Furthermore, the payback period of both teleophthalmic programs are well within the estimated seven year life span of the equipment, making it an extremely attractive proposal.

A single unit teleophthalmic screening service is shown to be more cost-effective than having two separate teleophthalmic teams in our separate cost-effectiveness analysis. This reflects the population differences across the Top End, where the greater proportion of the rural and remote population resides in the Katherine Region. It would be cost-effective to have two teleophthalmic screening teams if we were to provide the service to urban Darwin, which would include a further 2,500 diabetic patients.

It is also very important to note that the teleophthalmic program has only been functional for the past 18 months, as compared to the longer operational time frame of the ophthalmologist.

Table 9.4. Sensitivity analysis of capital change for teleophthalmic screening service

Sensitivity Analysis					
Change	**0%**	**+ 10%**	**+ 20%**	**+ 50%**	**+ 240%**
Pay-back period (years)	2.5	2.8	3.1	3.9	6.3
NPV @ 5% (AUD)	111,121	111,121	94,245	68,930	– 7,012
IRR	62.66%	51.52%	43.06%	26.33%	3.66%

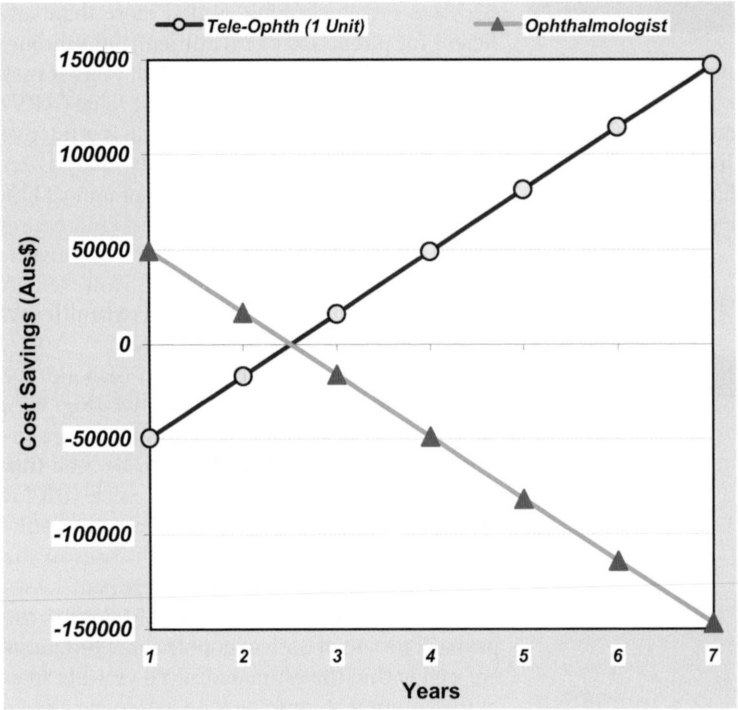

Fig. 9.3. Cost savings comparisons of ophthalmologist and teleophthalmic diabetic eye screening programs

We believe that in time with the continuation, familiarity and acceptability of this teleophthalmic program, its efficiency would increase and a conservative estimate of 1,000 screenings per year could be easily achieved. One thousand screenings per year equates to a diabetic screening coverage rate of approximately 75%. Our experience has shown us that achieving a screening rate of up to 85% is well within limits, and at that level of screening, teleophthalmology will prove to be even more cost-effective than it is currently.

Finally, all economic analyses must be appreciated in tandem with the understanding of the service provision in each community. We can see that not only is it cost-effective to have a teleophthalmic diabetic eye screening service, but that it also provides the benefits of increased screening rates, education of patients, and most importantly, of local health workers.

References

1. Javitt JC (1995) Cost-savings associated with detection and treatment of diabetic eye disease. PharmacoEconomics 8(suppl):33–39
2. Javitt JC, Aiello LP (1996) Cost-effectiveness of detecting and treating diabetic retinopathy. Ann Intern Med 124(2):164–168
3. Laupacis A, Feeny D, Detsky AS, Tugwell PX (1992) How attractive does a new technology have to be to warrant adoption and utilisation? Tentative guidelines for using clinical and economic evaluations. Can Med Assoc J 146:473–481
4. Parsonage M, Neuburger H (1992) Discounting and health benefits. Health Econ 1:71–76

Chapter 10

Economic Evaluations in Teleophthalmology

10

Johanna Lamminen, Heikki Lamminen, Ville Voipio

This chapter addresses the following

Key Concepts:

- Investments in telemedicine should either produce cost savings or improve service quality.
- When determining the potential benefits of telemedicine, all factors, not just cost factors, should be analyzed.
- Economic evaluation studies can be hard to generalize from industrial situations to health care systems.
- A balanced scorecard approach, which is a synthesis of financial accounting models and competitive capabilities, views organizational performance from four perspectives: financial, customer, internal business processes, and learning and growth.

10.1 Introduction

Economic issues have become increasingly important topics in health care in the industrialized world. Many western countries have development programs in their public health sectors that aim a better health care cost-efficiency by finding alternative ways of providing services. In this context, telemedicine is thought to have economic benefits, especially when providing health services to sparsely populated areas. It has been assumed that telemedicine can improve the health service chain and thus in some cases also enhance the quality and efficiency of health care [1]. It has also been suggested that the economic evaluation of telemedicine needs to be carried out to answer the key question, Should we do this [2]?

Literature shows that telemedicine can provide savings, especially for thinly settled where the distances to hospitals are great and when patients need special transportation, such as helicopter or ambulance [3]. Real-time video conferencing between a specialist and a general practitioner or a resident generally improves the health process and serves education purposes.

Economic evaluations in telemedicine should include at least two aspects: investment calculations and usage cost (i.e., studying medical processes).

10.2 Economic Evaluations in Telemedical Investments

All investments need to be carefully analyzed. There should always be stated objectives and goals for the investment: "Why should we invest in this?" Objectives are different in each case, and cost savings are not always the main target.

Investments in telemedicine should either produce cost savings or improve service quality. There are several methods that can be used to analyze whether the investment has brought the estimated financial benefits. All decision makers have to demand investment calculations and benefit analyses before making a decision.

The most commonly used methods for analyzing the investment decision from a financial point of view are *economic lifetime* and *return on investment*. The factors contributing to economic calculations may be classified into two categories: *soft* and *hard factors*. The hard factors – direct expenses, time, quantities, etc., are straightforward to evaluate. However, the soft factors – customer experience, organizational learning, etc. are usually very difficult to express in financial terms; therefore, their presence adds considerable uncertainty to investment calculations.

10.3 Economic Evaluations in Medical Processes

In medicine the main goal is always to provide high quality services for patients. The best knowledge and capabilities should always be available to ensure that all patients are treated equally. Such considerations encourage discussions about the quality of health care, which requires competent people, as well as effective processes and work methods. The findings from economic evaluation studies are hard to generalize [4]. One reason is that treatment processes can vary. Most financial calculation methods have been developed for industrial use, where processes are constant and quantities are high. In addition, *manufacturing* time and expenses, which are easy to measure and quantify, can be easily identified. What is less clear is how well these models can be used in health care. A particular challenge is how to analyze the results.

It is widely accepted that in health care two important key factors are *time* and *quality of services*. This means it is essential to make prompt diagnoses and to treat the patient in the right place at the right time. In health care, the treatment process can be long, especially for chronic diseases. In such cases, often several different parties will take part in the process. Given this, a key goal in health care is to improve the efficiency of that process; indeed, maintaining and improving the efficiency of these processes should be the focal point in managing health care organizations. The success of health care depends not only on how well each department and/or organization performs its work, it also depends on how well the various departmental and organizational activities are coordinated.

10.4 Analyzing Health Care Services

In the following subsections we will discuss key methods for analyzing health care services.

10.4.1 Balanced Scorecard

A key tool for analyzing health care services is the *balanced scorecard* method, which is a synthesis of financial accounting models and competitive capabilities. By using the balanced scorecard method it is possible to take both the hard and the soft factors into account. Balanced scorecard is also useful, because it expands the set of business objectives beyond the summary of financial measures. In our articles, we have also used normal cost calculation methods, while at the same time, proving that investment in telemedicine is logical [3]. The number of patients has been the key driver; we have also tried to determine the break-even point, where there are enough patients to justify the telemedicine investment.

10.4.2 Telemedicine Consultation Expenses

Presently, our studies have concentrated solely on historical information. As such, we have calculated expenses by comparing expenses incurred in traditional workflow with those incurred using telemedicine. The telemedicine consultation between specialist and general practitioner may in the long run save much more than expected. These extra savings come from the improved quality of the health care, as patients receive correct diagnoses immediately and timely treatment saves costs in the long run. This aspect, however, has not been taken into account in our studies.

10.4.3 Organizational Performance Perspectives

The objectives and measures view organizational performance from four perspectives: financial, customer, internal business processes, and learning and growth [5].

10.4.3.1 Finance

Financial perspective links the strategy with the long-term financial objectives. When investing in telemedicine, there should always be a long-term vision of what the organization should achieve with the investment. Investments in telemedicine are often rationalized by potential cost savings, without backing up this claim with solid data. To make better informed decisions, telemedicine cost analyses should be presented in a manner that enables easy tailoring of the method to suit other operating environments and patterns of care [2].

When analyzing the financial benefits, future operating expenses need to be taken into account as well. When comparing telemedicine with traditional methods, it is very important to identify the real expenses of the existing systems. This is because a service may be clinically competent and cost-effective in one context, but highly ineffective when viewed in another context wherein accessibility and quality of local services are higher.

10.4.3.2 Customer

In health care, needs of medical consumers need to be viewed differently from customers of a typical corporate business. In medicine, along with the service, it is important also to consider patient's experience of the health service. For example, patients usually find the treatment options provided via telemedicine very convenient [6]. In most cases it is quite natural that telemedicine will bring added value to the patient, since the patient does not need to travel long distances.

It may be challenging to discuss medical consumers of health services, because these individuals often receive health care services for which they are not directly paying. In such cases, the customer may be either the patient or the party that is paying for the service. For instance, this may occur with a public health program or an insurance company. Either way, fiinancially, the interests of these different parties may conflict in some cases. Therefore, when undertaking any analyses, it is important to define clearly the exact meaning of the word *customer*.

10.4.3.3 Internal Business Processes

Processes in health care are not as easy to standardize as are typically corporate, internal business processes. The question to consider is, which processes are the most important core processes? Our studies have indicated that telemedicine has improved these processes [6]. The quality of operations can also be measured in this category, and when evaluating processes, the quality factor must not be omitted.

There are many different management strategies that have been applied to process management. Six management programs can be identified: total quality management, time-based management, supply chain management, activity based management, lean management, and business process redesign.

Cost of quality is one of the key measurements in total quality management and in lean management. In time-based management, the key measurement is production time, which is also an important key measure in business redesign. In supply chain management and in activity-based management, minimizing cost and maximizing profit is the main aim; in this model, quality has only a tool value, and is not as important.

Which of these management programs can be chosen in the context of health care? Time varies with each patient, and patients need to be investigated and helped no matter how much time each takes. Cost of quality and customer satisfaction are naturally the key measurements. Quality is the key issue in services, and with the help of telemedicine, quality can be improved. This makes total quality management a very useful tool in health care management. The key theme in total quality management is not the cost of each phase of the process, but making things right across the whole process.

In ophthalmology, particularly for efficient screening processes for diabetic retinopathy or emergency cases, the whole process can be improved with telemedicine. In those cases, good process quality results in finding treatable cases in time to avoid later costs and human suffering, which is difficult to calculate in economic terms. Delayed diagnosis may also adversely change the level of impairment and cause high indirect costs to society.

10.4.3.4 Learning and Growth

In medicine, constant learning is also a key factor, as medical knowledge can become dated quickly. A key concern is how to keep the organization and each individual practitioner up-to-date in medical knowledge, and in the core competencies of health care.

Competencies address the ability to bundle skills as a result of organizational learning [7]. In practice it means the ability to combine different technical and operational skills. Core competencies do not wear out with use. Unlike physical assets, which deteriorate with time, information-based competencies are enhanced when applied and shared. Telemedicine makes the work of medical professionals more visible to peers and colleagues. At the same time, it also offers opportunities for colleagues to learn from each other, to eliminate inadequate practices, as they cannot go unnoticed indefinitely.

10.5 Ophthalmologic Frame

Ophthalmology has unique features compared to other medical specialties. For instance, for general practitioners (GPs) unfamiliar with a biomicroscope, the basic ophthalmologic examination is difficult to perform. Most GPs have a limited knowledge of ophthalmology, which primarily covers conjunctivitis and allergic diseases. Because, in most countries, patients with chronic eye care problems as well as other eye diseases are managed by private ophthalmologists, limited knowledge can be problematic in terms of optimal care – especially because it has been estimated that 7% of a GP's acute patients have eye problems. This is a big challenge for health care processes, because eye conditions requiring emergency care, such as acute glaucoma, endophthalmitis, and keratitis, can threaten vision.

In addition, ophthalmology requires skills in imaging and other specific diagnostic techniques that are essential for making diagnoses, and for following up on chronic diseases, such as diabetic retinopathy, glaucoma, and macular degeneration.

In ophthalmology, telemedicine can be used for chronic diseases by transmitting fundus photographs and other patient information, and in emergency situations, by using real-time solutions, especially in cases when expensive emergency transportation by ambulance or helicopter can be avoided [3]. In addition to improved treatment results, telemedicine can offer economic savings in both cases.

10.6 Balance Scorecard in Teleophthalmology

Investments in telemedicine can be evaluated by calculating savings in travel expenses, more efficient investment usage, and saved vision. However, care of the medical consumer is probably the most important issue. If the patient is seen as a customer, their opinions should be evaluated frequently. It must be kept in mind, however, that from the perspective of patients, it is not easy to compare various service alternatives if they have not experienced all of them.

Internal business processes can be done more efficiently with telemedicine. The information travels instead of the patient. Immediately after a patient's diagnosis is made, for example, laser treatment, scheduling, and follow-up can be arranged more efficiently. In addition, diagnoses and treatments can be connected from both a process and patient point of view, and every real-time and store-and-foreword consultation acts as continuing education for the medical professional.

Figure 10.1 shows one example of how to create the balance scorecard for a health care organization.

10.7 Conclusion

When analyzing the potential benefits of telemedicine, all factors – in addition to and including cost factors – need to be weighed. Telemedicine can improve health care services and also leverage the knowledge within an organization. There are often situations where improvements in processes that create new and better ways of doing things will automatically also save costs.

In health care, human resource expenses are the most significant cost factor. To ensure

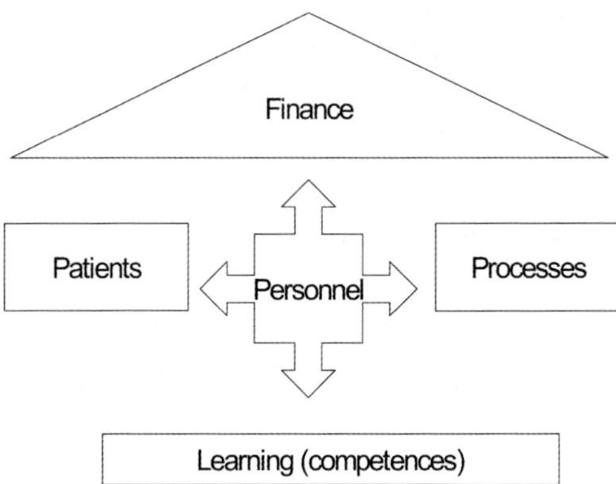

Fig. 10.1. Balanced scorecard for health care organization

smooth adoption of new processes such as telemedicine, personnel need to know the goals of the changes. Otherwise the collective concern about the possibility to lose employment or benefits may counteract the positive aspects of the new process.

In terms of operational aspects, the biggest challenges involve the optimal usage of surgical facilities and large diagnostic investments (such as imaging equipment). Additionally, those who invest in health care believe that telemedicine will lead to more effective health care by enhancing skills of personnel, and increasing usage of all other investments.

Digitalization of medical diagnostic equipment and integration with patient information systems, along with the a lack of resources, are the key reasons why telemedicine will have a bigger role in the health sector than is generally acknowledged today. It seems that in the future, telemedicine will be the only way to offer health services with higher quality within given financial constraints.

When managing and leading a health care organization, it is essential to notice how corporate management methods can be applied to health care. Due to the unique features of health care, industrial methods are not directly applicable. However, they can be used beneficially if their strengths and weaknesses are properly identified.

References

1. Lamminen H, Voipio V, Ruohonen K (2001) Telemedicine framework and applications in dermatology and ophthalmology. Ann Med 33(4):222–228
2. Mair FS, Haycox A, May C, Williams T (2000) A review of telemedicine cost-effectiveness studies. J Telemed Telecare 6(1):38–40
3. Lamminen H, Lamminen J, Ruohonen K, Uusitalo H (2001) A cost study of teleconsultation for primary-care ophthalmology and dermatology. J Telemed Telecare 7(3):167–173
4. Witten P, Mair F, Haycox A, May C, Williams T, Hellmich S (2002) Systematic review of cost-effectiveness studies of telemedicine interventions. Br Med J 324:5
5. Kaplan R, Norton P (1996) Translating strategy into action, the balances scorecard. Harvard Business School Press, Boston, MA
6. Lamminen H, Salminen L, Uusitalo H (1995) Teleconsultations between general practitioners and ophthalmologists in Finland. J Telemed Telecare 5(2):118–121
7. Prahalad C, Hamel G (1990) The core competence of the corporation. Harv Bus Rev May–June:79–91

Part II

Looking for Problems and Solutions – Telescreening

II

Chapter 11

Teleophthalmology Assessment of Diabetic Retinopathy

11

Ingrid E. Zimmer-Galler

This chapter addresses the following

Key Concepts:

- Diabetic retinopathy is a leading cause of blindness in working-age adults, but appropriate treatment can significantly reduce the risk of vision loss.
- Teleophthalmology programs based on digital retinal imaging show great promise to increase rates of evaluation for diabetic retinopathy.
- The recommendations of the *Telehealth Practice Recommendations for Diabetic Retinopathy* divide programs into four areas of care: image acquisition, image review and evaluation, patient care supervision, and image and data storage.
- Teleophthalmology assessment of diabetic retinopathy includes personnel, equipment and data transfer, legal requirements, program validation, and quality control.

11.1 Introduction

Diabetic retinopathy is a leading cause of blindness in working age adults [1]. Multiple prospective randomized clinical trials have demonstrated that appropriate treatment can significantly reduce the risk of vision loss from diabetic retinopathy [2–5]. The clinical benefits of regular examinations to establish the presence of treatable diabetic retinopathy have long been recognized [20, 22]. It has been estimated that programs resulting in detection and appropriate treatment of diabetic retinopathy could potentially save over 400 million USD in health care costs in the United States annually [6].

In spite of well-established guidelines for recommended eye examinations, a large number of patients with diabetes do not undergo such examinations [7, 8]. It is estimated that 50% or more of patients with diabetes in various populations do not follow recommendations for regular eye examinations [9]. Reasons for poor compliance are numerous, and include lack of visual symptoms in the early stages of the disease, socio-economic factors, geographic restrictions, and lack of patient and provider education about the need for regular retinal examinations for diabetic retinopathy [10].

Diabetic retinopathy is readily detected by examination and retinal imagery is regularly used to document retinal findings. In recent years, digital retinal photography has been used as a tool to assess patients with diabetic retinopathy both in the clinical and research setting. Teleophthalmology programs based on digital retinal imaging show great promise to increase rates of evaluation for diabetic retinopathy. Diabetic retinopathy is an ideal model for telemedicine initiatives, and evaluation for diabetic retinopathy is one of the most common uses of telemedicine in ophthalmology.

In the past decade, a plethora of diabetic retinopathy assessment programs on both large and small scales have been initiated. Many health care providers are interested in utilizing such programs to increase compliance with the recommendations for diabetic eye examinations. Designing, building, and implementing a teleophthalmology diabetic retinopathy program may be challenging. In conjunction with the

American Telemedicine Association (ATA), Ocular Telehealth Special Interest Group (OT-SIG), and the National Institute of Standards and Technology (NIST), a working group formulated a guide for leadership and staff to develop coherent, effective, and sustainable ocular telehealth diabetic retinopathy programs [11]. In this chapter the *Telehealth Practice Recommendations for Diabetic Retinopathy* will be reviewed.

11.2 Mission and Goals

When designing, building, and implementing a teleophthalmology diabetic retinopathy program, a clear mission statement and goals are essential. No one single system can fill all the needs and requirements of every program. It is less important, for example, whether an individual program uses a mydriatic or non-mydriatic camera, stereo or non-stereo images, single field or multiple fields, captures color or monochromatic images, etc. More importantly, specifics regarding the type of teletechnology to be used must be tailored to each individual program's needs.

The mission of a teleophthalmology diabetic retinopathy program is typically to increase access and adherence to established standards of care among patients with diabetes. Goals specific to diabetic retinopathy programs may include (1) improving access to the diagnosis and management of retinopathy, (2) reducing the incidence of vision loss, (3) improving cost-effectiveness, and (4) enhancing efficiency and clinical effectiveness of diabetic retinopathy diagnosis and management. Programs may target specific populations of patients, or be implemented on a large scale, or over a large geographic area.

11.3 Requirements to Implement Four Elements of Care

The *Telehealth Practice Recommendations for Diabetic Retinopathy* divides diabetic retinopathy telehealth programs into four elements of care: image acquisition, image review and evaluation, patient care supervision, and image and data storage. Each of these components requires personnel with specific duties and qualifications, equipment and data transfer, legal requirements, validation, and quality control.

11.3.1 Personnel

Image acquisition personnel who acquire retinal images often are not licensed eye care professionals. In fact, images are frequently obtained in settings where a licensed physician is not physically available. Therefore, image acquisition personnel must possess an appropriate knowledge base and demonstrate necessary skills to allow independent imaging. Such personnel must be able to communicate with patients to obtain informed consent, whether written or oral, and must be able to provide basic patient education. If pupillary dilation is utilized for imaging, the imager should have an understanding of angle closure glaucoma and appropriate actions to take if angle closure is suspected.

Image readers review and evaluate images for retinal lesions and to determine levels of diabetic retinopathy. Any trained, non-licensed readers must undergo in-depth training to acquire the required knowledge and skills specific to the needs of the ocular telehealth program, including performing official gradings and interpretation of retinal images. Specific protocols for initial and recurrent training and certification need to be established and documented. Such readers should also be under the direct supervision of a licensed eye care provider with expertise in the evaluation and management of diabetic retinopathy. The licensed provider is ultimately responsible for the image gradings.

Finally, telehealth programs for diabetic retinopathy should include information specialists who are image and data management specialists. Such personnel should be responsible for the integrity of stored images and data, and for the coordination of system-wide maintenance.

11.3.2 Equipment and Data Transfer

Equipment requirements are directly related to the applications they support, which, depending on the program's goals, necessitates different medical peripherals, communication technology, and support personnel. Hardware and software are used for medical information capture, transmission and display. Performance levels of teletechnological equipment should match clinical requirements.

11.3.2.1 Requirements

Equipment used in telehealth systems must conform to the requirements of local and federal regulatory agencies, such as the United States (US) Food and Drug Administration (FDA). Teletechnology equipment specifications and needs will vary widely depending on individual program goals. The diagnostic accuracy of any imaging system to be used must be validated (see Section 11.3.2.4 Validation) and the technology used should adhere to standards of Digital Imaging and Communications in Medicine (DICOM).

11.3.2.2 Data

Data compression is frequently used to facilitate transmission and storage of large data files (such as for retinal imagery). Compression algorithms must undergo thorough clinical validation, as well as periodic review, to ensure appropriate image quality and diagnostic accuracy.

Retinal image analysis technology is emerging to enhance image quality and also to automatically identify specific lesions of diabetic retinopathy [12]. Any such image processing algorithms, especially when used to assess levels of diabetic retinopathy, must undergo rigorous validation to ensure diagnostic accuracy. In the US, such technology must also be approved by the FDA before implementation in the clinical setting is possible.

Data communication and transfer should be individualized to each program's requirements. However, transmission systems should include robust error-checking systems to preclude loss of clinical information. Conformance with DICOM standards, and HL7 standards if interfacing with other health information systems, is recommended.

Computer display monitors for evaluation of retinal images should be of high quality and capable of high resolution. Display monitors used for diagnostic purposes should also be validated for accuracy of clinical diagnosis, realizing that display capabilities and characteristics may change over time.

Other issues to consider include the need for storage capacity, and policies on archiving and retrieving digital images in accordance with any applicable local or federal regulations. Similarly, security protocols need to be clearly defined to protect patient confidentiality, including 128-bit encryption and two-point authentication technology to safeguard data integrity. In the US, teleophthalmology systems must conform with Health Insurance Portability and Accountability Act (HIPPA) requirements. Finally, system and data reliability and redundancy policies, as well as a backup disaster plan should be considered.

11.3.2.3 Legal Requirements

Legal requirements relating to the practice of teleophthalmology are generally similar to those for other telemedicine modalities, with licensure issues varying from state to state (and country to country). Typically, all criteria must be met for licensure in every state or region where a telemedicine program is implemented, as well as in the location of the reading center where images are evaluated. Patients should be informed about the telehealth program and be allowed to decide whether to participate. As a part of informed consent, patients need to be advised that a teleophthalmology retinal examination does not replace a comprehensive eye examination. Signature consent is not necessarily a requirement, since ocular telehealth procedures are considered low risk and within commonly accepted standards of practice [13]. However, program outcomes should be continuously monitored to ensure that they meet or exceed current standards of care for retinal examination.

11.3.2.4 Validation

The *Telehealth Practice Recommendations for Diabetic Retinopathy* considers validation of diabetic retinopathy programs essential. ETDRS

(Early Treatment Diabetic Retinopathy Study) 30°, seven-field, stereo color 35 mm slides [14] are considered the gold-standard for evaluation of diabetic retinopathy. Since currently there are no widely accepted standard criteria for the use of digital imaging for evaluation of diabetic retinopathy, telemedicine programs for diabetic retinopathy should demonstrate an ability to compare favorably with ETDRS film photography.

Validation studies should include kappa values for agreement of diagnosis, false positive and false negative readings, positive predictive value, negative predictive value, and sensitivity and specificity of diagnosing levels of diabetic retinopathy, including macular edema. Classification schemes other than ETDRS, such as the proposed International Clinical Diabetic Retinopathy Disease Severity scale [15], may also be used for grading diabetic retinopathy. Ocular telemedicine protocols should state the standards used for validation, as well as relevant data sets for comparison.

In diabetic retinopathy telehealth programs, inability to obtain adequate images should be considered a positive finding, since the presence or absence of disease cannot be determined. Patients for whom adequate images are not obtained or are unreadable should be referred for evaluation by an eye care specialist.

Four categories of validation for diabetic retinopathy telehealth programs using ETDRS 30°, seven-field, stereo, standard, color fundus photographs as the reference standard are recognized by the *Telehealth Practice Recommendations for Diabetic Retinopathy*:

- Category I validation indicates a system that can separate patients into those who have no or very mild non-proliferative diabetic retinopathy (ETDRS level 20 or below) and those with more severe levels of diabetic retinopathy (ETDRS level 35 or worse). Functionally, this allows identification of patients with no or minimal diabetic retinopathy and those who have more than minimal diabetic retinopathy. A Category 1 validated program is designed so that all patients with greater than minimal diabetic retinopathy are referred for further evaluation.
- Category 2 validation indicates a system that can accurately identify patients with sight-threatening diabetic retinopathy and those without sight-threatening disease. Sight-threatening diabetic retinopathy includes any level of diabetic macular edema, severe non-proliferative disease (ETDRS level 53 or worse), and proliferative diabetic retinopathy (ETDRS level 61 or worse). Patients with sight-threatening disease require prompt referral for possible treatment such as laser photocoagulation.
- Category 3 validation allows patient management with decisions that match recommendations based on a dilated clinical retinal examination. This category of validation indicates a system that can identify levels of non-proliferative diabetic retinopathy, proliferative diabetic retinopathy, and macular edema with sufficient accuracy to determine appropriate disease management strategies. Additionally, this level of validation also requires the ability to detect clinically significant macular edema.
- Category 4 validation indicates a system that has been shown to match or exceed the ability of ETDRS photographs to identify lesions of diabetic retinopathy in order to determine levels of retinopathy and macular edema. Functionally, Category 4 validation indicates that a program can replace ETDRS photographs in any clinical or research setting. Although the quality of digital imaging systems is approaching that of film photography, to date, no digital imaging system has been conclusively shown to match or exceed ETDRS stereo fundus photographs for the detection of diabetic retinopathy lesions. Currently this is a theoretical rather than a practical validation category.

11.4 Quality Control

All telehealth programs should have specified policies and procedures in place to monitor and to continuously evaluate system performance [16]. Various elements of the program that include – but are not limited to – image acquisition, image transmission, and image evaluation functions, need to be re-evaluated at regular intervals. Program outcomes also need to be regularly and formally reviewed to assure sustained quality care. Outcome review and problem identification should be used to guide corrective interventions.

Telehealth Practice Recommendations for Diabetic Retinopathy lists examples of quality control measures that include standardized training for key personnel, such as imagers and readers. Training can include structured self-study and curriculum training with methods to assess skills proficiency. Initial certification should be considered provisional, followed by full certification, based on experience with a specified number of clinical encounters over a specified period of time. Levels of proficiency should be documented with a formal quality assurance review of a specified number of cases. Certification should be time-limited, requiring re-certification based on specified time periods, the number of patients, and proficiency as measured by formal reviews.

Imagers and readers should have ongoing performance reviews by random sampling of image quality and image interpretations. Outcome analyses can be used to assess proficiency, provide opportunities for program improvement, identify the need for changes in training, or identify the need for additional training.

Continuing education is an integral component of any quality assurance program and is considered a fundamental method to facilitate current competency and recurrent training. Continuing education programs do not need to follow a specific format but should be geared to achieve the desired outcome with maximal efficiency and effectiveness.

11.5 Program Examples

A number of telehealth programs have been validated against the gold-standard stereo seven-field fundus photographs for detection of diabetic retinopathy. Several of these programs have been implemented on a wide scale, with large numbers of patients with diabetes imaged to date. Two of these programs will be briefly reviewed.

11.5.1 DigiScope

An example of a diabetic retinopathy program validated at a Category 1 level is the DigiScope diabetic retinopathy risk assessment program by EyeTel Imaging, Inc. (Columbia, Maryland USA). This program is unique in that it utilizes a proprietary semi-automated fundus camera, the DigiScope [17] (Fig. 11.1), which is placed in the offices of primary care physicians.

Patients with diabetes who have not been evaluated by an eye care specialist in the past year are imaged with the DigiScope by office staff. Only minimal training is required to obtain high quality images. The device captures multiple high contrast images and estimates visual acuity. Data is encrypted and automatically transmitted overnight to a central expert reading center for review by trained, certified readers under the direction of a retinal specialist (Fig. 11.2).

The images are captured through a dilated pupil to maximize the number of gradable images. Referral is recommended for any level of diabetic retinopathy greater than microaneurysms only (modified ETDRS level 35 or worse retinopathy). A report is returned to the primary care physician with recommendations for referral or re-image in 12 months.

A validation study of 111 patients was performed against seven-field stereo photographs

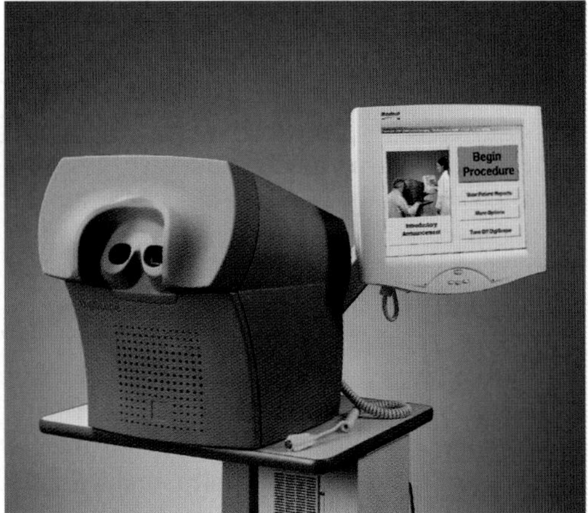

Fig. 11.1. The DigiScope, an Internet-based semi-automated fundus camera, is placed in primary care physicians' offices for diabetic retinopathy assessment

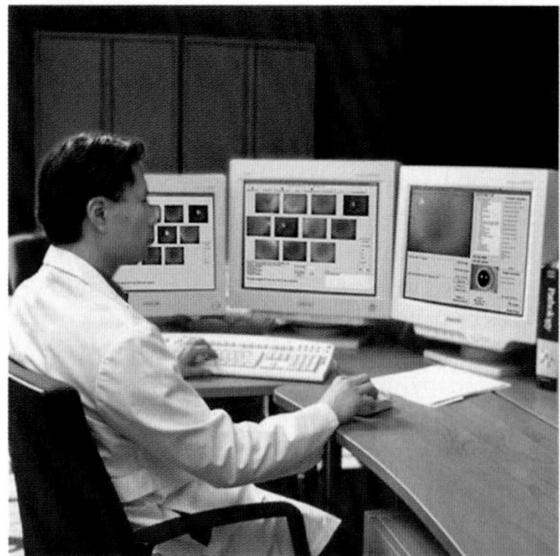

Fig. 11.2. Reading center for evaluation of DigiScope images by trained, certified readers with retina specialist supervision

[18]. Agreement based on the ability of the DigiScope to identify patients with diabetic retinopathy greater than minimal non-proliferative disease was very good (K = 0.83, sensitivity = 0.84, and specificity = 0.97) [19]. To date, more than 22,000 patients with diabetes have been imaged with the DigiScope system.

11.5.2 EyeTel Imaging

The EyeTel Imaging, Inc. business model is based on placement of the DigiScope in the offices of primary care physicians for only a nominal set up fee and monthly maintenance fee. Imaging fees are based on the standard charge for fundus photography with interpretation. Reimbursement is shared between EyeTel Imaging, Inc. and the primary care physician, who provides the office space and staff for the imaging procedure. Reimbursement has been successful, but depends on agreements negotiated by EyeTel Imaging, Inc. with individual health insurances (including Medicare) and health maintenance organizations (HMOs). A standard national reimbursement policy for diabetic retinopathy assessment programs is not in place in the US, and reimbursement issues remain a major hurdle to successful implementation of these programs.

11.5.3 Joslin Vision Network and Other Programs

The Joslin Vision Network has a diabetic retinopathy assessment program validated at a Category 3 level [19]. This system can be used to determine the clinical level of diabetic retinopathy, timing of the next appropriate retinal evaluation, and necessity of referral to an ophthalmologist. The Joslin system utilizes a commercially available non-mydriatic fundus camera optimized for low-light-level retinal imaging with remote image capture capability, and subsequent transmission of data to a central reading center for interpretation.

A validation study of 54 patients with diabetes demonstrated substantial agreement ($\kappa = 0.65$) between the clinical level of diabetic retinopathy assessed from Joslin Vision Network images compared to seven-field stereo photographs [19]. Agreement was excellent ($\kappa = 0.87$) for recommended referral to an ophthalmologist [19].

The Joslin Diabetes Eye Health Care Model is a program to facilitate diabetes management and provide quality eye care for all people with diabetes. The program is designed to assess the retina and diagnose the level of diabetic retinopathy in patients with diabetes every year to ensure timely treatment as indicated, while also managing diabetes medically and warehousing data at the Joslin Diabetes Center for education and population-based and clinical outcome studies. The Joslin Vision Network telemedicine initiative provides a technology platform for facilitating treatment and management of diabetic retinopathy. The Joslin Vision Network diabetic retinopathy assessment program has been implemented in numerous locations across the United States.

Other examples of diabetic retinopathy programs with Category 3 validation include Inoveon's Diabetic Retinopathy 3-DT System [20] and the northern Alberta community program [21]. Both of these systems are described in greater detail in other chapters in this book.

11.6 Conclusion

Implementation of telemedicine systems for diabetic retinopathy surveillance has the potential to significantly increase access to appropriate retinal care. The *Telehealth Practice Recommendations for Diabetic Retinopathy* provide guidelines for the design and implementation of a diabetic retinopathy telemedicine care program, and form the basis for evaluation of diabetic retinopathy telehealth techniques and technologies. Future studies are still needed to evaluate outcome data to assess the effectiveness or limitations in providing quality eye care with teleophthalmology.

References

1. Harris M, Hadden WC, Knowler WC, Bennett PH (1987) Prevalence of diabetes and impaired glucose tolerance and plasma glucose levels in US population ages 20–74 years. Diabetes 36:534–534
2. The Diabetic Retinopathy Study Research Group (1981) Photocoagulation treatment of proliferative diabetic retinopathy: clinical application of Diabetic Retinopathy Study (DRS) findings; DRS report number 8. Ophthalmology 88:583–600
3. Early Treatment Diabetic Retinopathy Research Group (1991) Early photocoagulation for diabetic retinopathy; ETDRS report number 9. Ophthalmology 98:766–785
4. Early Treatment Diabetic Retinopathy Research Group (1985) Photocoagulation for diabetic macular edema; ETDRS report number 1. Arch Ophthalmol 103:1796–1806
5. The Diabetic Retinopathy Vitrectomy Study Research Group (1988) Early vitrectomy for severe proliferative diabetic retinopathy in eyes with useful vision. Results of a randomized trial; DRVS report number 3. Ophthalmology 95:1307–1320
6. Javitt JC, Aiello LP, Chiang Y, Ferris FL, Canner JK, Greenfield S (1994) Preventative eye care in people with diabetes is cost-saving to the federal government. Implications for health-care reform. Diabetes Care 17:909–917
7. Kraft SK, Marrero DG, Lazaridis EN, Fineberg N, Qiu C, Clark CM (1997) Primary care physicians' practice patterns and diabetic retinopathy: current levels of care. Arch Fam Med 6:29–37
8. Lee PP, Feldman ZW, Ostermann J, Brown DS, Sloan FA (2003) Longitudinal rates of annual eye examinations of persons with diabetes and chronic eye diseases. Ophthalmology 110:1952–1959
9. Brechner RJ, Cowie CC, Howie LJ, Herman WH, Will JC, Harris MI (1993) Ophthalmic examination among adults with diagnosed diabetes mellitus. JAMA 270:1714–1718
10. Schoenfeld ER, Greene JM, Wu SY, Leske C (2001) Patterns of adherence to diabetes vision care guidelines: baseline findings from the Diabetic Retinopathy Awareness Program. Ophthalmology 108:563–571
11. Cavallerano J, Lawrence MG, Zimmer-Galler I, Bauman W, Bursell S, Gardner WK, Horton M, Hildebrand L, Federman J, Carnahan L, Kuzmak P, Peters JM, Darkins A, Ahmed J, Aiello LM, Aiello LP, Buck G, Cheng YL, Cunningham D, Goodall E, Hope N, Huang E, Hubbard L, Janezewski M, Lewis JW, Matsuzaki H, McVeigh FL, Motzno J, Parker-Taillon D, Read R, Soliz P, Szirth B, Vigersky RA, Ward T, American Telemedicine Association Ocular Telehealth Special Interest Group, National Institute of Standards and Technology Working Group (2004) Telehealth practice recommendations for diabetic retinopathy. Telemed J E Health 10:469–482
12. Hansen AB, Hartvig NV, Jensen MS, Borch-Johnsen K, Lund-Andersen H, Larsen M (2004) Diabetic retinopathy screening using digital non-mydriatic fundus photography and automated image analysis. Acta Ophthalmol Scand 82:666–672
13. Stanberry B (2001) Legal ethical and risk issues in telemedicine. Comput Meth Programs Biomed 64:225–233
14. Early Treatment Diabetic Retinopathy Study Group (1991) Grading diabetic retinopathy from stereoscopic color fundus photographs – an extension of the modified Airlie House Classification; ETDRS report 10. Ophthalmology 98:786–806
15. Wilkinson CP, Ferris FL, Klein RE, Lee PP, Agardh CD, Davis M, Dills D, Kampik A, Pararajasegaram R, Verdaguer JT, Global Diabetic Retinopathy Project Group (2003) Proposed international clinical diabetic retinopathy and diabetic macular edema disease severity scales. Ophthalmology 110:1677–1682
16. Eliasson A, Poropatich R (1998) Performance improvement in telemedicine: the essential elements. Mil Med 8:530–535
17. Zeimer R, Zou S, Meeder T, Quinn K, Vitale S (2002) A fundus camera dedicated to the screening of diabetic retinopathy in the primary care physician's office. Invest Ophth Vis Sci 43:1581–1587
18. Schiffman RM, Jacobsen G, Nussbaum JJ, Desai UR, Carey D, Glasser D, Zimmer-Galler IE, Zeimer R, Goldberg MF (2005) Comparison of a digital retinal imaging system and seven-field stereo color fundus photography to detect diabetic retinopathy in the primary care environment. Ophthal Surg Las Im 5:46–56

19. Bursell SE, Cavallerano JD, Cavallerano AA, Clermont AC, Birkmire-Peters D, Aiello LP, Aiello LM, Joslin Vision Network Research Team (2001) Stereo nonmydriatic digital video color retinal imaging compared with Early Treatment Diabetic Retinopathy Study: seven standard field 35-mm stereo color photos for determining level of diabetic retinopathy. Ophthalmology 108:572–585
20. Fransen DR, Leonard-Martin TC, Feuer WJ, Hildebrand PL, Inoveon Health Research Group (2002) Clinical evaluation of patients with diabetic retinopathy: Accuracy of the Inoveon Diabetic Retinopathy-3DT system. Ophthalmology 109:595–601
21. Tennant MT, Greve MD, Rudnisky CJ, Hillson TR, Hinz BJ (2001) Identification of diabetic retinopathy by stereoscopic digital imaging via teleophthalmology: a comparison to slide film. Can J Ophthalmol 36:187–196
22. The American Academy of Ophthalmology Quality of Care Committee Retina Panel (1989) Diabetic retinopathy: preferred practice patterns. San Francisco, CA

Chapter 12

Diabetic Retinopathy Screening: Which Model is Appropriate?

12

Chris J. Barry, Ian L. McAllister, Ian J Constable, Kanagasingam Yogesan

This chapter addresses the following

Key Concepts:

- Diabetic retinopathy screening by health professionals other than ophthalmologists is now an accepted adjunct to standard clinical practice in many countries world-wide.
- With the advent of affordable digital imaging technology, screening programs can become more centralized, allowing data auditing and automatic recall systems.
- Three separate governmental health agencies supervise health delivery in the one State in Austrailia, which can be a deterrent to a unified screening service, because cultural, bureaucratic, political, and remuneration complications remain hurdles to gaining a unified approach.
- The rural and remote diabetic screening model can also be applied to glaucoma, amblyopia, trachoma and optometric services.
- Telemedicine and digital screening will play an increasingly vital role in the delivery and assessment of screening programs.

12.1 Introduction

Screening diabetics for retinopathy is now commonplace for optometrists, physicians specializing in diabetes, ophthalmic photographers, ophthalmologists, and allied health professionals. Recently, there has been a major shift in screening delivery, with fewer ophthalmologists to more health professionals – a shift that is potentially increasing the detection and treatment of diabetic retinopathy. Non-mydriatic retinal cameras, which are now in use in many countries as a screening tool, have become simple to operate, requiring only limited training relative to other screening modalities.

Diabetic retinopathy screening by health professionals other than ophthalmologists, is now an accepted adjunct to standard clinical practice in many countries world-wide. The screening methodology chosen is dependent on the availability and experience of personnel, and on whether the target population is metropolitan, rural, or remote-based. Screening programs are usually managed on a local or city-centric model. With the advent of affordable digital imaging technology, screening programs can become more centralized, allowing data auditing and automatic recall systems. These idealistic scenarios are yet to realize their full potential, but are the screening goals in many locations.

Not surprisingly, the latest information and up-to-date discussion papers are Web-based documents rather than scientific journal reviews. In particular, the United Kingdom (UK) screening protocol evaluations are well underway in a search for a nationwide approach for both metropolitan and rural models, along with detailed assessments of the various methodologies.

Following is an overview of diabetic retinopathy screening models, with information obtained from Web-based discussion documents, the scientific and medical press, and our own observations and experience, which covers three decades of metropolitan, rural and remote diabetic retinopathy screening programs in Western Australia.

12.2 Rationale for Screening

The four World Health Organization (WHO) principles for medical screening programs state that (1) the condition should be an important health problem with a recognizable pre-symptomatic state, (2) it should be an appropriate screening procedure that is acceptable both to the public and health care professionals, (3) treatment should be safe, effective and universally approved, and (4) the economic cost of early diagnosis and treatment should be considered in relation to total expenditure on health care.

Diabetic retinopathy is a complication of both insulin dependent (type 1) and non-insulin dependent (type 2) diabetes. The prevalence of retinopathy is strongly linked to the duration of diabetes. After 20 years of diabetes, nearly all patients with type 1 diabetes and over 60% of patients with type 2 diabetes have some degree of retinopathy; up to a fifth of newly diagnosed diabetics have been found to have some retinopathy.

Additionally, diabetics are 25 times more likely to go blind than a person in the general population [1, 2].

Following are other statistics on diabetes and related ailments:

- Estimates on the prevalence of diabetes vary from 2–4% of the population, and are considerably higher in some ethnic and indigenous groups.
- Ten to fifteen percent are type 1 diabetics; the remainder have type 2 diabetes.
- Ten years after diagnosis, the prevalence of retinopathy is 40 to 50%.
- Twenty years after diagnosis, the prevalence of retinopathy is 90%.
- Diabetic retinopathy remains the most common cause of blindness in the working age population in many countries, including Australia, the UK and the United States (US).

The Diabetic Retinopathy Study (DRS) [3] and the Early Treatment of Diabetic Retinopathy Study (ETDRS) [4] are two major studies that have contributed to understanding the natural course of diabetic retinopathy, as well as risk factors for visual loss; they also provide guidelines for the management of diabetic retinopathy. The DRS established that panretinal photocoagulation could improve the visual prognosis of proliferative retinopathy, while the ETDRS and other studies established the benefit of focal laser photocoagulation in eyes with macular edema.

Several studies have reported the cost-effectiveness of screening for retinopathy [5, 6], by establishing that screening saves vision at a relatively low cost, and that this cost is many times less than the disability payments provided to people who go blind in the absence of a screening program.

In 1983 the annual cost of treating a diabetic at risk of blindness was estimated in the UK to be £387 (GBP), compared with welfare benefits paid to a blind person in the amount of £3,575 (GBP) per annum. Laser treatment facilities for diabetic retinopathy are available in most western countries and a screening program is a suitable adjunct to treatment facilities with the promise of reaching a far higher proportion of the target population.

12.3 Screening Modalities

Many different types of screening programs that are currently used are dependent on the local availability of facilities. Variables include the number of available ophthalmologists, other trained healthcare professionals, geography, equipment, and the resources available for screening.

The gold standard for identifying and grading retinopathy is a retinal examination that uses indirect biomicroscopy by an ophthalmologist or seven field stereoscopic photographs of each eye interpreted by experienced readers.

Potential screening methods for diabetic retinopathy are:

1. Ophthalmoscopy
   a. Ophthalmologists
   b. Optometrists
   c. Diabetic physician
   d. General practitioner
2. Photography
   a. Large city centers
   b. Mobile rural
3. A combination of ophthalmoscopy (1) and photography (2)

12.3.1 Ophthalmoscopy

Mass screening for diabetic retinopathy by indirect ophthalmoscopic fundal examination and slit lamp biomicroscopy by ophthalmologists is the preferred screening method, because it maintains a high level of sensitivity and specificity detection rates. Treatment can be scheduled after examination, reducing the number of patients that do not receive appropriate management or follow-up. However, the number of ophthalmologists per patient population varies dramatically between countries, and with city, rural or remote locations. Therefore, other screening modalities may be used to supplement this lack of personnel.

Optometrists are generally accessible from the patient's home or workplace in a metropolitan or rural setting. Facilities for slit lamp biomicroscopy are available at most practices and some optometrists are already performing indirect ophthalmoscopy on a slit lamp. Others can easily be trained to acquire this skill. It has been shown that with appropriate training, they are able to detect diabetic retinopathy and make the correct decision about whether to refer the patient for secondary care. Optometrist-based screening schemes are successfully in operation in many places [7].

Diabetic physicians can provide eye screening as a part of the total package of diabetic care; they are experienced in this field and check the patient at regular intervals. However a large proportion (40–60%) of diabetics are not seen by a diabetes specialist, but, instead, are cared for by their general practitioners. This is because general practitioners (GPs) are easily accessible to many patients, and thus are well-positioned to do screening in communities – even though direct ophthalmoscopy is the usual screening tool of GPs, which may not be as sensitive as other screening modalities [8, 9].

12.3.2 Photography

The gold standard of seven field 30° stereophotographs is not practical in mass screening programs due to cost and the time it takes to photograph, collate, and read the images. Non-mydriatic retinal cameras usually have a 45° angle of view, and screening protocols use either a single image of the posterior pole per eye, two images (macula centered, disc centered), or stereo images either in color or monochrome red-free.

Recording and archiving of images have traditionally been done using 35 mm photographic slides or Polaroid prints. The role of newer technology in the form of digitally computerized imaging offers the prospect of immediate high quality images that can easily and quickly be transferred from the screening camera to a central reading center if sufficient band width telecommunications are available.

12.3.2.1 Mobile Retinal Photography

Studies have shown that a mobile retinal photography service can provide an acceptable screening service [10]. The photographs can be taken by a mobile unit with a camera and a technician, and are later assessed by a trained reader or an ophthalmologist. Non-mydriatic retinal cameras are now simple to operate and require only minimal photographic training for successful results to be obtained (Fig. 12.1). As this method is well suited to serve rural communities where the number of diabetics may be small, trained nurses, trainee doctors, photographers or trained health workers can operate the camera (Fig. 12.2). Strangely, the promise of non-mydriatic imaging from scanning laser ophthalmoscopy has not been realized in any known major study

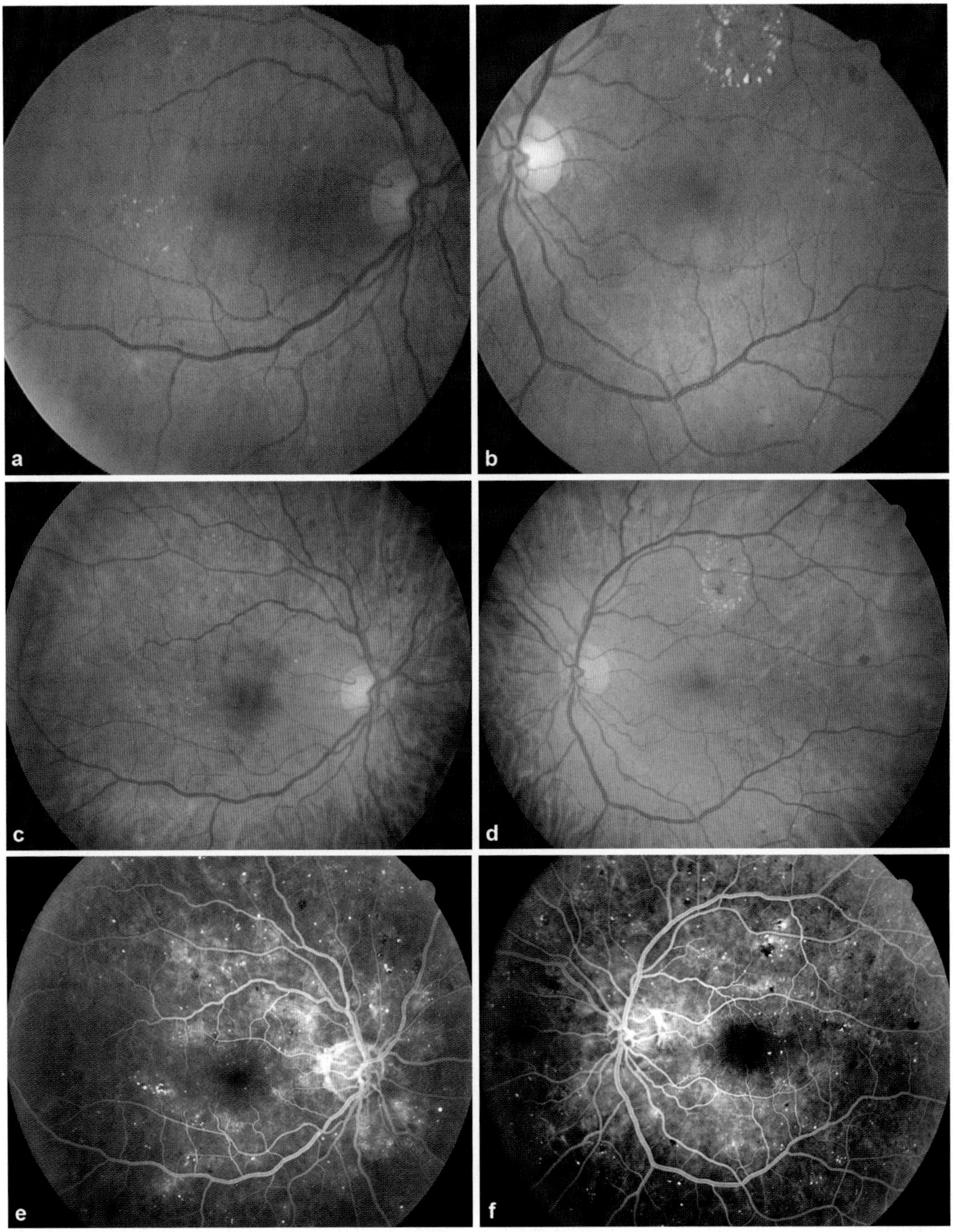

12

Fig. 12.1. Comparison of screening images with clinic-based investigation. **a** and **b** are Polaroid images taken by a health worker using a non-mydriatic camera. **c–f** were taken using a Canon 60UVi mydriatic camera of the same patient. Although more information is available with conventional, clinic-based images, the screening photographs are adequate for retinopathy assessment and treatment

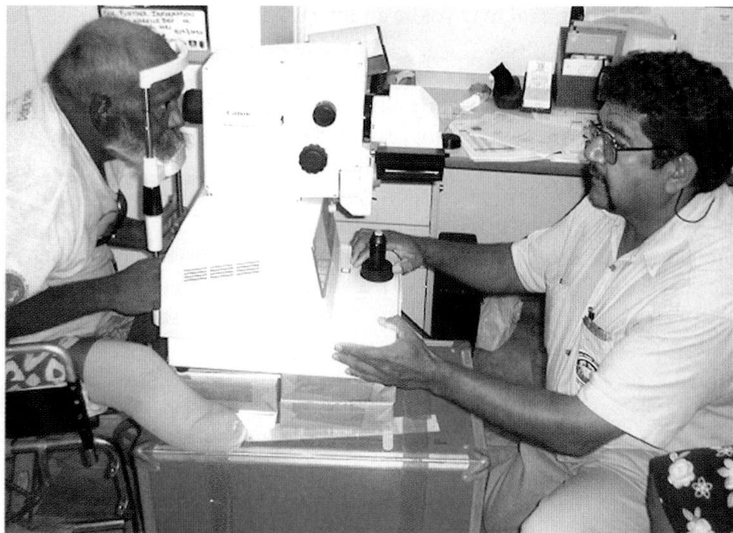

Fig. 12.2. Screening venues may not always be perfect. Here the camera travel case is used as a table (photo provided by Shelley Walters)

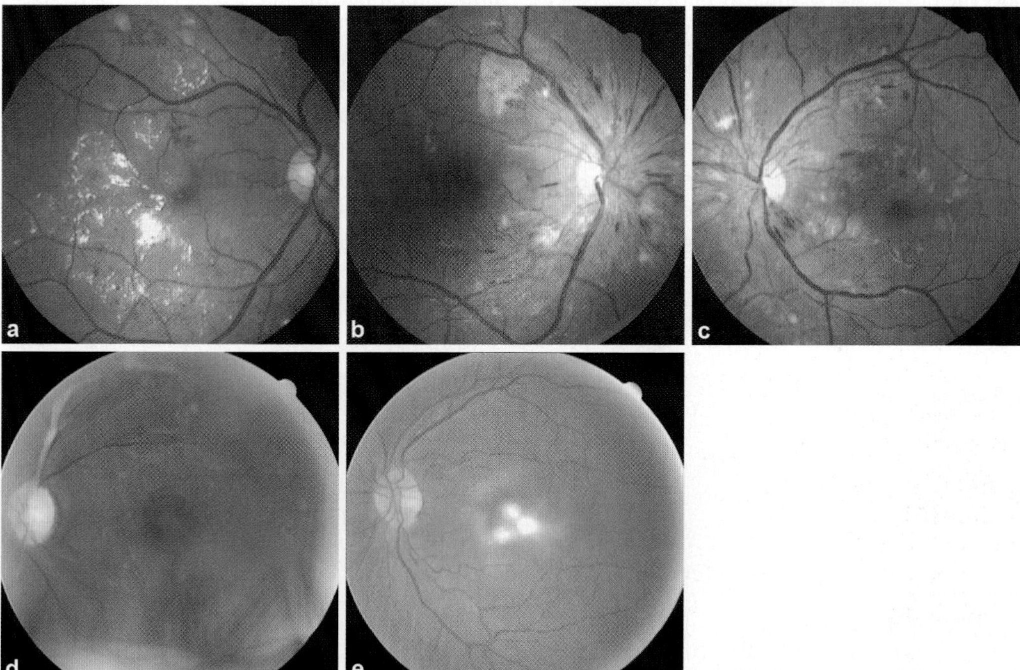

Fig. 12.3. Good quality images (**a–c**), although **b** has some fall-off due to a small pupil. **d** image is graded as adequate, with eyelashes interfering with image; however, scar tissue and previous laser are visible. **e** image is graded as unacceptable, because artifacts on the front surface of the lens obscure the macula

of rural screening, and may yet be an instrument of interest in this process.

To achieve near universal coverage, the screening method has to be community-based and the point of delivery must be within easy reach of the population. A central database, in the form of a diabetic register, which generates recalls is useful to ensure that people at risk do not *slip through the net* and is also valuable for auditing the effectiveness of the program [11].

12.3.2.2 Mydriatic Agents

The use of mydriatic agents to improve screening performance remains a contentious issue, particularly with non-medical personnel. With photography, the proportion of unusable images is lowered when mydriasis is used. Studies report the proportion of unclear photographs (Fig. 12.3) that cannot be assessed vary from 3 - 26%, [12] although recent data suggests that a technical failure rate well within the 5% Diabetes UK (BDA) Audit Standard is achievable in routine practice when mydriasis is used [13].

Additionally, some patients resist being dilated, because they will be unable to drive afterward. However, if retinal images cannot be obtained even with mydriasis, a fundal reflex (red reflex) photograph can give the reader information on of either lenticular or corneal opacities. Combined with visual acuity (Fig. 12.4), the use of red reflex photography decreases the number of unusable images (Fig. 12.5).

12.4 Current Screening Provisions

In the following subsections we will describe screening provisions in the UK, the US, and Australia.

12.4.1 United Kingdom and United States

There is inconsistency in service provision for diabetic retinopathy screening in the UK, with services ranging from centralized services that utilize and offer the latest cost-effective technology and recording program outcomes, to ad hoc services with no central organization and no recording of service outcomes [7]. The proportion of people with known diabetes screened in a year ranges from 38–85% across districts, and from 14% to 9% across general practices [13]. Similar data has also been published from the US [14]. For instance, when 4410 diabetic adults in upstate New York were studied, 34% of patients were screened in 1993. The probability of screen-

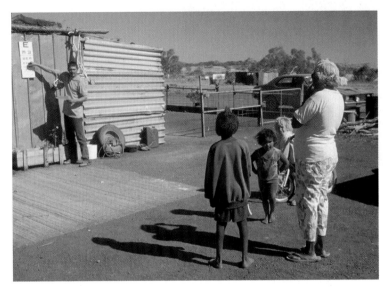

Fig. 12.4. Visual acuity is an important part of the screening process, although conditions may not be perfect. Note that an E chart is used so that illiterates are not embarrassed

ing was significantly higher for older, female, white patients, though only 16% of diabetic patients received an annual screening for two consecutive years (1992 and 1993). The low rate of diabetic retinopathy screening raises quality of life issues for patients with diabetes, and other concerns such as long-term costs of caring for them, and social costs due to lost productivity.

12.4.2 Australia

In Australia, three separate governmental health agencies supervise health delivery in the one State. This is not unique to Australia, and can be a deterrent to a unified screening service. Separate databases exist for the diabetic population, dependent upon the delivery agency. Cultural, bureaucratic, political and remuneration complications remain hurdles to gaining a unified approach. However, in some remote areas, bi-annual attendance for retinal photography is higher than city-based models.

Indigenous Health Workers ensure appointment attendance and that follow-up treatment is similarly supervised. This model has many benefits where non-compliance is considered high. Locally based, culturally sensitive, trained personnel are able to assist with all levels of information dissemination, transport and appointment attendance.

In addition, it is more appropriate that ethnic and indigenous peoples feel at ease throughout the screening and treatment process, particularly where the prevalence of diabetes can exceed 25%. The use of portable diode lasers in rural centers with no resident ophthalmic services has greatly improved attendance for treatment, and is cost-effective where expensive patient travel can be reduced. Ultimately, the availability of resources and infrastructure together with local remunerative practices will dictate the choice between these screening modalities.

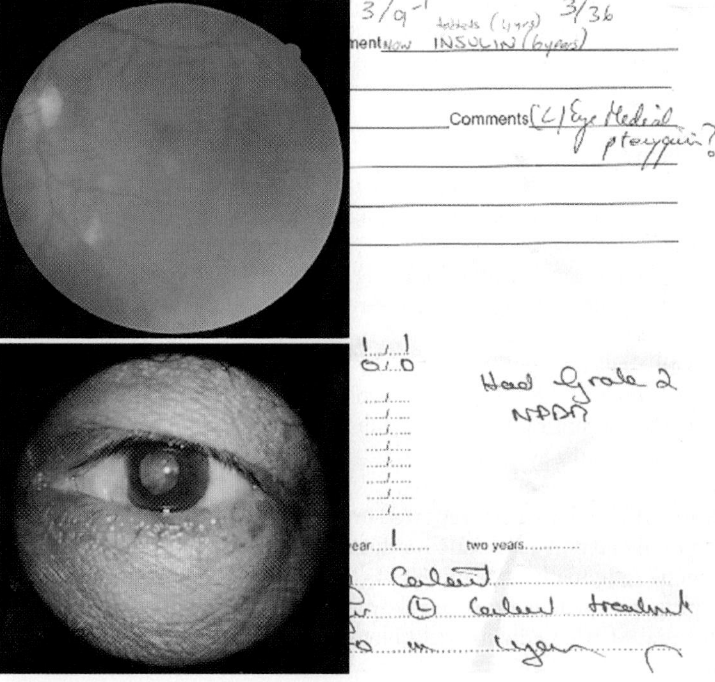

Fig. 12.5. Section of a remote area screening data sheet. The fundus image has poor quality although hemorrhages and exudates can be identified. Visual acuity (OS) was assessed as 20/200. A red reflex photograph using the non-mydriatic camera identifies a presumed cortical cataract, partially explaining the reduced visual acuity

12.5 Telemedicine

Telemedicine, or the exchange of medical data via electronic communication, can encompass the transfer of basic patient information, the transfer of images, videos and patient interviews over telecommunication networks. A major barrier in ophthalmology is that high-resolution color images are required to capture the fine detail of the eye. Image files can be large, and therefore transmission of these high-resolution images can be time intensive.

12.5.1 Advantages

With the store-and-forward method of image transmission, images can be captured, compressed, and stored in the computer for transmission at a later stage. This is a cost-effective mode that utilizes low bandwidth and can that can send high-resolution images. Therefore, it is more suitable for ophthalmology, particularly eye screenings.

The advantages of digital photography and therefore of telemedicine include:

12

- Ease of image acquisition and storage
- Low running costs compared to film
- Patient-comfort with the lower flash intensity of digital camera systems
- Ability to review images with patients, and potentially educate them
- Immediate assessment of image quality, with the option of re-taking the image, if necessary
- Archiving, storing, manipulating, and transmitting digital images to another location for review
- Utilizing the potential for in-built audit systems to help the systems evolve usefully, while preventing treatable patients from being lost in the system

Several studies have been reported on the validation of digital non-mydriatic fundus cameras for diabetic retinopathy screening [14–19]. However, programs to date have been slow to realize the potential of telemedicine technology, primarily due to the lack of remuneration for reading and referral services.

12.5.2 Digital Cameras

Digital cameras are useful in either rural or city-based screening models, but remote digital screening has been less successful to date. Digital cameras add a greater degree of complexity for unskilled operators. They have a greater chance of breakdown (particularly the older video capture systems) where mobile services are required. If good communication and transmission lines are unavailable, Polaroid film remains a useful alternative.

12.5.3 Remote Areas

We are currently assessing commercial digital cameras attached to non-mydriatic cameras in remote areas. Early trials suggest that this new generation of digital cameras are capable of crossing rough terrain and unsealed roads although further remote trips will be needed to fully trial all aspects of digital imaging in these locations.

Screening remote indigenous Australian aborigines requires long distance travel over rough terrain to communities with small populations. However, diabetes is a major health problem among aborigines, and maintaining ophthalmic care is a high priority.

In Western Australia, both government and non-government agencies carry out diabetic retinopathy screening under the umbrella supervision of the Lions Eye Institute. The findings from one group for 2004 are shown in Table 12.1 from a mainly aboriginal population living in a rural setting and were assessed by the same observer. From Table 12.1 it can be seen that 26.2% of those screened need ongoing ophthalmic follow-up. This reinforces the need for the continuance of screening programs. All images were taken by Aboriginal Health Workers after a short training program with Canon non-mydriatic cameras using mainly Polaroid film.

Table 12.1. Results of diabetic retinopathy screening for 2004 by a rural-based aboriginal program

NPDR grade 1	2.1%
NPDR grade 2	13.7%
NPDR grade 3	2.1%
PDR grade 1	2.1%
Maculopathy 1	0.6%
Age-related macular degeneration	0.6%
Cataract (requiring treatment)	0.6%
Cupped discs	1.3%
Old branch retinal vein occlusion	1.3%
High BP (copper wiring)	0.6%
Benign intra cranial hypertension?	0.6%
Unknown blood disorder	0.6%
Total	**26.2%**

12.5.4 Implementation Studies

There are very few implementation studies on telemedicine screening of diabetic retinopathy reported in the literature [20–23]. Digital eye screening in a prison has been successfully tested by our group [24–26]. Of note is one prison in Western Australia, where four of six inmates with hospital outpatient appointments could be diagnosed as not needing follow-up appointments after telemedicine consultations. There was a cost saving of 220 USD per inmate (year 2000 values).

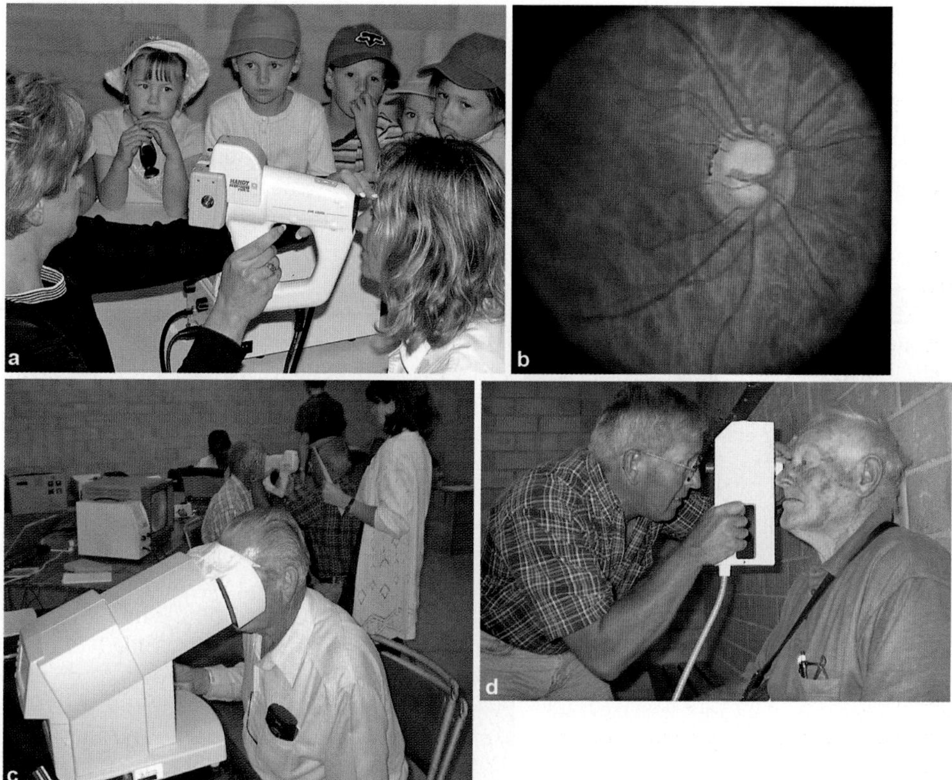

Fig. 12.6. Glaucoma can be screened by imaging the optic disc (a–b) with a hand held non-mydriatic camera, frequency doubling perimetry (c) and pneumatic tonometry (d).

12.6 What Does the Future Hold?

Screening of known diabetics by non-ophthalmologists is now generally accepted as an alternative to conventional eye examinations for diabetic retinopathy. It can further be argued that a similar approach can be applied to other eye conditions, particularly in areas where resident ophthalmic services are unavailable. The rural and remote diabetic screening model can also be applied to glaucoma, amblyopia, trachoma and optometric services. Significant eye problems with a presymptomatic state will benefit from improved access to screening programs, and decreasing treatable blindness rates in remote communities (Figs. 12.6, 12.7, and 12.8). Coupled with the powerful and emerging technology of telemedicine, there are endless possibilities for moving the primary eye examination away from the office to locations where services are less than adequate, albiet without large infrastructure costs.

Telemedicine and digital screening will play an increasingly vital role in the delivery and assessment of screening programs. A significant component of any screening program is that it must be readily available to the entire target group. Mobile screening services coupled with telemedicine data transfer, and high quality control levels that ensure timely treatment are all prime requisites.

12.7 Conclusion

Annual or bi-annual dilated fundus examination is desirable for screening diabetic retinopathy. Although the importance of this schedule is widely accepted, this objective continues to elude about half the patients with diabetes mellitus. A good start has been made in organizing diabetic retinopathy screening, but in order to provide a sensitive, cost-effective, and easily accessible screening service that achieves universal coverage, more programs must be initiated, funded, and audited.

Key issues in the future will be the training of screening personnel, and finding funds for screening. At the same time, newer technologies, including digital imaging, may reduce the cost of

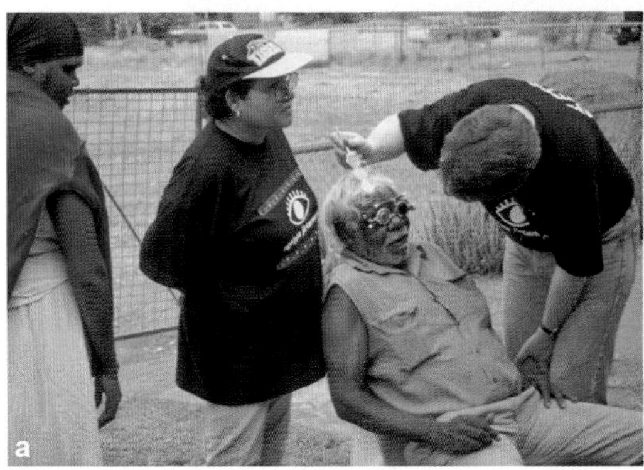

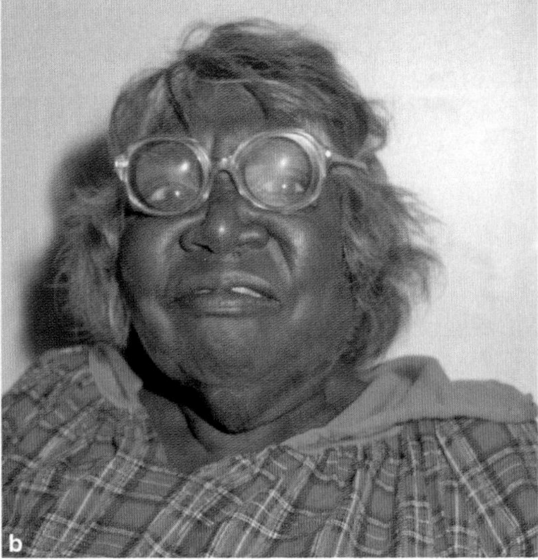

Fig. 12.7. Simple refraction test that can often improve vision. This female (**b**) has had an intracapsular cataract operation in the past without IOL insertion, requiring her to wear thick corrective glasses that have literally been sandblasted by the desert. A new pair of glasses returned vision to normal

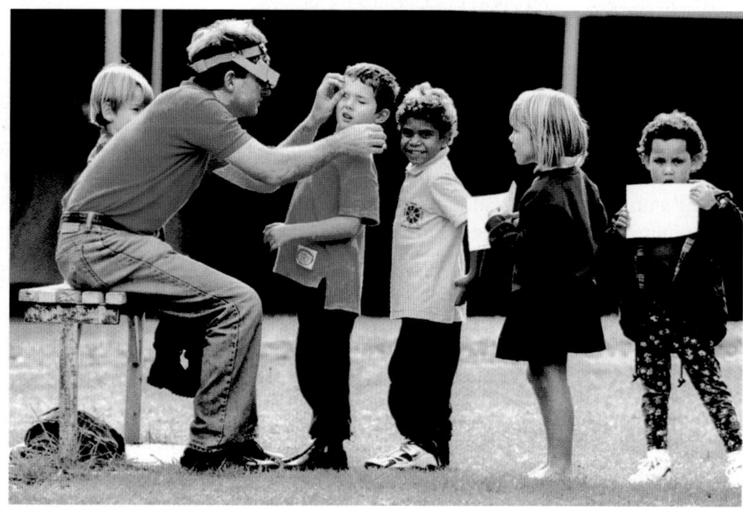

Fig. 12.8. Everting the eyelid to look for trachoma, a severe, chronic, contagious conjunctival and corneal infection often associated with dry hot climates where personal hygiene may be restricted. Photo: Courtesy West Australian

screening. Nationwide diabetic registers will play an important role in ensuring attendance, and continuing audit will ensure further improvements.

References

1. Prasad S (1999) Screening for diabetic retinopathy: an overview. http://www.priory.com/med/eye.htm. Cited 4 Oct 2005
2. Ophthalmic Research Network (2005) Screening for diabetic retinopathy. http://www.diabetic-retinopathy.screening.nhs.uk/overview-of-screening-models.html. Cited 4 Oct 2005
3. Early Treatment of Diabetic Retinopathy Study Group (1985) Photocoagulation for diabetic macular edema (Early Treatment Diabetic Retinopathy Study). Arch Ophthalmol 103(12):1796–1806
4. Early Treatment of Diabetic Retinopathy Study Group (1991) Grading diabetic retinopathy from stereoscopic color fundus photographs: an extension of the modified Airlie House classification; ETDRS report number 10. Ophthalmology 98(5):786–806
5. Matz H, Falk M, Gottinger W, Kieselbach G (1996) Cost-benefit analysis of diabetic eye disease. *Ophthalmologica* 210(6):348–353
6. Lairson DR, Pugh JA, Kapadia AS, Lorimor RJ, Jacobson J, Velez R (1992) Cost-effectiveness of alternative methods for diabetic retinopathy screening. Diabetes Care 15(10):1369–1377
7. Bagga P, Verma D, Walton C, Masson EA, Hepburn DA (1998) Survey of diabetic retinopathy screening services in England and Wales. Diabet Med 15:780–782
8. Taylor DJ, Fisher J, Jacob J, Tooke JE (1999) The use of digital cameras in a mobile retinal screening environment. Diabet Med 16:680–686
9. Buxton MJ, Sculpher MJ, Ferguson BA, Humphreys JE, Altman JFB, Spiegelhalter DJ, Kirby AJ, Jacob JS, Bacon H, Dudbridge SB (1991) Screening for treatable diabetic retinopathy: a comparison of different methods. Diabet Med 8:371–377
10. Pugh JA, Jacobson JM, Van Heuwen WA (1992) Screening for diabetic retinopathy: the wide angle camera. Diabetes Care 16:889–895
11. Aldington SJ, Kohner EM, Meuer S, Klein R, Sjølie AK (1995) Methodology for retinal photography and assessment of diabetic retinopathy: the EURODIAB IDDM complications study. *Diabetologia* 38(4):437–444
12. Walters S, Mak D, Barry CJ, McAllister IL (2003) Screening for diabetic retinopathy in the Kimberley region of Western Australia. J Ophthalmic Photogr 25(1):36–39
13. Grimshaw GM, Baker R, Wilson AD, Thompson JR, Atkinson M (1999) Report of the Inter-College Audit of Diabetic Retinopathy Screening. Leicester University, Leicester
14. Diamond JP, McKinnon M, Barry C, Geary D, McAllister I, House P, Constable IJ (1998) Non-mydriatic fundus photography: a viable alternative to funduscopy for identification of diabetic retinopathy in an Aboriginal population in rural Western Australia? Aust N Z J Ophthalmol 26:109–115

15. Young S, George J, Lusty J, Owens DR (1997) A new screening tool for diabetic retinopathy: the Canon CR5 45NM retinal camera with Frost Medical Software RIS-Lite digital imaging system. J Audiov Media Med 20:11–14
16. Lim JI, LaBree L, Nicholos T, Cardenas I (2000) A comparison of digital nonmydriatic fundus imaging with standard 35-millimeter slides for diabetic retinopathy. Ophthalmology 107:866–870
17. Yogesan K, Constable IJ, Barry CJ, Eikelboom RH, McAllister IL, Tay-Kearney ML (2000) Telemedicine screening of diabetic retinopathy using handheld fundus camera. Telemed J 6(2):231–235
18. Constable IJ, Yogesan K, Eikelboom RH, Barry CJ, Cuypers M (2000) Digital screening for eye disease. Clin Exp Ophthalmol 28:129–132
19. Bursell SE, Cavallerano JD, Cavallerano AA, Clermont AC, Birkmire-Peters D, Aiello LP, Aiello LM, Joslin Vision Network Research Team (2001) Stereo nonmydriatic digital-video color retinal imaging compared with early treatment diabetic retinopathy study seven standard field 35-mm stereo color photos for determining level of diabetic retinopathy. Ophthalmology 108:572–585
20. Tennant MTS, Rudnisky CJ, Hinz BJ, MacDonald IM, Greve MDJ (2000) Teleophthalmology via stereoscopic digital imaging: A pilot study. Diabetes Technol Ther 2(4):583–587
21. Cummings DM, Morrissey S, Barondes MJ, Rogers L, Gustke S (2001) Screening for diabetic retinopathy in rural areas: The potential of telemedicine. J Rural Health 17(1):25–31
22. Marcus DM, Brooks SE, Ulrich LD, Bassi FH, Laird M, Johnson M, Newman C (1998) Telemedicine diagnosis of eye disorders by direct ophthalmoscopy: a pilot study. Ophthalmology 105(10):1907–1914
23. Liesenfeld B, Kohner E, Piehlmeier W, Kluthe S, Aldington S, Porta M, Bek T, Obermaier M, Mayer H, Mann G, Holle R, Hepp KD (2000) A telemedical approach to the screening of diabetic retinopathy: digital fundus photography. Diabetes Care 23(3):345–348
24. Tang RA, Appel D, Caswell H, Campbell A, Jennische M (2000) Managing eye disease behind bars: how we handle consultations and referral screening triage. Telemed J 6:188
25. Barry CJ, Henderson C, Kanagasingam Y, Constable IJ (2001) Working towards a portable teleophthalmic system for use in maximum security prisons: a pilot study. Telemed J E Health 7(3):1–5
26. Yogesan K, Henderson C, Barry CJ, Constable IJ (2001) Online eye care in prisons in Western Australia. J Telemed Telecare 7(2):63–64

Chapter 13

Digital Detection of Diabetic Retinopathy – Screening From an American Perspective

13

Lawrence M. Merin

This chapter addresses the following

Key Concepts:

- More than 40 million American citizens have impaired glucose tolerance (so-called *pre-diabetes*).
- We face an unprecedented healthcare crisis: a huge increase in people at risk for the worst complications of chronic illness, with too few specialists to provide regular screening and timely intervention.
- For many in underserved areas, or who do not recognize the risks, or who do not have the financial ability to pay for care, diabetic retinopathy threatens to deprive them of their vision.
- Digital detection of diabetic retinopathy uses high-resolution retinal imaging as a technological means to reach patients who would not otherwise obtain dilated retinal examinations, and offers an efficient method of shepherding those patients with treatable diabetic eye disease toward the ophthalmic specialist care they need to preserve their sight.

13.1 Introduction

We live in dangerous times, caused by a unique confluence of factors that include economic stress associated with an increase in relatively low-paying service industry jobs, health care system breakdown caused in large measure by huge increases in pharmaceutical costs, ethnic and racial health disparities, increasingly sedentary lifestyle, poor nutrition, increasing obesity [1], and more than 43 million Americans who lack health insurance. Thus, it is not surprising that new cases of chronic illnesses like diabetes are on the rise [2, 3]. Taken singularly, each of these health issues represents a severe public health problem. In concert, they form a perfect storm that threatens millions of people with permanent disability, and poses a great danger to the physical and economic well-being of society [4, 5].
In the case of diabetes, the following statements are uncontroversial:

1. The longer a patient has diabetes and the more severe the disease, the greater the chance of developing diabetic retinopathy.
2. Diabetic retinopathy has a well-understood natural history with a prolonged asymptomatic early stage.
3. Early treatment results in improved visual outcomes.

Strategies to detect and treat diabetic retinopathy have been proposed and subsequently validated by numerous multicenter clinical trials, which have been translated into evidence-based patient care. When applied rigorously, annual dilated retinal examinations combined with laser photocoagulation reduce the risk of vision loss and can preserve useful vision. However, the recommended care standards are not universally obtained by known diabetics. Education and affluence are associated with better health, and patients who fit those metrics are more likely to be examined and treated regularly. People who live in major metropolitan areas have greater choice of providers. Patients who are indigent [6], elderly [7], poorly schooled, members of an ethnic or racial minority [8, 9], or who live in a rural area are less likely to obtain annual eye examinations and thus are more likely to suffer the consequences of untreated disease.

Remote detection of diabetic retinopathy through the use of digital imaging and telemedicine, is a useful addition to conventional physician-provided screening [10]. It overcomes time, money and logistical constraints, improves access, reduces disparities, provides equity of care, and improves outcomes – and it may also be beneficial even in light of today's unprecedented increases in newly diagnosed cases of diabetes.

13.2 Materials and Methods

In countries with a centralized health care authority, programs that extend screening opportunities to most known diabetic patients have already been established. For instance, both England [11] and Scotland [12] have developed extensive background documentation, program descriptions, protocols, and quality assurance schemes, and have made these documents readily available on the World-Wide Web.

Several approaches to diabetic retinopathy screening are evolving in the United States (US), a country that lacks centralized health care management and has a long history of ad hoc, market-driven health care delivery approaches. These vary in certain technical details, such as angle of view, stereo or monoscopic imaging, selected wavelength or full color, image resolution, use of dilating agents and the number of recorded fields. The one important similarity is that these programs offer screening opportunities in non-traditional (e.g., non-ophthalmological) settings, most often a general health care or primary care clinic.

This approach breaks with the historical model of eye care providers delivering specialty eye care services to patients who visit them in their own clinics. The new method consists of eye care providers delivering care remotely to patients in primary care clinics, with technology serving as a surrogate for the usual face-to-face physician-provided examination.

13.3 Vanderbilt Ophthalmic Imaging Center (VOIC) Screening Program

The following sections describe the approach used by the Vanderbilt Ophthalmic Imaging Center (VOIC) screening program.

13.3.1 Venue

At present, the VOIC network is comprised of five screening sites, four of which provide screening as a component of direct patient care; the fifth site acquires data for a research grant funded by an outside agency. Two of the patient care sites are community health centers, staffed by primary care physicians, nurse practitioners, residents, and allied health personnel. The other two screening sites are located within Veterans Administration medical centers, where they are situated close to primary care clinics.

The full-time availability of both the camera and screening personnel facilitates patient screening. Some of the sites make appointments for patients to return for screening at a later date, while others offer on-demand screening.

13.3.2 Screening Staff

Each of our participating clinics provides screening staff to the program. These individuals do not have ophthalmic photography backgrounds, but rather, are trained to perform screening according to the VOIC protocol. Our current screeners include licensed practical nurses, medical assistants, and research assistants. Training consists of an initial didactic presentation and practical demonstration, followed by continual monitoring of technical quality.

13.3.3 On-Site Hardware and Software

The screening encounter begins with visual acuity measurement. In the often cramped and always busy internal spaces of a community health center, we believed that the use of a wall-mounted self-illuminated test chart and 20 feet of unobstructed viewing space could not be reliably obtained. Instead, we elected to use a desktop visual acuity measurement device equipped with an ETDRS test target (Optec 800, Stereo Optical Company, Chicago, IL), similar to the LogMar unit in use in the UK and elsewhere (Fig. 13.1). This unit has a built-in illumination system and is equipped with a pinhole attachment to help overcome refractive errors. The results of this measurement are entered into the patient's database and thus become part of the electronic record.

13.3.3.1 Instruments

We use screening-type retinal fundus cameras, designed to produce a moderately wide angle view of the retina through a physiologically dilated pupil. These instruments are meant to be used in a darkened room, where the patient's pupils are expected to dilate sufficiently to admit the illuminating rays from the camera and to produce an artifact-free image. Screening cameras typically utilize an infrared focusing beam and a small video monitor. The screener adjusts composition and focus by watching the monitor, but the infrared illumination is virtually invisible to the patient and does not interfere with the dilating process. We use Canon CR6-45NM cameras (Canon Medical Products, Irvine, CA) in each of our screening clinics (Fig. 13.2), although we pharmacologically dilate all patients.

13.3.3.2 Images

The retinal images are captured on digital cameras that are attached to the fundus cameras. The first two camera sites were equipped with three megapixel cameras (the highest quality cameras then available in the so-called *prosumer* class.) Since then, six megapixel cameras have become affordably available and the more recent sites are equipped with them. Images are held temporarily in a laptop computer attached to the camera stand. The Dell Latitude C-600 series (Dell Computer Corporation, Round Rock, TX) is used throughout our network.

The resolution, bit-depth, and playback characteristics of the digital images are associated with the ability of the process to identify pathological conditions. As currently configured, our equipment records images that are 8.5 Mb in size. These large files are saved as portable network graphic (PNG) files, a lossless compression

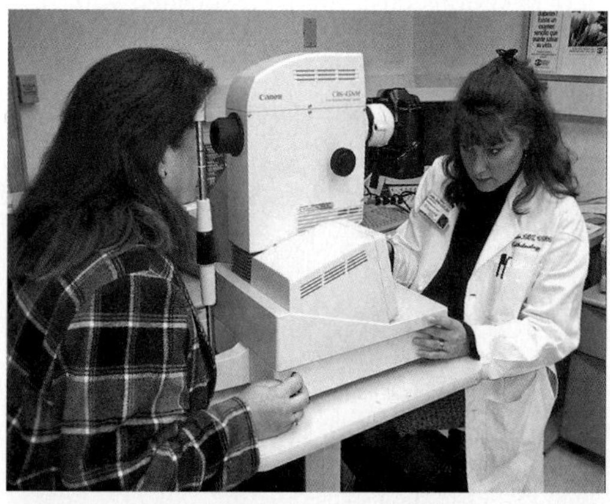

Fig. 13.1. Measuring device for optec visual acuity. This self-contained desktop unit incorporates its own illumination and optics. We use a log-mar test target based on the ETDRS target, providing measurements from 20/200 to 20/12. To overcome possible refractive errors, a pinhole attachment is inserted when the patient cannot read better than 20/50

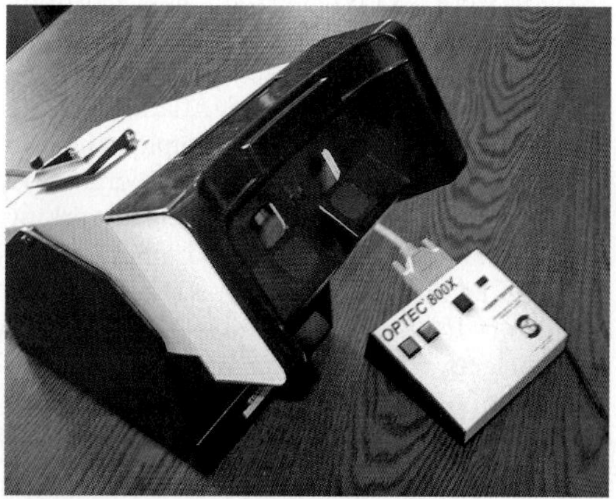

Fig. 13.2. Retinal screening camera in use. The screener (L) is able to compose and focus the image by observing the built-in monochrome screen attached to the camera. Our network uses the Canon CR6-45NM camera with pharmacologic dilation

algorithm that preserves image detail but slightly reduces the overall size.

The software for image acquisition and database entry is designed exclusively for retinal screening programs. The EyeQ Superlite program (Digital Healthcare, Cambridge, UK, available in the US from Canon Medical Products, Irvine, CA) is used at each capture station and interfaces with its counterpart review software in the VOIC Reading Center.

13.4 Telecommunications and Server

We use store-and-forward technology to transmit the digital images from the screening sites to our reading center. Because we do not need live motion or real-time interaction, we store the images and patient identifiers in the laptop computer temporarily, and then upload them at the end of the day's clinical activities. Each patient's file is at least 35 Mb in size and takes about 3.5 min to upload over our T1 broadband connection. This configuration is point-to-point (camera site to computer) and is considered secure, because it does not traverse the Internet.

T1 lines are affordable only within fairly short distances. Alternatives include frame relay, various DSL iterations, and the use of Virtual Private Network (VPN) software and hardware solutions. We established a strategic partnership with our local telecommunications service provider (BellSouth Corporation, Atlanta, GA) to facilitate the correct design and implementation of this crucial component of our program. We urge new programs to establish a close working relationship with their local telecommunications provider, and believe that such a relationship is mandatory to ensure that data is handled safely and efficiently. These vendors should also be fully aware of federal regulations mandated by the Health Insurance Portability and Accountability Act in the US.

We use a Dell PowerEdge server configured in a Redundant Array of Independent Discs, which offers the safety associated with multiple disc drives. The server is configured so that incoming images are held in a working directory. After review and grading, the images are archived in the same machine. We use digital data tape to back up the server every day. As storage capacity nears, we plan to consider off-site automatic data backup using a Storage-Area Network (SAN).

13.5 Analysis and Grading

Our review stations are equipped with Mitsubishi Diamond Pro 2060U 22 inch CRT monitors (NEC-Mitsubishi Electric Visual Systems; Tokyo, Japan), configured to display 2,048×1,536 pixels (Fig. 13.3). We are thus able to display each image in its entirety on the screen. Use of the review software permits additional magnification of either the entire image or selected portions as needed.

The software also permits a variety of image processing tools, including red-free viewing and adjustment of contrast and brightness. These tools help elucidate ambiguous lesions and enhance the viewing of retinal pathology when the patient has media changes. None of these enhancements permanently alter the original file, however. They are used only to improve our understanding of findings that may require referral for more thorough analysis by an ophthalmologist.

We use a customized grading form that uses checkboxes to denote the presence of a wide variety of lesions customarily associated with dia-

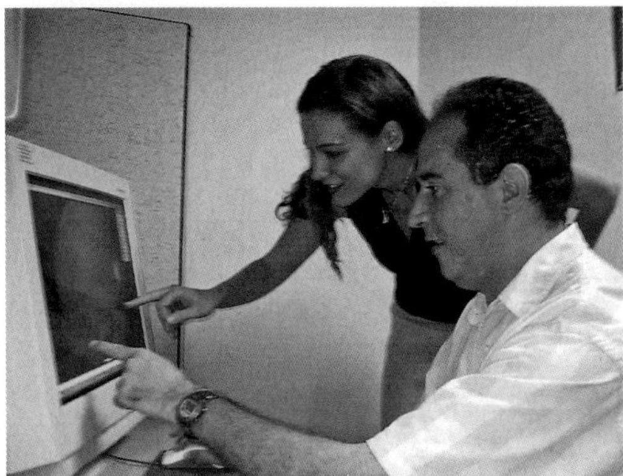

Fig. 13.3. Image grading. Drs. Cynthia Recchia, *left*, and Kamel Guentri *right*, use Mitsubishi CRT 22 inch monitors, set at 2,048×1,536 pixels, to review screening images

betic retinopathy. The form also includes boxes for optic nerve cupping, hypertensive changes, and text boxes for the entry of comments. It features suggestions for referral exhibited as three options: rescreen in one year, non-urgent referral, and urgent referral, each of which is based on the severity of diabetic and other retinal lesions detected upon review.

We use multiple graders that review images in masked fashion. The first level grader reviews every image and marks the grading form as needed. The intermediate grader reviews all image sets that exhibit any pathological changes as well as a percentage of normal images. The senior grader reviews a portion of all previously graded images for quality assurance, and also adjudicates disagreements that stem from ambiguous lesions, or those in which a clear referral strategy is in question.

Since the original design of our grading form, we have incorporated a new grading scheme into our program. The recently proposed international classification system for diabetic retinopathy [13], derived from the various levels of severity described in the ETDRS, is a streamlined method of description that facilitates communication between ophthalmologists and primary care physicians. As such, it is a boon to a program like ours wherein the managing physician or nurse practitioner prefers to receive a simple description of the patient's current retinal status and direct clinical management suggestions to optimize patient care.

13.6 Reporting and Archiving

Unlike conventional physician-provided examinations in which the patient is told about their condition directly, our program conveys clinical information directly to the supervising primary care physician. In effect, this process gives the primary physician another tool with which to take care of patients. Responsibility for the screening encounter and the interpretation is delegated to the screening program, and the results are then conveyed back to the primary care physician. Referral for ophthalmic follow-up care is done by the primary care physician, using local providers. In the case of Veterans Administration (VA) patients, the VA eye clinic manages patients who need further specialist care.

Some of our participating clinics still use paper charts, and for these we print out a copy of the grading sheet, then we mail, fax, or hand-deliver the report. For clinics using electronic medical records, the grading form is used as a worksheet in order to enter the findings and recommendations as an electronic consultation report. We do not include copies of the retinal images with the report, but if a clinician requests it, we can burn images to Compact Dics (CD) as JPEGs or TIFFs.

Turnaround time is short. Typically, all patient images arrive at our server during the evening and are fully graded by noon the next day. Thus, the final report is available within 24 h of the screening visit.

After the report has been generated, we archive the image and data package in our server. Archiving makes the images permanent and no further changes can be applied to the grading sheet. At present, we use digital tape to create daily back up records of the archives; within the next year we plan to outsource this function to a company that provides an automatic data storage and disaster recovery product.

13.7 Economic Considerations

A key attribute of effective population-based screening initiatives is economic sustainability [14]. The test must be affordable in order to be used. By using a technology-based solution, and staffing the program with screeners who function well but who lack in-depth ophthalmic and/or imaging experience, we are able to deliver this model of care for a unit price far below that of conventional physician-provided face-to-face care [15]. Funds thus saved may be re-allocated to help defray the costs of laser treatments that will be required by screen-positive cases.

13.8 Results

Our screening initiative has now been in operation for 24 months. It began with a single camera, and has now grown to five units in metropolitan

Nashville and Middle Tennessee. Participating clinics include community health centers, primary care clinics and Veterans Administration medical centers.

To date, we have screened more than 6,000 patients. Of all patients screened, approximately 60% were found to be within normal limits, or with mild background diabetic retinopathy below the threshold for referral. Each of these *normals* obtained the dilated retinal examination recommended for all people with diabetes.

Aggregate data from all participating sites shows that 30% were non-urgently referred for evaluation of findings that may lead to vision loss. Most of these were found to have vision of 20/50 or worse with pinhole correction. The next largest number of non-urgent cases were people whose optic nerves demonstrated a cup-to-disc ratio of 0.6 or greater.

Finally, 10% were referred urgently, primarily for presumed clinically significant macular edema, appearing in these non-stereo images as exudates within one disc diameter of the center of the fovea. Other reasons for urgent referral included optic nerve pallor or disc edema, proliferative diabetic retinopathy with or without high-risk characteristics, vitreous hemorrhage and inflammatory lesions such as toxoplasmosis. A small but significant subset of patients was found to have retinal thromboembolic lesions, and we immediately alerted their primary care physicians so that appropriate medical evaluation could be ordered without delay.

Although the primary reason for this screening initiative is the discovery of lesions associated with diabetes, we analyze every image for the presence of any pathology whatsoever, even if it is unrelated to hyperglycemia, and we diligently report those findings so that the patient can obtain proper follow-up care.

13.9 Discussion

There are many barriers to conventional physician-provided dilated retinal examinations, including cost, geographic location, and the time required to travel back and forth, as well as time waiting for the provider. By placing the screening encounter within a familiar health care setting, retinal imaging can occur during a routine clinic visit. This simplifies the process for elderly and infirm patients who may require public transportation. For the working poor who may not be given time off for multiple medical appointments, integrating the screening opportunity into an already-scheduled visit reduces the time away from work.

The use of visual acuity measurements and the decision to refer patients who cannot read better than 20/50 with correction produces a significant over-referral, since many of these patients may have amblyopia or simply need a careful refraction. However, we believe that each screening encounter could be a once in a lifetime opportunity, especially when working with indigent patients in safety net clinics. For this reason, we would rather over-refer than ignore a problem that may have an easy remedy and would enhance the visual capability of the individual.

13.9.1 Simple Implementation

Screening-type retinal cameras are designed to be easy to operate, and they incorporate various optical components that simplify alignment and focus. By observing the image on the attached monitor, these instruments provide an indication of the real image, rather than forcing the screener to work through the challenge of aerial image focusing customarily encountered in clinical fundus cameras. This simple instrument allows the use of screeners with non-traditional backgrounds, and thus the labor costs associated with this program are economically sustainable.

In our model, the actual salary and fringe benefits are paid by the participating institution rather than by us. This enables screeners to perform other tasks in the clinic when there are no patients to be photographed. We usually train two people at each site to perform screenings, as this provides for lunch breaks, vacation and sick time without incapacitating patient flow.

13.9.2 Digital Imaging

The specific acquisition and playback parameters we use for digital imaging are based on the nature of diabetic lesions and the need for a robust, easily replaceable instrument. The resolution of the entire system (camera and review station) should be sufficiently high to resolve very small subject detail while simultaneously being compact enough to be transmitted in a reasonable interval over telecommunications links [16]. To understand the morphology of an unknown lesion, we believe at least four to six pixels should contribute to the image, providing an indication of area and color variation. The minimum standards recommended by the UK National Health Service stipulate 1,300×1,000 pixels. The least sensitive camera in our system offers a resolution of 2,160×1,440, while the most sensitive digital back provides 3,072×2,048 pixels. This issue is essential to running an accurate screening program, because higher image quality translates into greater opportunities to correctly identify subtle lesions that are important indicators of the patient's status. To understand whether a yellowish spot is a drusen body or an exudate, or whether a very faint reddish area on the optic nerve is a tiny tuft of proliferative tissue, we must use the highest level of technology.

13.9.3 Creating Quality Files

Furthermore, we must ensure that the integrity of these large files is protected from the moment of exposure until they are archived. Lossless file compression is mandatory, and the PNG algorithm provides us with a modest reduction in non-essential background information while simultaneously reducing total file size of each individual image to 8.5 Mb.

Our current telecom network uses T1 lines, but even these high-bandwidth connections require lengthy uploads. For a typical patient set of four images along with a small packet of patient identifiers, the 35 Mb file takes 3.5 min to upload to our server. Other telecom variants will result in slower speeds (Fig. 13.4).

We dilate every patient with a short-acting mydriatic agent. Tropicamide 1%, used alone, is not associated with systemic side effects or an increased risk of angle-closure glaucoma [17, 18]. However, it significantly improves the optical performance of the camera by permitting uniform retinal illumination even when the patient's iris is no longer capable of adequate physiological dilation.

13.9.4 Stereoscopic versus Monoscopic Imaging

One somewhat controversial aspect of retinal screening concerns the issue of stereoscopic versus monoscopic imaging. Clinicians who are used to viewing clinical images in stereo may question the effectiveness of a non-stereo image in denoting macular thickening. However, we have found high sensitivity with single image recording, and rely on a combination of visual acuity measurement [19] and the use of surrogate markers (typically lipid exudates) within one disc diameter of the fovea to represent presumed retinal edema. It is also much easier to produce a single high-quality image as compared to stereoscopic views, especially when the screener is not a professional ophthalmic photographer (JDM Gass, 2002, personal communication).

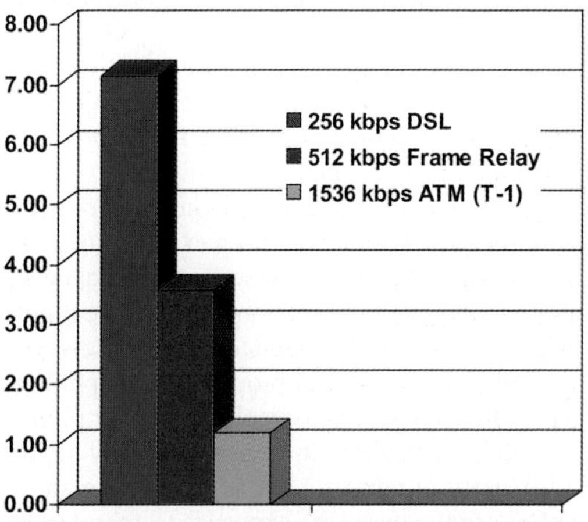

Fig. 13.4. Set of four full resolution retinal images is 35 Mb in size. Average upload times (in hours) for 25 screening studies @ 35 Mb. Although a simple DSL may be used, upload times are shortened significantly with broadband connections. We suggest that screening programs work closely with local telecommunications service providers to design a network that has adequate bandwidth and is cost-effective

13.9.5 Imaging Protocol

Our program uses a modified EuroDiab imaging protocol [20], in which the first image is created with the fovea in the center; the second image centers the optic nerve in the recorded field. While some believe that a single 45°, fovea-centered image should be sufficient for screening, the large numbers of patients who may be at risk for glaucoma necessitated the addition of the second image [21]. Because our software can very precisely calculate discrete anatomical areas and thus compute cup-to-disc ratios, we elect to acquire a centered, *en-face* view of the optic nerve for each eye, thus providing a geometrically true frontal image that does not exhibit any perspective distortion. We manually trace the on-screen outlines of the disc and use color and vessel configuration to approximate the edge of the cup, and then the program calculates areas and ratios.

13.9.6 Demographic Considerations

Screening programs may change the demographics of the typical ophthalmic clinical practice. Using typical numbers, about half of the known diabetics in a service area obtain conventional physician-provided examinations. Of these (based on ethnicity, race, disease duration, and hemoglobin A1c levels), most are normal, while about a third require intervention for retinopathy. For practices associated with a digital screening program, normal diabetics may no longer attend the clinic for routine screening exams. However, many more patients will be screened in that geographic area, and proportionately more patients will be referred to the practice for care. However, virtually all of these will require fundus photography, fluorescein angiography and laser photocoagulation, resulting in commensurately higher third-party reimbursement as well as the application of the physician's expertise to many more patients who require it.

Digital screening is not intended to be a replacement for a comprehensive eye examination. Indeed, issues concerning any eye findings *not* including the retina (such as motility, lids, cornea, tear film, Intraocular Pressure (IOP), refraction, lens opacities and the like) cannot be addressed with fundus image-based retinopathy detection. What these programs do most effectively, however, is to extend access to people who otherwise would never obtain any ophthalmic care at all.

13.10 Economic Issues

For the most part, American health care is designed and delivered according to market forces. While the federal Department of Health and Human Services (DHHS) helps regulate reimbursement of specific procedures through its Centers for Medicare and Medicaid (CMS), the Bureau of Primary Health Care supports a system of community health clinics for the underserved, with the vast majority of care paid for by private insurance companies, along with copayments by their subscribers.

For a variety of complex and historical reasons, CMS does not have a national policy that permits reimbursement for image-based retinopathy screening. Because private insurers look to CMS to provide policies and standards, they too have been reluctant to provide funding. At present, much retinopathy screening in the United States is funded either through grants and philanthropy. For certain community health centers and the Veterans Administration, funding is obtained through a re-allocation of monies already assigned to primary health care or diabetes care. possible remedy is through legislative action; with this in mind, a bill has been drafted that addresses this issue.

13.11 Summary

For many health care consumers, on-demand screening in the primary care clinic saves weeks or months of waiting for an appointment at an eye care facility for a traditional physician-provided dilated eye examination; indeed, for some, digital imaging is their first experience obtaining ophthalmic health care. For those patients found to have vision-threatening disease, digital screening brings them one step closer to obtaining the expert ophthalmic treatment they require to preserve their vision and to remain productive members of society.

We believe that every patient screening encounter represents an improvement in health care delivery. Each screening can overcome racial, ethnic and economic disparities. Each contributes to equity of care. Each is a victory over apathy, ignorance, and lack of access to high quality health care – barriers that far too often lead to blindness for people with diabetes.

References

1. Mokdad AH, Ford ES, Bowman BA, Dietz WH, Vinicor F, Bales VS, Marks JS (2003) Prevalence of obesity, diabetes, and obesity-related health risk factors, 2001. JAMA 289(1):76–79
2. National Center for Chronic Disease Prevention and Health Promotion, Centers for Disease Control and Prevention (2004) National diabetes fact sheet. http://www.cdc.gov/diabetes/pubs/estimates.htm. Cited 3 Feb 2004
3. US Department of Health and Human Services, Agency for Healthcare Research and Quality (2003) National Healthcare Disparities Report 2003. http://qualitytools.ahrq.gov/disparitiesReport/download_report.aspx. Cited 3 June 2004
4. Saadine JB, Narayan KMV, Vinicor F (2003) Vision loss: a public health problem? Ophthalmology 110(2):253–254
5. Verma L, Prakash G, Tewari HK (2002) Diabetic retinopathy: time for action. No complacency please! Lett Bull World Health Organ 80(5):419
6. Centers for Disease Control and Prevention (2002) Socioeconomic status of women with diabetes – United States, 2000. MMWR Morb Mortal Wkly Rep 51:147–148, 159
7. Munoz B, West SK, Rubin GS, et al. (2000) Causes of blindness and visual impairment in a population of older Americans: the Salisbury Eye Evaluation Study. Arch Ophthalmol 118:819–825
8. West SK, Klein R, Rodriguez J, Munoz B, Broman AT, Sanchez R, Snyder R (2001) Diabetes and diabetic retinopathy in a Mexican-American population. Diabetes Care 24:1204–1209
9. Bonds DE, Zaccaro DJ, Karter AJ, Selby JV, Saad M, Goff DC (2003) Ethnic and racial differences in diabetes care: the Insulin Resistance Atherosclerosis Study. Diabetes Care 26:1040–1046
10. Villalpando CG, Villalpando EG, Diaz SM, Martinez DR, Perez BA, Andrade SI, Stern MP (1997) A diabetic retinopathy screening program as a strategy for blindness prevention. Arch Med Res 28(1):129–135
11. National Health Service, National Screening Committee. Preservation of sight in diabetes: a risk reduction program. http://www.diabetic-retinopathy.screening.nhs.uk/diabetic-retinopathy.html. Cited 4 Feb 2004
12. Cummins E, Facey K, Macpherson K, Morris A, Reay L, Slattery J (2001) Health technology assessment of organization of services for diabetic retinopathy screening. Health Technology Board for Scotland, Glasgow
13. Wilkinson CP, Ferris FL, Klein RE, Lee PP, Agardh CD, Davis M, Dills D, Kampik A, Pararajasegaram R, Verdaguer JT (2003) Proposed international clinical diabetic retinopathy and diabetic macular edema disease severity scales. Ophthalmology 110(9):1677–1682
14. Wilson JMG, Jungner G (1968) Principles and practice of screening for disease; public health paper number 34. World Health Organization, Geneva
15. James M, Turner DA, Broadbent DM, Vora J, Harding SP (2000) Cost-effectiveness analysis of screening for sight threatening diabetic eye disease. Br Med J 320:1627–1631
16. Merin LM, Reeves D (2003) Technical issues in retinopathy screening (letter). Diabetes Care 26(3):965–966
17. Patel KH, Javitt JC, Tielsch JM, Street DA, Katz J, Quigley HA, Sommer A (1995) Incidence of acute angle-closure glaucoma after pharmacologic mydriasis. Am J Ophthalmol 120(6):709–717
18. Pandit RJ, Taylor R (2000) Mydriasis and glaucoma: exploding the myth: a systematic review. Diabet Med 17(10):693–699
19. Broadbent DM, Harding SP, Gillibrand WP, Vora JP (1997) Visual acuity detects CSMO? The value of visual acuity measurement in screening for diabetic maculopathy; the Liverpool Diabetic Eye Study. Diabet Med 14(l1):S65
20. Aldington SJ, Kohner EM, Meuer S, Klein R, Sjolie AK for EURODIAB IDDM Complications Study Group (1995) Methodology for retinal photography and assessment of diabetic retinopathy: the EURODIAB IDDM Complications Study. Diabetologia 38:437–444
21. Stellingwerf C, Hardus PLLJ, Hooymans JMM (2001) Two-field photography can identify patients with vision-threatening diabetic retinopathy. Diabetes Care 24:2086–2090

Chapter 14

Improved Screening for Retinopathy of Prematurity (ROP) – Demonstration of a Telemedical Solution

14

Heike Elflein, Birgit Lorenz

This chapter addresses the following

Key Concepts:

- Improvement in neonatal intensive care has increased the survival rates of premature infants world-wide.
- Neonatologists and ophthalmologists now have to face disorders due to immaturity, particularly retinopathy of prematurity (ROP).
- In 2001, a telemedical program using a digital retinal camera system was started that connected five neonatal intensive care units (NICUs) with the reading center at the Department of Pediatric Ophthalmology and Opthalmogenetics at the University of Regensburg, which was designed to evaluate the potential of telematics in ROP, and to improve screening modalities of prematures at risk for ROP.

14.1 Introduction

At present, approximately 5% of infants with a birth weight below 1,250 g will develop threshold disease [1]. Once threshold disease is reached (ROP Stage 3+, Zone I or II), it will first lead to retinal detachment in as many as 50% of the children, and then to severe visual impairment or blindness, if left untreated [2]. Zone I disease usually presents in a more aggressive way. Therefore, the recommendation from Germany for treating Zone I disease is treatment at an earlier stage (prethreshold disease in Zone I) [3]. Timely laser photocoagulation will stop the disease in at least 95% of infants [4]. The optimum time for treatment, though, is a subject for debate and discussion. Following the results of the Early Treatment for Retinopathy of Prematurity (ETROP) Study, treatment at an earlier, prethreshold stage – even in Zone II – might improve anatomical and functional outcome [5]. Timely detection of treatment-requiring disease is crucial. Ophthalmologists who have specialized in pediatric retina provide the best screening, with dilated binocular indirect visualization being the current standard examination.

The cost of failure in screening or treatment is very high. When an infant becomes blind in Germany, direct pension costs can come to 300,000 EUR, based on the actual rates that have been calculated for a period of 50 years. Consequently, even a few failed screenings or treatments, when multiplied by the high cost of failure, present a compelling economic reason to support screening and treatment programs – apart from the personal tragedy of the afflicted baby.

Providing ROP screening by expert pediatric ophthalmologists or retina specialists for repeated exams is not broadly feasible. The low incidence of treatment-requiring stages also makes it difficult to gain sufficient experience with treatment-requiring ROP. For instance, of the babies selected for screening, only about 5% will need treatment [1].

Each child generally receives two visits or more from an ophthalmologist, but the incidence of the ophthalmologist prescribing treatment after an examination is less than 3% of the visits. This suggests that the screening process is a low incidence activity, and that the challenge of maintaining a high attention level during a difficult exam with low incidence is well known.

Every ophthalmologist dealing with pre-term infants and ROP is aware of late referrals, i.e., babies presenting with retinal changes that are beyond the stage that offers the best chance for inducing regression of disease with good anatomical and functional outcome. Visual prognosis is then severely reduced with the risk of blindness that could have been avoided.

14.2 The Bavarian ROP – Telemedicine Project

With the advent of telemedicine, improved ROP screening appears to be possible with the use of hand-held (Fig. 14.1) and cart-based (Fig. 14.2) digital wide field, and transmission of the images for expert evaluation. In 2001, the first author initiated the installation of digital widefield cameras (RetCam 120) in five NICUs (Bayreuth, Deggendorf, Passau, Regensburg, and Weiden) in Bavaria over a distance of 200 km, connected to the reading and treatment center of the Department of Pediatric Ophthalmology and Ophthalmogenetics at the University of Regensburg, Germany (Fig.14.3) [6, 7].

Informed consent is obtained from all parents after explaining the examination method. According to the German screening guidelines [3], images of all premature infants at risk for ROP (gestational age <32 weeks; birthweight <1,500 g; gestational age ≥32 weeks <36 weeks and supplemental oxygen >3 days) are taken with the RetCam 120, using the ROP nosepiece, which images 130° of the retina at once.

The children are imaged and examined by a general ophthalmologist, as this is the convention in Germany. In other countries, imaging is also performed by nurses or ophthalmic photographers [8, 9]. In order to document an eventual, persisting, and dilated tunica vasculosa lentis as an indicator of acute ROP, anterior segment imaging is done in all instances with the RetCam in non-contact mode. Thereafter, the ophthalmologists are advised to take nine images from the retina of each eye using a coupling gel in contact mode.

The images are sent electronically (appropriately masked for confidentiality) to the reading center for evaluation. Follow-up examinations are recommended according to the stage of ROP, image quality, pediatric data, and the German guidelines for screening for ROP. Image evaluations are based on the presence of a persistent dilated tunica vasculosa lentis, extent of retinal vascularization, and on the existence of vascular dilatation and tortuositas at the posterior fundus pole (Plus' disease). Figure 14.4 shows a child at threshold stage; Fig. 14.5 shows the same child

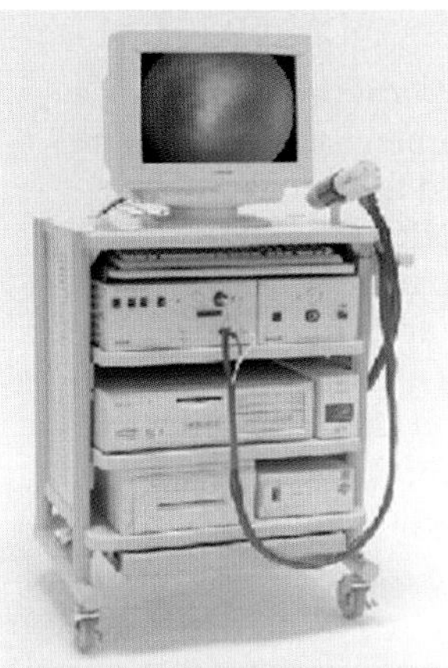

Fig. 14.2. Image capture system is cart based and contains light source for camera, real-time display system, and digital capture means

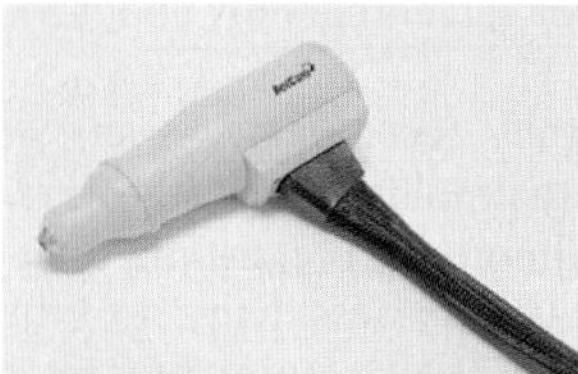

Fig. 14.1. Hand-held image capture unit for RetCam contains optics, focusing motor, megapixel CCD, and connecting cable to cart

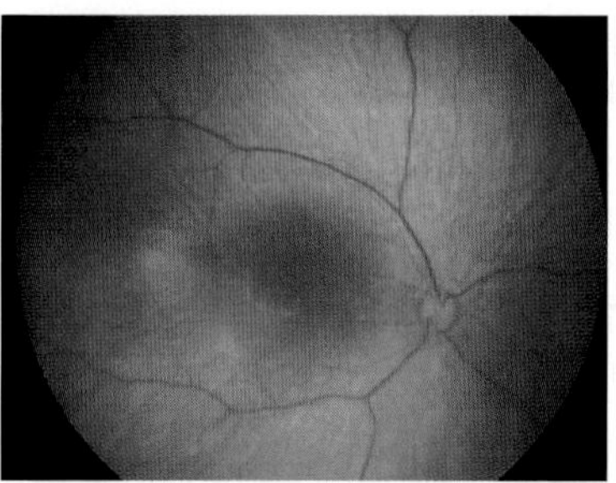

Fig. 14.3. Fundus of premature baby without pathology; GA: 30 weeks, birth weight 1,125 g. Postmenstrual age at examination 36 weeks

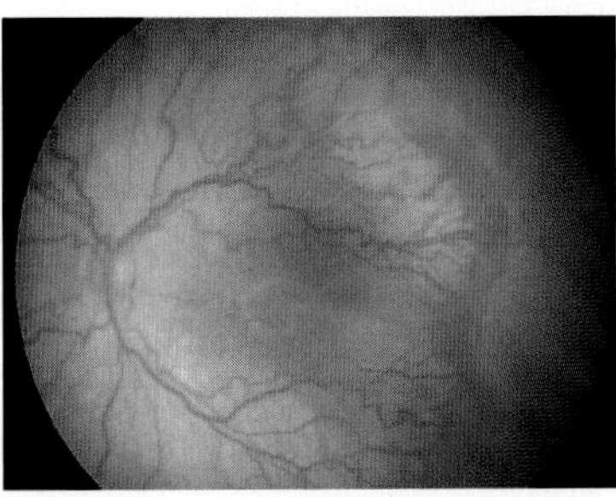

Fig. 14.4. Course of acute ROP, stage 3+ requiring DLC in a premature baby, GA 27 weeks, birthweight 980 g. This baby is at threshold disease in Zone II

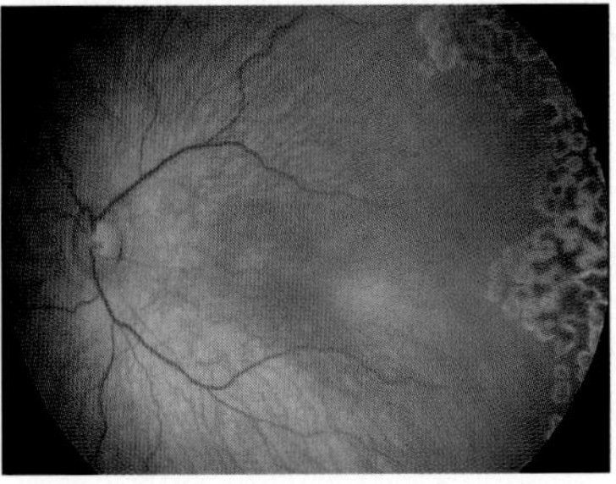

Fig. 14.5. Same child after treatment, with complete resolution of the acute ROP

after treatment, with complete resolution of the acute ROP.

In the case of a possible treatment-requiring stage, binocular indirect ophthalmoscopy (BIO), which is the gold standard for ROP screening, is performed by a staff member of the reading center to verify the findings. Treatment, if required, is performed onsite or at the reading center, depending on availability of anesthesia in the NICUs.

14.3 Screening and Treatment Results

To date, we have examined more than 600 babies, with no incidents of missing treatable disease, nor have there been late referrals for exams done through the RetCam. About 4% of the babies were treated as a result of the RetCam referral. According to the availability of prolonged anesthesia, about half of the treatment procedures could be performed onsite at the respective NICUs, without high risk or expensive transportation to the reading center that is also the treating institution.

14.3.1 Overcoming Limitations

Retinal images with the RetCam are of lower contrast and resolution than visualization using BIO. About 5% of the imaging sessions do not generate sufficiently high quality images to evaluate the actual risk. In cases of insufficient image quality, we order the exam to be repeated within a week or less, according to the disease severity.

Very small infants can be difficult to image peripherally, but most of these – even the tiniest babies – can be imaged posteriorly, which is generally sufficient for risk assessment if follow-up examinations are advised until vascularization is complete in peripheral Zone II.

Difficulties in imaging the more peripheral parts of the retina are overcome only in part by the slimmer nosepiece of the ROP lens compared to the standard lens used in earlier studies [10, 11], but if the guidelines of screening for ROP are followed, additional signs, such as dilation of the retinal vessels at the posterior pole (Plus' disease), will detect significant disease.

14.3.2 Interpreting Images

Interpreting the images is a finely honed skill. As compared with BIO, a three-dimensional view is not available. Being familiar with both the funduscopic aspect and the RetCam image is crucial for correct interpretation of the images. With these precautions, the RetCam 120 is very well suited as a screening tool.

The transmission of image data and pediatric data usually causes no problems. Trouble in data delivery generates an error message, making it necessary to send the data a second time. Problems making data delivery impossible, even after a couple of attempts, have never occurred.

14.4 Using RetCam120 for Imaging

Several studies have investigated the benefits and limitations of using the RetCam 120 for imaging ROP. In a study by Schwartz, et al. [12], the authors compared conventional BIO evaluations and recommendations with telemedical evaluations and recommendations from RetCam 120 images. All but one set of the examined 19 pairs of eyes had severe ROP at least at the prethreshold stage, according to the international classification of retinopathy of prematurity (ICROP) definition. A weak aspect of the study is that the results particularly highlighted the intra-clinic differences in treatment decisions. However, the main point is that all children noted to have severe ROP by the on-site group were also noted to have at least pre-threshold ROP by the remote group.

Roth and coworkers also compared conventional screening with RetCam 120 examinations [11]. In this study, the sensitivity to stage one or stage two ROP located in peripheral Zone II or III via RetCam images was low. However, in those missed cases ROP regressed spontaneously. The authors stated that they were using an early version of the camera nosepiece and a broad-bladed lid speculum, and that these mechanical limits severely constrained the view of the periphery. By using the special, smaller nosepiece for preterm babies those problems can be solved, at least in part. Looking at the results regarding detection of cases requiring treatment, the success rate of the RetCam was 100%.

14

Yen, et al. [8, 9] reported that in a specific screening design, i.e., only two examinations, one at 32 to 34 weeks and one at 38 to 40 weeks, the RetCam examination had insufficient sensitivity to be recommended as a substitute for indirect ophthalmoscopy in screening for ROP. In contrast to the RetCam examinations, the indirect ophthalmoscopy screening was continued at least every two weeks according to the actual guidelines. Our recommendation of course is to follow-up the infants with the RetCam according to the guidelines, until retinal maturity or complete resolution of any acute ROP stage is documented.

In another study, a French group reported on their results with RetCam screening for ROP [13]. The study focused on one neonatal intensive care unit (NICU), with RetCam images of 145 prematures at risk who were evaluated by neonatologists and by ophthalmologists. The authors stated an exact correlation between observers in all cases of acute ROP. In a Canadian study [14], the sensitivity to detect severe ROP was also shown to be 100% when comparing the RetCam to binocular indirect ophthalmoscopy in 44 prematures who were at risk.

14.5 Prospects

Our telemedical project has been operating successfully for more than four years. Unfortunately, a comparison of the RetCam images with the findings from the gold standard for ROP screening (BIO) is not possible in the peripheral NICUs, since examinations are performed by a single local ophthalmologist. Nevertheless, there is no indication that treatment-requiring stages were missed with the RetCam.

We did, however, compare BIO versus digital imaging at the local NICU in Regensburg, where more than 100 infants had received dual examinations. Digital imaging using the RetCam 120 was successful in detecting all referral-warranted ROP stages, with no false negative and no false positive results, i.e., the sensitivity and the specificity to detect severe ROP that might require treatment were both 100%.

Advantages of digital imaging of ROP include better communication with parents and between pediatric physicians or nurses, more uniform evaluation, medical/legal documentation, rapid training of junior ophthalmologists, and access to expert assessment. From a scientific point of view, digital examination allows objective evaluation of the time course of the disease, which gives new insight into the evolution and resolution of ROP, which will help evaluate actual and future treatment modalities.

The authors do not have any financial interest or proprietary interest in the digital RetCam120 camera system (Massie Research Laboratories, Dublin, CA, USA), or in Massie Research Laboratories, Dublin, CA, USA.

References

1. Reynolds JD (2001) The management of retinopathy of prematurity. Paediatr Drugs 3:263–272
2. Cryotherapy for Retinopathy of Prematurity Cooperative Group (1990) Multicenter trial of cryotherapy for retinopathy of prematurity; one-year outcome: structure and function. Arch Ophthalmol 108:1408–1416
3. Clemens S, Eckardt C, Gerding H, et al. (1999) Augenärztliche Screening – Untersuchung von Frühgeborenen. Ophthalmologe 96:257–263
4. Seiberth V, Linderkamp O, Vardarli I, et al. (1996) Diodenlaserkoagulation der Retinopathia praematurorum Stadium 3+. Ophthalmologe 93:182–189
5. Good WV, Hardy RJ (2001) The multicenter study of early treatment for retinopathy of prematurity (ETROP). Ophthalmology 108:1013–1014
6. Lorenz B (2006) Screening for Retinopathy of Prematurity. In: Lorenz B, Moore AT, eds. Pediatric Ophthalmology, Neuro-Ophthalmology, Genetics. Essentials in Ophthalmology. Krieglstein GK and Weinreb RN, series eds. Springer Berlin Heidelberg New York
7. Lorenz B, Elflein H (2002) Preventing blindness in premature infants: A telemedical solution gains acceptance. Neonatal Intensive Care 15:42–48
8. Yen KG, Hess D, Burke B, et al. (2000) The optimum time to employ telephotoscreening to detect retinopathy of prematurity. Trans Am Ophthalmol Soc 98:145–151
9. Yen KG, Hess D, Burke B, et al. (2002) Telephotoscreening to detect retinopathy of prematurity: preliminary study of the optimum time to employ digital fundus camera imaging to detect ROP. J AAPOS 6:64–70
10. Seiberth V, Woldt C (2001) Weitwinkelfundusdokumentation bei Retinopathia praematurorum. Ophthalmologe 98:960–963
11. Roth DB, Morales D, Feuer WJ, et al. (2001) Screening for retinopathy of prematurity employing the RetCam 120: sensitivity and specificity. Arch Ophthalmol 119:268–272
12. Schwartz SD, Harrison SA, Ferrone PJ, Trese MT (2000) Telemedical evaluation and management of retinopathy of prematurity using a fiberoptic digital fundus camera. Ophthalmology 107:25–28
13. Sommer C, Gouillard C, Brugniart C, et al. (2003) Depistage et suivi de la retinopathie du premature par camera de retine (Retcam 120) : experience d'une equipe de neonatalogistes a propos de 145 cas. Arch Pediatr 10:694–699
14. Ells AL, Holmes JM, Astle WF, et al. (2003) Telemedicine approach to screening for severe retinopathy of prematurity: a pilot study. Ophthalmology 110:2113–2117

Chapter 15

Visual Rehabilitation Consultations through Telemedicine

15

Jade S. Schiffman, Gina G. Wong, Rosa A. Tang, Randy T. Jose

This chapter addresses the following

Key Concepts:

- As the population ages, a growing number of people will require low vision or visual rehabilitation services.
- An infrastructure and protocols have been used for a low vision telemedicine consultation pilot program.

15.1 Introduction

As the population ages, a growing number of people will require low vision or visual rehabilitation services. In the United States (US) in 2000, about 0.78% of those older than 40 years old were blind, and 2.4 million or 1.98% had low vision [1]. The US definition of blindness is 20/200 or less, and for low vision it is less than 20/40 in the better-seeing eye. Based on studies in the US, Europe and Australia, Congdon et al. predict that by the year 2020, the number of blind people older than 40 in the US will increase 70% to 1.6 million, and the number of people with low vision will be 3.9 million [1].

The leading causes of blindness are age-related macular degeneration, glaucoma, and cataracts. In people younger than 40 years old, the leading cause of blindness is diabetic retinopathy; about 4.1 million Americans have diabetic retinopathy [2]. Pollard et al. found that the barriers to accessing low vision service are the limited geographic distribution of clinics and transportation to get services [3]. Visually disabled individuals could function more independently if they had access to visual rehabilitation, thus increasing their quality of life.

15.2 Requirements for a Low Vision Telerehabilitation Model

Access to low vision rehabilitation is often difficult for patients in rural areas; therefore, a model for visual rehabilitation through telemedicine was developed. In Houston, TX, in the US, the Center for Sight Enhancement at the University of Houston College of Optometry offers patients visual rehabilitation and access to eye care specialists. Because the university also has access to other specialists, such as neuro-ophthalmology, a team approach is possible.

15.2.1 Access to Care Pilot Project

A Texas Infrastructure Telemedicine Board grant was awarded to the University of Houston in 1999 to set up a pilot project to increase access to care via telemedicine. The grant provided funding for the infrastructure without providing funds for people who would work with telemedicine.

A telemedicine model for visual rehabilitation was developed to provide low vision consultations at a rural hospital in Matagorda. Throughout this chapter, we discuss expected reimbursement for telemedicines or basic low vision consultation visits, the infrastructure used, remote/consult site paperwork requirements, protocol for a telemedicine low vision consultation, and we'll give an example of one case.

15.2.1.1 Reimbursement

Telemedicine reimbursement generally uses the same current procedural technology codes and international classification of diseases (ICD-9) codes used during normal eye exams or consultation visits. At this time in the US, Medicare will only reimburse for real time, face-to-face telemedicine consultation, and will not reimburse for store-and-forward consultations, except in two states: Alaska and Hawaii [4]. The telemedicine remote site is able to bill for the visit and then the consultant can bill when a real-time consultation is completed. The Benefits Improvements and Protection Act (BIPA) of 2000 allowed a facility fee to be charged by the originating or remote site of 20 USD or more [4]. If the telemedicine site is in a hospital, an additional room fee can also be billed. In addition, the patient can generally purchase the visual aids from the consultant site.

15.2.1.2 Infrastructure

The infrastructure was selected after much research and analysis. Telemedicine software capable of interfacing with electronic medical record software was chosen. Both software companies were flexible in trying to develop capabilities that were not initially available. All software was password protected, all activity within the software was time and date stamped, and the data was encrypted for transmission. The telemedicine software allowed creation of episodes or exam visits with patients incorporating paper exam scanned data, video and audio clips, and still images or photos. These episodes could be accessed from the electronic medical record created for each patient.

15.2.1.3 Paperwork and Protocol

Typewritten data also could be created and sent from either the telemedicine software or the electronic medical record. The telemedicine software was capable of real-time consultations or store-and-forward transmission. Patient episodes of video clips, audio, and still images create large files. T1 lines were chosen as the fastest route to transmit the large files and allow better quality real-time consultations. A mobile telemedicine cart with various peripheral devices was chosen to increase flexibility and access to other specialists via telemedicine. The computer, flat screen monitor, flat bed scanner with automatic document feeder, 8 mm camcorder with tripod, microphone, speakers, and a projector were mounted on the cart (Figs. 15.1a and 15.1b). A non-mydriatic fundus camera was selected to allow visualization of the fundus by the low vision specialists and potential use for diabetic screenings. The projector on the mobile cart allowed for tele-educational sessions. A mobile cart of low vision aids such as magnifiers, telescopes and low vision acuity charts was set up for the remote site (Fig. 15.2).

The project and consent forms created were reviewed by the University of Houston human subjects committee and institutional review board, and the rural hospital's committee. Approval was given by both organizations, although the rural hospital developed its own consent form as well.

Eye care providers or specialists are required to be licensed in any state to practice telemedicine. As remote site telemedicine consultations were done at the hospital, all practitioners had to be credentialed at the rural hospital as well.

15.2.2 Data Gathering

A model of how exam data was to be gathered and transmitted to the low vision specialist was developed. The low vision specialists suggested the details of the exam that would be helpful for them to view and hear, so audio and video clips of parts of the exam were captured.

15.2.2.1 The Exam

As the patient's eye health diagnosis and retinal or nerve status is considered when suggesting visual aids or devices, photos of the fundus were to be captured for review. Flow charts outlining the basic low vision exam, and low vision exam forms were created, so the initial low vision exam could be performed by an untrained

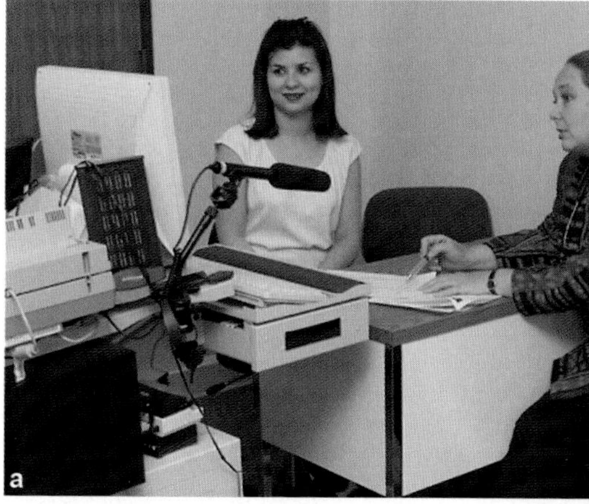

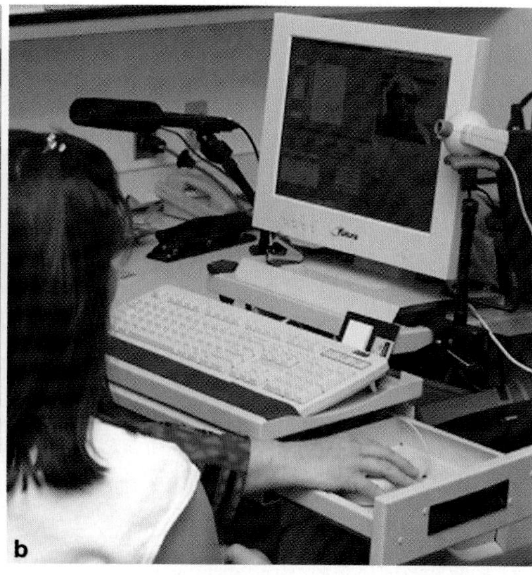

Fig. 15.1. **a** Telemedicine mobile cart with flat screen monitor (*left*). **b** Peripheral devices such as flat bed scanner with automatic document feeder, microphone, speakers, video camcorder with tripod, and projector (*right*)

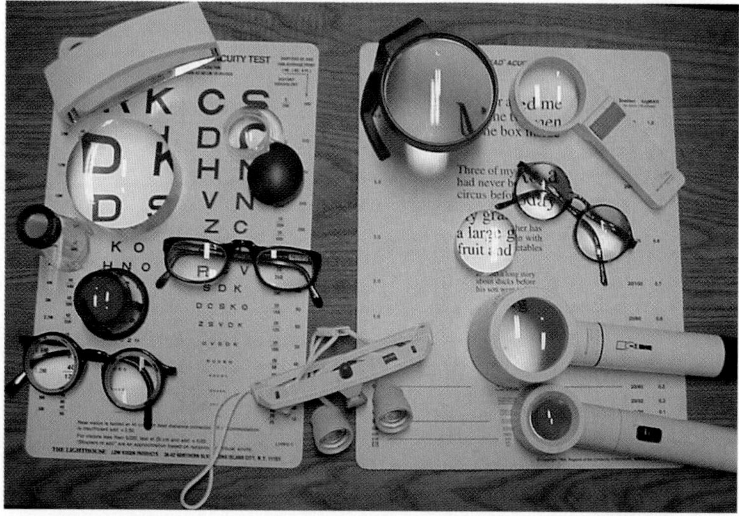

Fig. 15.2. Low vision acuity charts and assorted magnifiers and near devices available at the remote site

nurse or technical personnel at the remote site (Fig. 15.3). These charts specified what devices should be tried at distance and close up, and what data was to be videoed and scanned for the specialist. The exam findings with various devices or acuity charts were gathered and parts of the exam were simultaneously videotaped for review by the specialist. Patients were scheduled for two telemedicine visits over two weeks. The first visit or pre-consultation exam was to gather exam data and video clips for the low vision specialist. This data was then sent via store-and-forward for the consultant to review and make recommendations. A second visit allowed time for devices recommended by the specialist to be tried, followed up by a real-time video consultation between the patient and the specialist. (Table 15.1)

Table 15.1. Low vision protocol for exam testing, image and audio/visual video clip capturing for distance and near devices. Images needed: (1) Fundus picture of each eye with Topcon Nonmydriatic camera (2) Visual fields (3) Amsler grid (4) Low vision exam form (5) Low vision history form (6) Consent form

	Patient	Chart needed	Light on	Camera focus	Examiner audio	Patient audio	Cameral light on/ focus
1	Distance visual acuity	Feinbloom	Feinbloom chart	On patients face-eyes	Announce patients lowest VA read with difficulty or easily in Snellen, e.g., 10/20	Reading acuity chart lowest line	On/auto or manual
2	Telescope 2.2× for distance	Feinbloom	Feinbloom	Face close up	Announce patients lowest VA read with difficulty or easily	Reading acuity chart lowest line	On/auto or manual
	If patient can obtain equal to or better than 10/20 distance acuity (20/40) with the 2.2 FDTS, then skip the 4×12 demonstration						
3	Telescope 4×12 for distance	Feinbloom	Feinbloom	Face close up	Announce patients lowest VA read with difficulty or easily	Reading acuity chart lowest line	On/auto or manual
4	Near vision acuity with bifocal if has them	Single letter (OD and OS) and paragraph (OU) chart Allow patient to hold chart	Near light on paragraph chart or single letter chart	@ 45 – side view View of both the patient's face while reading and the chart	Announce patients lowest VA read with difficulty or easily in M notation at what distance, e.g., 2 M at 30 cm	Reading acuity chart lowest line	On/auto or manual
5	Near visual acuity with near optical device +5.00D over subjective refraction	Paragraph: if patient is unable to obtain paragraph acuity, then check VA with single letter chart	Near light on	Side view of patient holding near chart and reading lowest line can read easily and lowest line read with difficulty	Announce patients lowest VA read with difficulty or easily in M notation at what distance, e.g., 1 M at 5 cm	Reading acuity chart lowest line	On/auto or manual
	If patient obtains a near acuity (paragraph) of 1 M or better with the +5D lens over demonstration distance correction, then skip the +10D demonstration						
6	Near visual acuity with near optical device +10.00D over subjective refraction	Paragraph or single letter chart	Near light on	Side view of patient holding near chart and reading lowest line can read easily and lowest line read with difficulty	Announce patients lowest VA read with difficulty or easily in M notation at what distance, e.g., 0.4 M at 5 cm	Reading acuity chart lowest line	On/auto or manual
7	Amsler grid each eye OD, OS, and OU Ask patient to find center dot, hold it, and draw defects in vision around fixation	Amsler grid	Amsler grid	Zoom in on patient eye movements	Announce whether patient eccentrically viewing, and describe abnormality found	Reading acuity chart lowest line	On/auto or manual

Images needed
1. Fundas picture af each eye with Tapoon Nonmydriatic camera
2. Visual fields
3. Amsler grid
4. Law vision exam form
5. Law vision history form
6. Consent form

15.2.2.2 Findings

Patients were referred for visual rehabilitation by a local ophthalmologist or optometrist.

Local eye care providers were asked to send copies of the most recent eye exam findings, including visual fields. They presented the concept of consultation via telemedicine, the consent forms, and low vision questionnaire to the patient. The eye care provider faxed or mailed the forms and exam data to the remote site presenter, who scanned the data into the telemedical electronic file. An appointment was made with the low vision remote presenter. Following the flow chart, exam data, video clips with audio, and scanned images were obtained and sent via store-and-forward to the consultation site for review. The telemedicine software was able to page or e-mail the specialist when there was a patient episode or electronic file for review. The telemedicine software could be accessed from any location, so the consultant was not forced to go to the designated telemedicine room. A review version of the telemedicine software could also be installed on the consultant's computer. This allows the consultant the convenience of reviewing and making audio or written recommendations from any location.

15.3 Case Study

A patient was referred for visual rehabilitation through telemedicine. He was legally blind due to macular degeneration, and wanted to be able to read again. He also wished to be able to help his wife read signs in the distance, and watch his grandson play baseball. This patient, who reported problems with glare as well, was seen for the initial telemedicine pre-consultation visit, and store-and-forward data was sent for consultant review. Next, the visual rehabilitation consultant made recommendations to address the patient's visual goals. During the second visit, the patient tried various devices for near and distance activities, after which he met the low vision consultant via a real-time telemedicine video connection.

The initial part of the second visit allowed the patient to try the visual devices recommended. With a handheld illuminated magnifier, he was able to read small print again, although slowly, and he was educated that with practice he could improve. A hand-held monocular telescope allowed him to help his wife spot distance signs or watch his grandson. However, a head-mounted Beecher telescope system was more comfortable and convenient for long periods of distance viewing. Glasses with filters were recommended, and helped to cut glare outdoors and increased contrast.

During the second half of the consultation visit, he was able to meet face-to-face with the low vision consultant via telemedicine. The patient and consultant were able to discuss any questions or problems with the devices tried, and any additional visual goals not addressed that could be addressed with another consultation visit.

This patient was very happy to be able to read print again, and see the faces of his wife and family. He and his wife no longer had to dread the time required to drive hours to Houston and then to fight the heavy metropolitan traffic. In many ways, on many levels, they were both satisfied with the telemedicine visual rehabilitation project.

15.4 Summary

Telemedicine can be beneficial in providing excellent low vision care. Ideally, other specialists could be consulted via telemedicine in the rural hospital to increase the viability of telemedicine. A dedicated telemedicine presenter-coordinator would have been helpful. The grant did not provide funding for personnel involved with the telemedicine project, so the remote site presenter and consultants had normal duties with the additional burden of telemedicine activities. This model has the potential to be self-sustaining. In addition to reimbursement for the telemedicine consultant services, there would be income from visual aids purchased by the patients.

References

1. Congdon N, et al. (2004) Causes and prevalence of visual impairment among adults in the United States. Arch Ophthalmol 122(4):477–485

2. Congdon NG, Friedman DS, Lietman T (2003) Important causes of visual impairment in the world today. JAMA 290(15):2057–2060
3. Pollard TL, Simpson JA, et al. (2003) Barriers to accessing low vision services. Ophthal Physl Opt 23(4):321–327
4. Office for the Advancement of Telehealth (OAT), The Center for Telemedicine Law (2003) Telemedicine reimbursement report, pp 1–56

Part III

The World View – Global Experiences in Teleophthalmology

III

Chapter 16

Teleophthalmology in Canada

Matthew T. S. Tennant, Chris J. Rudnisky,
Marie Carole Boucher, David Maberley

16

This chapter addresses the following

Key Concepts:

- Canada is a country well suited for teleophthalmology due to geography, burden of disease, and shortage of eye care specialists.

- Teleophthalmology in Canada is cost-effective when compared to the conventional eye examination.

- Government funds are available for teleophthalmology projects throughout Canada, reimbursement for physician services is provided in some provinces.

- Canadian teleophthalmology systems incorporate:

  1. Visual acuity
  2. Intraocular pressure measurement
  3. Mydriatic and non-mydriatic retinal camera systems
  4. Pupil dilation and no pupil dilation
  5. Stereoscopic and non-stereoscopic imaging.

1.1 Introduction

Canada is a country well suited to benefit by the introduction and utilization of teleophthalmology. Barriers to conventional delivery of eye care can be overcome by the electronic capture and transmission of eye photographs, as well as other health information. The section addresses three key barriers to optimal ophthalmic care, geography, burden of disease and shortage of eye care specialists, and reviews how teleophthalmology could bring benefits.

The majority of people living in Canada live in large urban centers, located primarily in the southern part of the country. The remainder of the population (approximately 10 million people) live in smaller rural communities spread out across an area of some 10 million km^2 [1]. Many communities are accessible only by air, with road access that is limited during winter months when ice highways are possible.

In northern Canada, people of Aboriginal, Metis or Inuit ancestry make up a large part of the population. In recent history, the prevalence of diabetes has increased in each of these groups [2–5]. The complications of diabetes, including eye disease, are now becoming evident. For instance, in one community in northern Alberta, diabetic retinopathy was found in 47% of patients who attended a diabetic eye screening clinic [6]. In another community in northern Ontario, 38 % of the diabetic population was found to have some level of diabetic retinopathy [7].

Eye trauma is another cause of vision loss for individuals living in northern communities. In Nain, Labrador, 11% of the resident population are legally blind from eye trauma [8]. Glaucoma and macular degeneration are two other causes of vision loss in people living in remote communities.

In urban populations, diabetic retinopathy is also prevalent [9]. A recently implemented diabetic retinopathy screening project in urban communities in the province of Quebec found a 32% prevalence of diabetic retinopathy [10]. Fifty-three percent of patients screened had never had an eye examination, and 86% had not been examined in the past two years.

There is a limited number of eye care specialists in many parts of Canada [11]. In many communities, residents must travel as far as 1,000 km to be assessed by an ophthalmologist. This barrier to eye care delivery has led to inadequate eye care for those in need. In British Columbia (BC), only 33% of First Nations individuals with diabetes living on reserves had undergone a yearly retinal examination [12]. In Nova Scotia, only 14% of diabetics had undergone an annual eye examination [13].

Although individuals living in the larger urban areas do not have to travel a great distance to see an ophthalmologist, waiting times for an eye exam can be lengthy. A study of a diabetic population in a Montreal suburb revealed only 19.8% of those screened had undergone a diabetic eye exam in the last two-and-a-half years while 10.1% of those screened had never had a diabetic eye exam [14]. Fourteen percent of the non-compliant group stated inaccessibility and difficulty in obtaining an appointment as the key reasons for not following up after a screening examination.

16.2 Teleophthalmology

Teleophthalmology provides numerous advantages when compared to a conventional eye examination. Digital imaging provides a permanent record of the eye, with the added benefit of data storage and transmission. As part of an electronic health record, teleophthalmology reports can be viewed by different members of the health care team at any location. In addition, subsequent analysis of a teleophthalmology database can assist in improving overall eye care.

16

Delivery of eye care by telemedicine is now a reality for many Canadians. The growth of teleophthalmology utilization has expanded from a few research centers five years ago, to the successful adoption of this technology in more than 100 communities across Canada today.

16.2.1 Reimbursement and Liability

Two provinces, Alberta and British Columbia, now offer a consultation fee code to ophthalmologists for a teleophthalmology examination. The fee code is on par with an in-person eye examination, but requires seven field, stereoscopic digital capture and review to qualify for reimbursement.

Informed consent by the patient is required for all teleophthalmology examinations across Canada. These consents emphasize the current shortcomings of mydriatic and non-mydriatic retinal cameras to image anterior to the equator.

Canadian physicians examining patients by teleophthalmology are covered by the Canadian Medical Protective Association. This mutual defense organization requires doctors to have liability coverage in the province where their practice is located, as well as in any other provinces where they may be providing care by telemedicine.

16.2.2 Cost-Effectiveness

For those living in remote locations, screening for eye disease by retinal photography is less expensive than a conventional eye examination by an eye care specialist. This is particularly true for diabetic retinopathy [15]. The five-year per person cost of a diabetic retinal examination in James Bay, northern Ontario was found to be $403 CAD for a retinal camera program as compared to $842 CAD for an examination by a retinal specialist [16].

16.2.3 Diabetic Retinopathy Teleophthalmology Screening

As the prevalence of diabetic retinopathy increases, more efficient methods are needed to identify treatable eye disease. In addition to providing accurate diagnosis and early treatment, the goal of an effective screening program for diabetic retinopathy lies in reaching as many at-risk diabetics as possible, in a simple and cost-effective manner as possible [17].

16.2.3.1 Quebec Solution

To satisfy this goal, two different teleophthalmology solutions have emerged within Canada. In urban communities as well as some rural communities, teleophthalmology screening systems are utilized. In Quebec, non-mydriatic, non-stereoscopic, three 45° field retinal photographs are captured without pupil dilation. Referral to an eye care specialist is based on the diabetic retinopathy presenting with ≥ ETDRS Grade 35 severity or with any diabetic retinopathy within one disc diameter of the fovea, making the sensitivity of these systems very high [10].

16.2.3.2 Rural/Remote Solution

In British Columbia, the First Nations on-reserve mobile diabetes project is a rural/remote program that utilizes a non-mydriatic, non-stereoscopic, digital, high-resolution (>3 Mb TIFF files) system with three-field photography [18].

In other remote, rural areas, teleophthalmology systems not only screen, but are able to diagnose treatable eye disease. These systems utilize seven 30° field, stereoscopic (7SF) digital imaging to identify ETDRS levels of diabetic retinopathy, age related eye disease study (AREDS) levels of macular degeneration, and cup-to-disc features of glaucoma. Only those patients who need further testing or treatment are referred [6].

16.3 Stereoscopic, Seven Field, Digital Photography

In the following subsections we will discuss clinical validation of stereoscopic, seven field, digital photography, and successful projects.

16.3.1 Clinical Validation

The University of Alberta's Department of Ophthalmology developed a novel teleophthalmology digital stereoscopic imaging system and validated the technology in a pilot project between Fort Vermilion, a small community in northern Alberta, and Edmonton. One hundred and twenty-one patients with diabetes underwent 7SF retinal photography with both digital and slide film media. The digital photographs were then transmitted by satellite to Edmonton to be read by a retinal specialist, while the slide film traveled by truck, to be developed prior to grading. All images were graded in a masked fashion with modified ETDRS grading protocol [19]. Correlation was high for severe NPDR (0.86), proliferative diabetic retinopathy (1.00) and CSME (0.97) [6].

To further clarify the role of digital stereoscopic imaging in the identification of CSME, another comparison study was performed between stereoscopic digital imaging of the macula and clinical examination with contact lens biomicroscopy. One hundred and twenty consecutive diabetic patients were enrolled. All eyes underwent a clinical examination, followed by digital photography. Exact agreement between the two diagnostic modalities was 84% when identifying CSME [20].

16.3.2 Current Projects

The success of this pilot project led to the expansion of teleophthalmology within Alberta to include all 44 First Nation Reserves (Fig. 16.1). One of two mobile units travels to each community with a photographer, nurse and nutritionist. Eye testing includes visual acuity, IOPs and 7SF retinal photography (Fig. 16.2) through a dilated pupil. In addition, blood testing (hemoglobin A1C, cholesterol, triglycerides, blood urea nitrogen, creatinine) and urinalysis are performed. Education includes nutritional support, foot care, and medication review. Retinal images are electronically packaged and encrypted, then transmitted over the Internet to a secure web server for review and ETDRS grading in stereo. Only those patients in need of treatment are referred to a tertiary care center. All other individuals are followed-up with repeat photography.

Additional stereoscopic teleophthalmology diabetic retinopathy screening projects are now a reality in many locations across Canada, including the provinces of Saskatchewan, Manitoba and Ontario.

In the Northwest Territories, retina consultation services are provided via the Internet. A

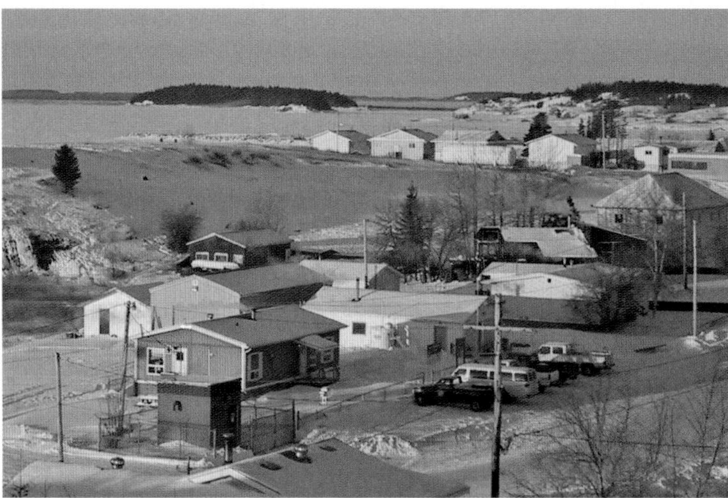

Fig. 16.1. Fort Chipewyan, Alberta: A First Nations community only accessible by airplane or by ice road during the winter

general ophthalmologist who works in Yellowknife refers patients to Edmonton for stereoscopic digital imaging. All images are reviewed by a retinal specialist. If laser treatment is required, patients are then transferred to Edmonton by plane, where they undergo a fluorescein angiogram prior to being seen in person by the specialist.

16.4 Non-Stereoscopic, Three-Field, Digital Imaging

In the following subsections we will discuss clinical validation of non-stereoscopic, three field, digital imaging, and successful projects.

16.4.1 Clinical Validation

The University of Montreal has been at the forefront of telemedicine screening for diabetic retinopathy in urban and semi-urban areas. Barriers to access have been reduced with this innovative program that improves patient comfort and compliance by utilizing non-mydriatic digital retinal cameras. A validation study was performed to demonstrate the effectiveness and safety of screening for diabetic retinopathy with two non-mydriatic digital images [21]. Additional research was performed to identify the number and positioning of fields necessary to screen for diabetic retinopathy [22].

The effectiveness and safety of screening for diabetic retinopathy with two 45° fields centered on the disc and the macula with a digital non-mydriatic camera was evaluated. Screening guidelines for the identification of screened patients needing referral to an ophthalmologist were developed following the completion of a prospective, masked, clinic-based cross-sectional diabetic retinopathy severity comparative study between digital images captured with a non-mydriatic camera, 7SF captured with slide film, and dilated ophthalmologic examination. Substantial agreement was found between imaging modalities by eye ($\kappa = 0.626 \pm 0.045$) as well as by patient assessment ($\kappa = 0.654 \pm 0.063$).

Three levels of screening threshold for patient referral to an ophthalmologist were chosen: very mild diabetic retinopathy (ETDRS severity level 20), mild diabetic retinopathy (ETDRS severity level 35), and moderate diabetic retinopathy (EDTRS severity level 43). Non-mydriatic camera screening with two field photography had a sensitivity 97.9%, 97.1%, and 53.3%, for each of the three screening levels, respectively, with a specificity of 81.3%, 95.5% and 96.9%. Chosen thresholds of very mild or mild diabetic retinopathy both correctly identified 100% of eyes with severe NPDR and/or proliferative retinopathy.

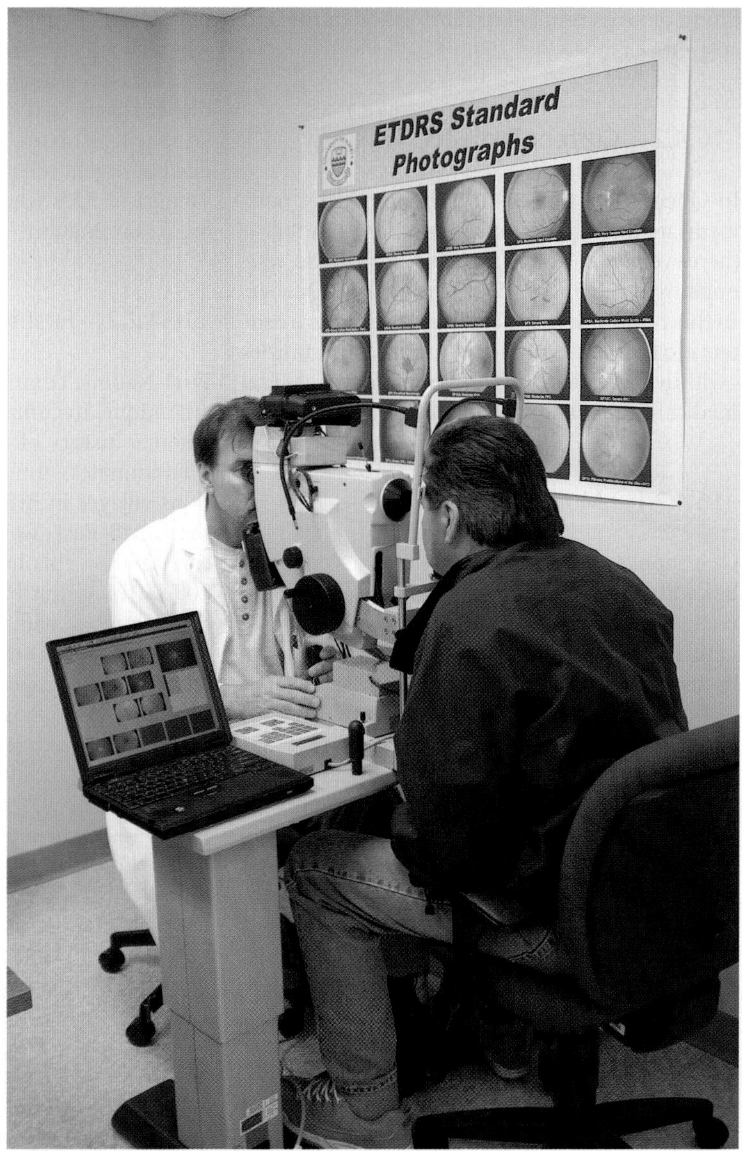

Fig. 16.2. University of Alberta Teleophthalmology Capture System (Zeiss FF450 retinal camera linked to Kodak DCS760 digital back)

In this selected population with a high prevalence (63.3%) of diabetic retinopathy, a two-image, non-mydriatic camera screening strategy with referral at mild diabetic retinopathy reduced the proportion of patients to be screened for diabetic retinopathy by an ophthalmologist from 100% to 55%.

The evaluation of the optimal number and positioning of 45° photographic fields necessary to screen for diabetic retinopathy was performed through a prospective, masked, cross-sectional, comparative study, that graded diabetic retinopathy in 98 patients (196 eyes), using two, three, and four non-mydriatic 45° fundus images, and compared to grading with the ETDRS 7SF captured on slide film [22]. No significant improvement in sensitivity or specificity was measured in detecting diabetic retinopathy when greater than two non-mydriatic 45° image fields centered on the disc and the macula were used, while the addition of fields resulted in diminished utility and cost-efficiency.

16.4.2 Current Projects

In Quebec, the success of the pilot digital non-mydriatic camera screening program has led to the development of a larger scale diabetic retinopathy screening project throughout Quebec. In this project, 13 permanent image capture centers are located in rural and urban communities –within pharmacies, optometrist offices, general medical clinics, and an endocrinology clinic.

16.4.2.1 Mobile Units

One mobile unit travels to different communities with a photographer and a nurse, who takes medical histories. A consent form explaining the nature of the telemedicine examination and its limitations is signed. Visual acuity is measured in both eyes, and then three 45° retinal photographs are taken, which include non-stereoscopic photographs of the disc, and capturing the macula and superior temporal quadrant–with an extra macular image taken to allow for stereo evaluation if indicated. The photographer verifies the quality of the images and repeats any photographs if necessary. Any inability to photograph the retina leads to referral to an ophthalmologist. At the same time, educational support is provided. Retinal images and clinical data are electronically packaged and encrypted, then transmitted without compression over the Internet to a secure Web server for review and non-stereo ETDRS grading. Stereo images of the macula are available and viewed if necessary. All images are reviewed, with and without image enhancing, by a retina specialist or a trained ophthalmologist.

Patients with diabetic retinopathy greater than ETDRS 35, or with any diabetic retinopathy within one disc diameter of fovea are referred to the closest treating ophthalmologist. All others are followed yearly with repeat imaging. After screening, all patients are contacted for follow-up and provided with a timely ophthalmologic appointment if needed. A report of the screening results with a picture of each eye is sent to all physicians involved in the care of the individual. All data, which is archived for 10 years, is available for epidemiological studies. To date, overall diabetic retinopathy was detected in 30% of the screened diabetics, with 10% of all screened in need of urgent referral. Screening provided a net savings of 83% when compared to ophthalmologic examination.

16.4.2.2 First Nations

First Nations communities in British Columbia are unique. In comparison to the rest of Canada, where a history of displacement to reservations predominates, almost all pre-existing First Nations villages in British Columbia (except for in the North-East) were designated reserves in the early 1900s. This has resulted in approximately 200 distinct First Nations communities in British Columbia, with an average band size of 250. In comparison, Quebec has a total of 39 reserves with an average size of approximately 1,000. Given the rugged geography of British Columbia, smaller and more isolated bands are particularly at risk for not receiving adequate health care.

The British Columbia First Nations On-Reserve mobile diabetes project addresses this issue by providing tertiary diabetes care for all communities in British Columbia north of Williams Lake. A Canon non-mydriatic camera (CR6-45NM) with digital Canon (D30) camera back captures 3.0 megapixel TIFF color images. Four 45° field images are generated and stored on compact flash card with back up to an external hard drive on a laptop computer. An extra macular image is routinely taken to allow for stereo evaluation as necessary.

If diabetic pathology is identified by the photographer, images are JPEG 3:1 compressed and encrypted prior to being sent via modem to a retinal specialist. All other images are not compressed but are saved onto a CD for later transfer to the reading center. Images are graded on a 21 inch CRT monitor with a stereo magnifier if macular pathology is identified. Histogram contrast enhancement and brightness levels are adjusted to assist in the reading, but all images are initially evaluated without processing.

16.5 Age-Related Macular Degeneration Teleophthalmology Screening

AMD is a leading cause of legal blindness in North America [23]. Early detection and treatment has been shown to decrease the risk of vision loss [24]. Teleophthalmology can assist patients who might not otherwise have access to specialist eye care.

16.6 Stereoscopic, One-Field, Digital Imaging

In the following subsections, we will discuss clinical validation of stereoscopic, one field, digital imaging, and successful projects.

16.6.1 Clinical Validation

A clinical validation study was performed to test whether or not stereoscopic digital imaging of the macula was as sensitive and specific as stereoscopic slide film. One hundred and three patients were consecutively enrolled. All eyes were photographed with both digital (six megapixel) and film photography through a dilated pupil. Digital images underwent JPEG 16× compression and were uploaded onto a secure web server. Both image formats were graded with a modified AREDS classification. Correlation was found to be high for AREDS level 4b or greater ($\kappa = 0.83$ SE 0.05, PPV 0.81, NPV 0.98, Sensitivity 0.94, Specificity 0.94) [25].

An ongoing multi-center study (Quebec, British Columbia) is currently evaluating macular digital imaging through widely available digital non-mydriatic fundus cameras (980×1,200 resolution) for AMD. Using AREDS classification, it is assessing stereoscopic and non-stereoscopic digital imaging correlation with 35 mm film, clinical examination and optical coherence tomography examination. This study follows earlier work by Maberley et al., which looked at the sensitivity and specificity of photographic screening for age-related macular degeneration [26].

16.6.2 Current Projects

In Alberta, ophthalmic consultations for macular degeneration are performed by teleophthalmology. Optometrists send stereoscopic digital images of the macula and disc captured through a dilated pupil to retinal specialists located at a tertiary care center. Patients with evidence of choroidal neovascularization are then scheduled for fluorescein angiography on the day of their clinical examination. If clinical examination and fluorescein angiogram confirm choroidal neovascularization, laser treatment is provided that same day.

16.7 Teleophthalmology Systems

This teleophthalmology system at the University of Alberta is hardware independent. Currently, three different retinal cameras are being utilized at different sites across Canada (Table 16.1). Images are captured then transferred as encrypted and compressed digital files to the password protected secure web server. Patient files are protected with USB key two factor authentication. Images are then reviewed in digital stereo with LCD shutter glasses. Computer algorithms automatically calculate levels of eye disease such as ETDRS level, once images are graded by a retinal specialist.

16.8 Camera Systems

The teleophthalmology camera system at the University of Montreal (Table 16.2) can incorporate multiple retinal cameras. Currently only one camera is utilized at the different sites. Images are captured then transferred without any compression as encrypted and compressed digital files to the password protected secure web server. Patient files are protected with USB key two factor authentication. Images are reviewed without, then with image enhancing, non-stereoscopically, on a 19- or 21-inch high-quality display monitor and, when indicated, in digital stereo with LCD shutter glasses. The images are graded manually by a retinal specialist.

Table 16.1. University of Alberta camera systems

Retinal camera	Digital camera	Pixelresolution	Color	Compression	Fieldsize	Number of fields	Stereopsis	Pupil-dilation
Zeiss FF450	Kodak DCS760	3,040×2,008	24 bit	16× JPEG	30	7	Yes (fields 1 and 2 only)	Yes
Topcon NW6S	Nikon D100	3,008×2,000	24 bit	16× JPEG	45	9	Yes (fields 1 and 2 only)	Yes
Canon CR-DGi	Canon Eos 10D	3,072×2,046	24 bit	16× JPEG	45	9	Yes (fields 1 and 2 only)	Yes

Table 16.2. University of Montreal camera system

Retinal camera	Digital camera	Pixelresolution	Color	Compression	Fieldsize	Number of fields	Stereopsis	Pupildilation
Variable	Nidek NM 1000	1,280×960	24 bit	None	45	3	Not routinely Used for field 2 if indicated	None Dilation only if insufficient image quality

Table 16.3. University of British Columbia camera system

Retinal camera	Digital camera	Pixelresolution	Color	Compression	Fieldsize	Number of fields	Stereopsis	Pupildilation
Canon CR6-45NM	Canon D30	2,160×1,440	12 bit	JPEG 3:1 when transmitting by modem	45	4	Not routinely Used for field 2 if indicated	Yes

The teleophthalmology camera system at the University of British Columbia (Table 16.3) currently utilizes a Canon non-mydriatic camera. Images are captured in remote locations and sent by modem in an encrypted format. Images are not compressed except when sent via modem (when a JPEG 3:1 compression is used). Images are graded on a 21-inch CRT monitor with a stereo magnifier if macular pathology is identified. Histogram contrast enhancement and brightness levels are adjusted to assist in the reading, but all images are initially evaluated without processing.

References

1. Canadian Statistics (2001) www.statcan.ca/english/Pgdb/. Cited 19 Feb 2005
2. Bruce S (2000) Prevalence and determinants of diabetes mellitus among the Metis of western Canada. Am J Hum Biol 12:542–551
3. Pioro MP, Dyck RF, Gillis DC (1996) Diabetes prevalence rates among First Nations adults on Saskatchewan reserves in 1990: comparison by tribal grouping, geography and with non-First Nations people. Can J Public Health 87:325–328
4. Thouez JP, Ekoe JM, Foggin PM, Verdy M, Nadeau M, Laroche P, Rannou A, Ghadirian P (1990) Obesity, hypertension, hyperuricemia and diabetes mellitus among the Cree and Inuit of northern Quebec. Arctic Med Res 49:180–188
5. Young TK, Reading J, Elias B, O'Neil JD (2000) Type 2 diabetes mellitus in Canada's first nations: status of an epidemic in progress. Can Med Assoc J 163:561–566
6. Tennant MT, Greve MD, Rudnisky CJ, Hillson TR, Hinz BJ (2001) Identification of diabetic retinopathy by stereoscopic digital imaging via teleophthalmology: a comparison to slide film. Can J Ophthalmol 36:187–196
7. Maberley D, Cruess AF, Barile G, Slakter J (2002) Digital photographic screening for diabetic retinopathy in the James Bay Cree. Ophthalmic Epidemiol 9:169–178
8. Johnson GJ, Green JS, Paterson GD, Perkins ES (1984) Survey of ophthalmic conditions in a Labrador community: II Ocular disease. Can J Ophthalmol 19:224–233
9. Green C, Hoppa RD, Young TK, Blanchard JF (2003) Geographic analysis of diabetes prevalence in an urban area. Soc Sci Med 57:551–560
10. Boucher M (2004) Results of a new health service model utilizing telemedicine in screening for diabetic retinopathy. In: Proceedings of the 7th Annual Canadian Society of Telehealth, Quebec City, Canada
11. Persaud DD, Cockerill R, Pink G, Trope G (1999) Determining Ontario's supply and requirements for ophthalmologists in 2000 and 2005: Methods. Can J Ophthalmol 34:74–81
12. Kaur H, Maberley D, Chang A, Hay D (2004) The current status of diabetes care, diabetic retinopathy screening and eye-care in British Columbia's First Nations Communities. Int J Circumpolar Health 63:277–285
13. Kozousek V, Brown MG, Cottle R, Hicks VA, Langille DB, Dingle J (1993) Use of ophthalmologic services by diabetic patients in Nova Scotia. Can J Ophthalmol 28:7–10
14. Boucher M, Nguyen N (2005) Mass community screening for diabetic retinopathy using a non-mydriatic camera with telemedicine. Can J Ophthalmol (in press)
15. Martin JD, Yidegiligne HM (1998) The cost-effectiveness of a retinal photography screening program for preventing diabetic retinopathy in the First Nations diabetic population in British Columbia, Canada. Int J Circumpolar Health 57(1):379–382
16. Maberley D, Walker H, Koushik A, Cruess A (2003) Screening for diabetic retinopathy in James Bay, Ontario: a cost-effectiveness analysis. Can Med Assoc J 168:160–164
17. Taylor HR (1997) Diabetic retinopathy: a public health challenge. Am J Ophthalmol 123:543–545
18. Maberley D, Morris A, Hay D, Chang A, Hall L, Mandava N (2004) A comparison of digital retinal image quality among photographers with different levels of training using a non-mydriatic fundus camera. Ophthalmic Epidemiol 11:191–197
19. Early Treatment Diabetic Retinopathy Study Research Group (1991) Grading diabetic retinopathy from stereoscopic color fundus photographs: an extension of the modified Airlie House classification; ETDRS report number 10. Ophthalmology 98:786–806
20. Rudnisky CJ, Hinz BJ, Tennant MT, de Leon AR, Greve MD (2002) High-resolution stereoscopic digital fundus photography versus contact lens biomicroscopy for the detection of clinically significant macular edema. Ophthalmology 109:267–274
21. Boucher MC, Gresset JA, Angioi K, Olivier S (2003) Effectiveness and safety of screening for diabetic retinopathy with two nonmydriatic digital images compared with the seven standard stereoscopic photographic fields. Can J Ophthalmol 38:557–568
22. Perrier M, Boucher MC, Angioi K, Gresset JA, Olivier S (2003) Comparison of two, three and four 45° image fields obtained with the Topcon CRW6 nonmydriatic camera for screening for diabetic retinopathy. Can J Ophthalmol 38:569–574

23. Congdon N, O'Colmain B, Klaver CC, Klein R, Munoz B, Friedman DS, Kempen J, Taylor HR, Mitchell P (2004) Causes and prevalence of visual impairment among adults in the United States. Arch Ophthalmol 122:477–485
24. Bressler NM (2002) Early detection and treatment of neovascular age-related macular degeneration. J Am Board Fam Pract 15:142–152
25. Somani R, Tennant MT, Rudnisky CJ, Weis E, Ting A, Eppler J, Hinz BJ, Greve MD, De Leon AR (2005) Comparison of stereoscopic digital imaging to film in the identification of macular degeneration. Can J Ophthalmol 40(3):293–302
26. Maberley DA, Isbister C, MacKenzie P, Aralar A (2004) An evaluation of photographic screening for neovascular age-related macular degeneration. Eye19(6):611–616

16

Chapter 17

Internet-Based Electronic Eye Care Consultations: Patient Perspective

17

Sajeesh Kumar, Kanagasingam Yogesan, Beth Hudson, Mei-Ling Tay-Kearney

This chapter addresses the following

Key Concepts:

- Patient satisfaction and attitudes toward Internet-based eye care services are evaluated.
- Patients expressed a high degree of satisfaction with Internet-based eye examinations.
- Lack of in-person contact with an ophthalmologist is not a major concern to most patients.
- In general, patients did not express negative attitudes toward Internet-based teleophthalmology services.

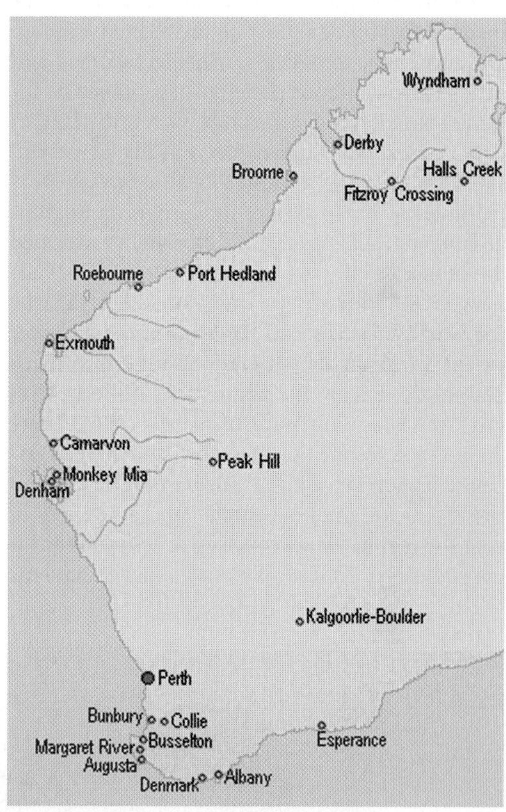

Fig. 17.1. Map of Western Australia (WA)

17.1 Introduction

As is typical in many large countries, Australia has a large landmass with a low population density, and providing the population with specialist eye care services is a major problem outside the major cities. The state of Western Australia (WA) (Fig. 17.1) has a land area of 2.5 million square kilometers, which is equivalent to one-third of the land mass of the United States (approximately two million kilometers).

Even though WA has a large land mass, 70% of people live in and around the capital city of Perth; the remaining 30% of the population lives in rural and remote WA. Therefore, when specialist ophthalmic care is required for people in remote areas, this need may remain unfulfilled for some time.

The fees for a single patient's eye care can run into thousands of dollars, when travel and accommodation for the patient (and usually a family member) is included; in addition, there is the intangible cost of taking people away from familiar surroundings, work, and community [1].

Internet-based eye care services have been proposed in WA as a means of improving access to specialist eye care [2]. A Web-based teleophthalmology service (www.e-icare.com) has been developed at the Center of Excellence in e-Medicine,(e-Med) and the Lions Eye Institute (LEI) in Perth [3]. This system, which stores and transmits multimedia data to a secure, central database, includes patients' data, such as demographic information, medical history, images, videos and audio files.

Before adoption into routine use, any new medical technology must be proved to be secure and acceptable to patients. Much is assumed and little is known about patients' acceptance of Internet-based eye care settings. Given the lack of data, e-Medicine undertook a study of patient satisfaction, using a trained health care worker-led Internet-based service in Carnarvon Regional Hospital (CRH) (Fig. 17.2), which is located in the heart of the Gascoyne Region of WA. Carnarvon is connected to the rest of Australia by the North West Coastal Highway and, to a lesser extent, by its airport. It takes about 2 h to fly or 11 h to drive from the nearest city of Perth (940 km). It has a population of 6,357 (1996). There are no eye specialist services available in the Gascoyne region on a full-time basis. The current practice is for an eye-specialist and a registrar to visit the region for a week, two times per year for consultations. In cases of emergencies, patients are airlifted to a hospital in the city by the Royal Flying Doctor Service (RFDS).

17.2 The Study

A trained teleophthalmology nurse-coordinator takes retinal photos and external eye pictures of patients at CRH with the equipment and technology developed at e-Medicine [3–6]. The equipment included (1) a portable slit lamp (e-Med), (2) a portable air-puff tonometer (Keeler Pulsair 3000, Japan), and a non-mydriatic digital fundus camera (Canon CR4-45NM, Japan).

These devices were connected directly to the online eye care system (www.e-icare.com) to transmit multimedia information to specialists in Perth. Each time a patient was screened at CRH, an automatic e-mail was sent to alert the specialist in Perth. The specialist reviewed the data, recorded image quality, diagnosed eye disease, and made recommendations for disease management and subsequent care. Specialist advice was returned to CRH within 24 h.

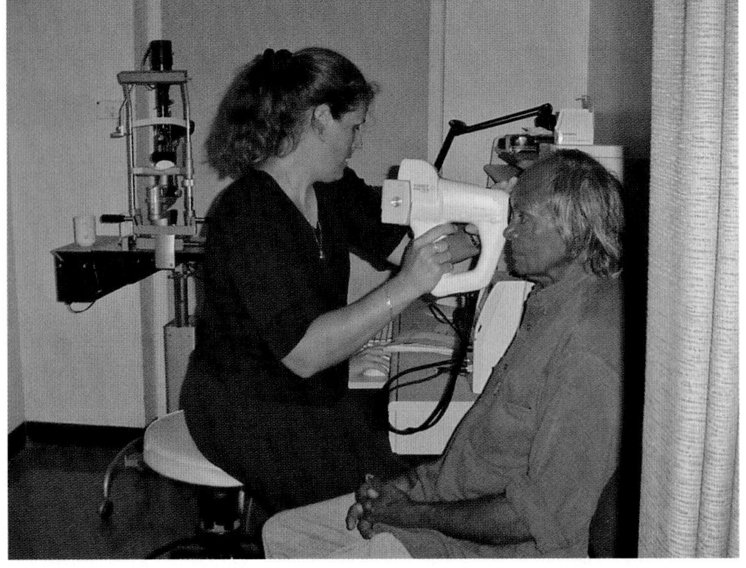

Fig. 17.2. Image of Carnarvon Teleophthalmology Center

17.2.1 Recruitment

The service was made available to patients referred from local general practitioners (GPs), as well as and walk-in patients. Patient participation was entirely on a voluntary basis. No fee was charged, and emergency cases were also seen. Media announcements on local radio stations and news services were also done.

In the meantime, a teleophthalmology protocol, which was primed for service, detailed the consultation criteria, and the technical and training requirements for people involved. It also specified the rights and responsibilities of the patients, prepared the patient for consultation, privacy and confidentiality issues, screening, referral and consultation procedures and other relevant information.

17.2.2 Questionnaires and Forms

Questionnaires were used to collect patient perceptions toward teleophthalmology. These were sent along with a stamped, self-addressed envelope to all patients after consultation. The responses were collected and analyzed. The questionnaire consisted of four closed-ended questions and nine questions on rating of the service (Fig. 17.3). The closed-ended questions were on service satisfaction, lack of direct physical contact with a distant clinician, privacy concerns and future use of the teleophthalmology service. The questionnaire asked the patient to rate various aspects of the teleophthalmology service such as physical comfort, psychological comfort, convenience, duration and timeliness of consultation, skills and attitude of consultant, skills and attitude of attending health care personnel and overall satisfaction with the Internet-based service. Samples of teleophthalmology protocol, patient information sheets, patient consent forms, patient evaluation forms, clinician perception forms, and the teleophthalmology service log sheet are attached as Appendices 2–7.

17.3 Results

During the study period (February–November 2003), 110 patients were presented via Internet-based teleophthalmology. Completed questionnaires were received from 45 patients (41%), of which 42% were from men and 58% from women (mean age 42 years, range 9–73 years). More than half of these patients (53%) came to the teleophthalmology center through local media announcements, while 36% were referred by health professionals in Carnarvon . A few of the patients (7%) became aware of the telemedicine service through their family or friends. Four percent of the patients used the service for consultations for eye disease treatment or care. Most of the patients (94%) used the Internet-based service for screening for eye diseases like glaucoma and diabetic retinopathy, while, 2% of the cases were for other purposes, including expert second opinion and post-operative follow up.

A majority of patients (98%) expressed satisfaction (Table 17.1) with Internet-based consultation and observed it as a convenient form of service. Lack of physical contact with the ophthalmologist was not a major concern to many patients (74%). While 88% were not apprehensive about privacy issues associated with teleophthalmology services, 98% of patients would

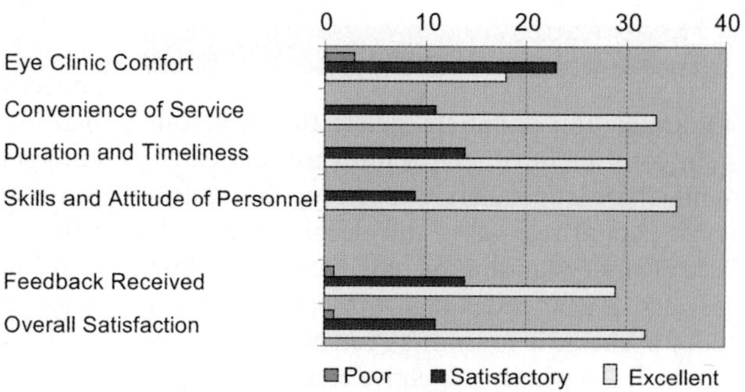

Fig. 17.3. Teleophthalmology patient rating with regard to service delivery

Table 17.1. Sample of patient comments about Internet-based teleophthalmology service

Patient Comments
– I am pleased to be provided with this service and would be happy for re-imagingmy eyes in January.
– A small room, rather than a curtained-off area would have been more suitable – mainly due to the light requirement.
– I was very happy to see the ad (advertisement) in the paper, as I would have to book in and wait for a GP referral otherwise.
– Was convenient and great use of technology, but still did not change anything in terms of treatment, as specialist was unable to offer a conclusive diagnosis, so chose to travel to Perth.
– The whole procedure was excellent and very friendly.
– Poor clinic area
– Personnel very helpful
– Quite happy with the service I received. Should be more of them
– Very friendly, convenient and helpful service
– Excellent service, saved us having to go to an Eye Specialist in Geraldton or Perth
– Unable to ask direct questions, as this was not a direct Telehealth service. Results took a week to come back.

prefer to use teleophthalmology in the future. Overall, the patients valued improved access to specialist services but had clear views as to the limitations of such a service.

The comfort level in the rural teleophthalmology center was rated poor to satisfactory by majority of patients, while the skills and attitude of the personnel at the telecenter were rated highly. The results of the evaluation also showed that trust between patients and treatment providers was of major importance in engendering positive attitudes.

GPs and other health care personnel in Carnarvon spoke favorably about using teleophthalmology, because they were able to get advice from colleagues and discuss alternative management strategies. Practitioners at e-Medicine found the experience informative and challenging.

17

17.4 Discussion

The evaluation of patient satisfaction is a common constituent of any health care service [1]. While there is speculation regarding the neutrality of patient responses and debate around the lack of understanding of how patients evaluate services, it is a mechanism through which attitudes of medical consumers can be usefully obtained. It is a wholly subjective assessment of the quality of service and, as such, is not a measure of final outcome of the technology used.

17.4.1 Patient Satisfaction Issues

Earlier evidence has suggested that patient dissatisfaction is mostly associated with non-compliance with instructions, delay in seeking further care, and poor understanding and retention of medical information [7]. This survey found at least 2% of the patients were not satisfied and may choose to refrain from future services. Another possible reason for dissatisfaction may be, as one patient stated, "convenient and great use of technology, but still did not change anything in terms of treatment." The Internet-based consultation was mainly used to provide diagnostic options, and not as a new treatment modality.

Few of the patients (5%) found the store-and-forward Internet-based service more time consuming than the conventional face-to-face method. It must be noted that, except in the emergency cases, the outcome reports of the Internet-consultation are sent by post to all patients within 24 h. Perneger et al., after comparing patient satisfaction in three treatment settings, suggested that satisfaction also reflects patients' characteristics and expectations, which are not related to quality of care [8].

17.4.2 Provider-Patient Communication Issues

In Carnarvon, patients had an opportunity to see the distant specialist in person on occasions of their regional visits once or twice a year. The Internet-based service was used mainly for monitoring or screening, post-operative follow-up, trauma and expert second opinion services. In this survey, at least one patient expressed concern about the inability to ask direct questions to a specialist, and 23% of the patients still preferred physical contact with the distant clinician. Data security over the Internet represents another aspect of the process, which is often overlooked. Seven percent of patients were concerned about the privacy issues associated with the security of information in an Internet environment.

17.4.3 Space Considerations

The Internet-based eye care system was deployed in Carnarvon Regional Hospital by accommodating the staff and equipment in the scarce space available within the hospital. In the absence of a dedicated room for telemedicine, a corridor area was curtained off to use as a teleophthalmology clinic. While this set-up was not comfortable for many patients, convenience in receiving eye care services in their familiar surroundings was perceived as a positive aspect of teleophthalmology (98%).

17.4.4 Perceived Benefits

Along with the convenience and cost savings associated with avoided travel to Perth, there were also indirect benefits to the family, which included increased access to clinical support, reduced risk associated with travel, and reduced disruption to family life.

The patients' response rate could have been higher in this study. This highlights the importance of finding other ways of working and organizing the communication network in order to increase the volume of response and follow-up from isolated, rural and remote patients. It was observed that a fair number of patients (7%) became aware of the telemedicine service through their family or friends, while a greater number of patients (36%) became aware through health care professionals in the locality, such as their general practitioners. Hence, general practitioners, family and friends, and other patients could be informed and encouraged to optimize the number of patients using telemedicine facilities and achieving better response rates. Despite a low volume of response from the patients, we may conclude that patients approve of Internet-based services, which is in compliance with protocols, as a feasible eye care modality in remote, rural areas. Patients surveyed during this study show no negative general attitudes toward Internet-based teleophthalmology services. From the patient perspective, the success of teleophthalmology has been overwhelmingly associated with time and cost savings associated with travel, convenience and increased access to services. The implementation of teleophthalmology projects may therefore have a positive effect within patient communities. As the use of Internet-based eye care service grows, patient perspective evaluations merit greater attention.

References

1. Sajeesh KR, Tay-Kearney M-L, Constable IJ, Yogesan K (2005) Internet based ophthalmology service: impact assessment. Brit J Ophthalmol (in press)
2. Sajeesh KR, Yogesan K, Constable IJ (2004) Should telemedicine in eye care be funded in Australia? Med J Aust 181(10):583
3. Yogesan K, Constable IJ, Morgan B, Soebadi DY (2000) International transmission of tele-ophthalmology images. J Telemed Telecare 5:41–44
4. Cuypers MJ, Constable IJ (1992) A new magnifying indirect stereo ophthalmoscope. Retina 12(2):141–146
5. Yogesan K, Barry CJ, Jitzkaia L, Eikelboom RH, van Saarloos, House PH, Morgan WH (1999) Software for 3-D visualization/analysis of optic-disc images. IEEE Eng Biol Med 18(1):43–49
6. Yogesan K, Constable IJ, Barry CJ, Eikelboom RH, McAllister IL, Tay-Kearney ML (2000) Telemedicine screening of diabetic retinopathy using a hand-held fundus camera. Telemed J E Health 6(2):231–235
7. Wilkin D, Hallam L, Doggett M (1992) Measures of need and outcome for primary health care. Oxford Medical Publications, Oxford, UK

8. Perneger TV, Etter J, Raetzo M, Schaller P, Stalder H (1996) Comparison of patient satisfaction with ambulatory visits in competing health care delivery settings in Geneva, Switzerland. J Epidemiol Community Health 50:463–468

Chapter 18

Teleophthalmology in India

18

Srinivasan Sanjay, V. Murali,
S. S. Badrinath, Rajiv Raman

This chapter addresses the following

Key Concepts:

- A telemedicine system has been developed in India, linking eye hospitals in Chennai and Bangalore, and providing remote ophthalmological care via a mobile bus.
- Rural patients undergo comprehensive eye screening and diagnosis in the remote bus, and receive awareness education about eye care and common eye diseases.

18.1 Introduction

Since 1990, India has made rapid strides in the fields of communication and information technology (IT). An important application of this is in the use of telemedicine to provide diagnostic and therapeutic medical care to the large, underserved areas of India. Telemedicine is most effective in India, which has a vast land area coupled with varied topography, such as the mountain regions of Himalaya, the desert of Rajasthan, far-flung areas of the North East, and the offshore islands of Andaman and Lakshadweep. With the majority of the population living in rural areas and most specialist doctors living in urban areas, telemedicine gives benefits, such as improved access, reduced cost, reduced isolation from doctors, and improved quality of health care.

The Indian Space Research Organization (ISRO) has played a vital role in providing the communication link for telemedicine activities in rural areas. Sankara Nethralaya, an Eye Hospital and Medical Research Foundation. In the city of Chennai was the pioneer in mobile teleophthalmology practice in India [1].

18.2 Setting Up a Telemedicine Unit

Setting up a telemedicine unit is a complex procedure that involves meeting requirements for hardware, software, communications, human resources, and consultations. The central hub requirements at Sankara Nethralaya included a room with air-conditioning, adequate lighting, comfortable seating, sound proofing to reduce background noise and audio echo, electricity with back-up, and the equipment necessary for receiving data and video conferencing.

The mobile unit requirements included the equipment necessary for comprehensive eye examination, facilities for equipment storage when not in use, seating for the patients, a power source for the equipment, and accessories like satellite tracking equipment, data and image capturing devices like digital cameras, scanners, etc.

The hardware requirements included a computer, video conferencing equipment, scanner, capture card, and color television.

The communications was through Local Area Network (LAN), Wide Area Network, Plain Old Telephone Service (POTS), or ISDN. Low-cost business terminals with small antennas (generally less than two meters in diameter), often termed Very Small Aperture Terminals (VSATs) were also used.

18.3 Sankara Nethralaya Experience: How It Began

A pilot project was started by Sankara Nethralaya, linking two of its eye care centers that were separated by a distance of 3 km. A junior ophthalmologist at the distant center examined about 100 patients, and had their medical information transferred to the Sankara Nethralaya main hospital by LAN over a fiberoptic cable. After looking at the images, a senior ophthalmologist at Sankara Nethralaya diagnosed and discussed the treatment modalities with the junior consultant.

The next step, which was accomplished in 2002, was to link Sankara Nethralaya Eye Hospital, Chennai, with Sankara Nethralaya Eye Hospital at Bangalore. The Bangalore branch, located 400 km away from Chennai, is headed by a vitreo-retinal consultant. The Indian Space Research Organization (ISRO) provided satellite connectivity for this service. Patients who required secondary consultations were subjected to routine examinations and their images were captured and sent to Sankara Nethralaya, Chennai. The senior super-specialty consultant discussed each case with the consultant and the patients in Bangalore, and offered advice and suitable management guidelines [2].

Following this, another unique teleophthalmology project was started in the villages within a 100 km radius of Chennai with a mobile bus offering primary eye care. It was inaugurated by Hon. President of India, Dr APJ Abdul Kalam in 2003. The key to the project was a mobile bus, designed by a team from Sankara Nethralaya with assistance from the ISRO. The total cost of this project, which was approximately 190,000 USD, was provided by ISRO and Sankara Nethralaya.

18.4 ISRO and Telemedicine

18

Established by the government of India in 1969, the prime objective of the ISRO has been to develop space technology and its application to various national tasks. The ISRO, which has a separate budget for the application of space technology for civilian purposes, started its ambitious telemedicine project in 2001 with a pilot project that ran for two years in the state of Madhya Pradesh.

The ISRO has initiated a number of telemedicine pilot projects that are very specific to development needs in India. ISRO telemedicine projects link hospitals in remote and inaccessible areas with super-speciality hospitals located in the city through Indian national satellite (INS). The cost of a telemedicine unit and very small aperture terminal (VSAT) communication is around 25,000 USD per site. Hospital staff are trained to utilize the telemedicine facilities by the telemedicine system vendors.

18.5 The Sankara Nethralaya Rural Mobile Teleophthalmology Project

The team members of the Rural Mobile Teleophthalmology project included one ophthalmologist stationed at Sankara Nethralaya, Chennai; two optometrists (traveling with the bus); a driver (who also doubled as a spectacle technician); four social workers (for planning, fundraising, enumeration, and counseling); and a technical advisor/ administrator to take care of human resources and equipment management.

The project currently serves seven districts around the city of Chennai. When a village is selected for screening, the social worker goes to the village three months prior to lay out the program details. Another visit is made to the village one month prior to the camp, to finalize the visit of the team, location, and the people who would benefit from the camp. Patients are first identified by the social worker who, by door-to-door enumeration, informs them of the day and date of the arrival of the bus. There are tandoras (drums) and auto rickshaw announcements about the camp three days prior to the camp. The day before the camp, awareness videos about common eye diseases are played in local languages to motivate people in the village to attend the camp. Patients at the camp site are registered and their detailed ocular and systemic history is noted. In the camp, patients undergo comprehensive eye screening by optometrists, and those with eye problems who require a consultation with an ophthalmologist are identified.

18.5.1 Vehicle Design

The Sankara Nethralaya mobile bus (Figs. 18.1 and 18.2) has three parts. The front portion of the bus is for the driver and staff during travel to remote areas. The middle portion is the main consultation room of the bus, which has ophthalmic and video conferencing equipment and seats for patients who wait their turn for teleconsultation. This part of the bus is fully air conditioned for optimal performance of the equipment. The ophthalmic equipment is mounted on a refraction unit which can be slid to use either the slit lamp or the non-mydriatic camera, and also includes the seating couch for the patient undergoing examination. There are storage compartments where the dismantled ophthalmic equipment is placed during travel.

The rear portion of the bus is for storage of one additional set of ophthalmic equipment, pamphlets, chairs, cleaning equipment and luggage of the teleophthalmology team; it also houses the generators (for captive power supply).

The satellite dish of the mobile bus is encased in a protective metal covering to prevent damage from natural causes, when not in use.

18.5.2 Ophthalmic, Teleconferencing, and Accessory Equipment Inside Bus

The ophthalmic equipment inside the bus (Figs. 18.3a and 18.3b) includes the following: video indirect ophthalmoscope, direct ophthalmoscope, video slit lamp imaging system, refraction unit, two portable slit lamps, three trial sets and vision drum, non-mydriatic fundus camera, four mirror gonioscope lenses, Schiotz tonometer, Nikon 2200 Digital Camera, and two battery operated and wall mounted streak retinoscopes.

Equipment in the bus used for teleconferencing (Fig. 18.4) includes the following: IP satellite console, antenna controller, P-4 computer with 512 Mb ram with flat bed scanner and ink jet printer, Sony™ video conferencing camera, and Vepro™ PACS cum tele-medicine software.

Accessories inside the bus include: a seating arrangement for patients, an air conditioner, a LCD projector, a laptop computer, a portable amplifier and cordless microphone, and an awareness video and CDs about cataracts, diabetic retinopathy, glaucoma, and eye donation.

Equipment outside the bus includes a 3 m dish antenna, two 5 KVA diesel generators, and a VSAT facility on top (Fig. 18.5).

18.5.3 Teleophthalmology Procedure

The selected patients have their slit lamp anterior segment, diffuse illumination, slit photos, and usually their non-mydriatic fundus photos taken inside the bus. Patients who subsequently have findings in the fundus are dilated and photographs are taken again. Patients who have squint or other extra-ocular problems are also photographed with a digital still camera capable of taking external photographs with zoom capability. Telecommunication between rural camp and Sankara Netralaya, Chennai is achieved by satellite connection through VSAT, which has a bandwidth of 384 Kb/s.

The ophthalmologist at Sankara Netralaya, Chennai examines the images received (Fig. 18.6) and comes to a provisional diagnosis. An anterior segment video may be requested in special situations. Demonstration of extra procedures like eye movements may also be requested. The ophthalmologist maintains electronic medical records of all patients, segregates interesting cases, maintains a file for discussion with peers or seniors, and is involved in the training of fellow ophthalmologists, paramedical ophthalmic assistants, and nursing staff in rural and semiurban areas. During the course of the teleconsultation, the ophthalmologist counsels the patient about familial eye diseases, preventive aspects and eye care.

18.5.4 Continuing Ophthalmic Tele-Education

Each month, through interactive lectures via video conferencing, the rural mobile teleophthalmology unit also conducts continuing ophthalmic tele-education for the ophthalmologists, physicians, nurses, and paramedical ophthalmic

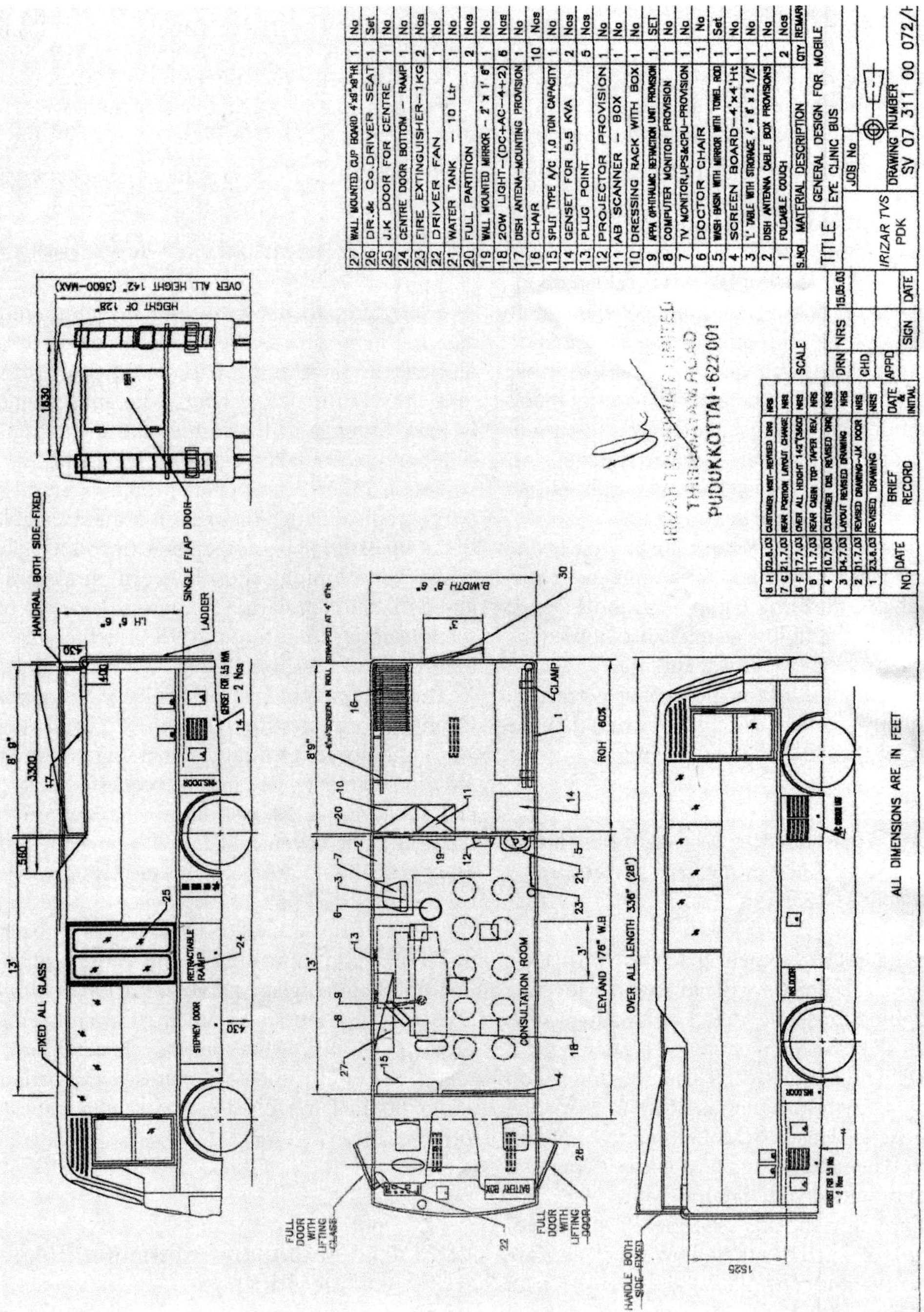

Fig. 18.1. Design of the teleophthalmology bus

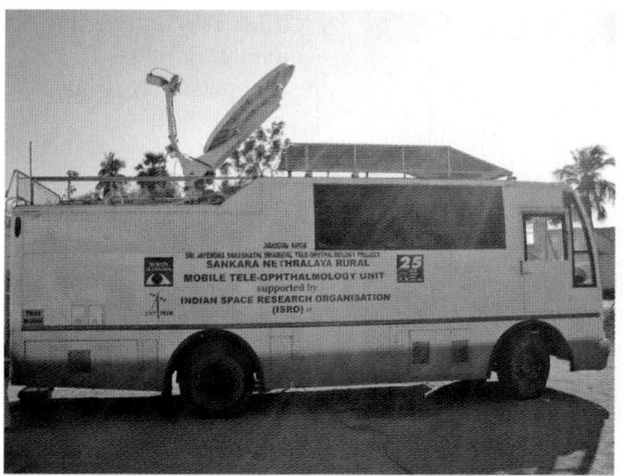
SANKARA NETHRALAYA RURAL
MOBILE TELE-OPHTHALMOLOGY UNIT
supported by
INDIAN SPACE RESEARCH ORGANISATION
(ISRO)
25

Fig. 18.2. Exterior of the teleophthalmology bus

assistants involved in eye care in rural and sub-urban areas.

The clinical ophthalmic grand rounds, which are a part of the academic activities of Sankara Nethralaya, Chennai, are beamed to different parts of India and also to Sultan Qaboos university, Oman for interactive sessions (Fig. 18.7).

18.5.5 Problems Associated with Implementation of the Project

The main problems that occurred throughout the entire project, which were mainly bus-related,

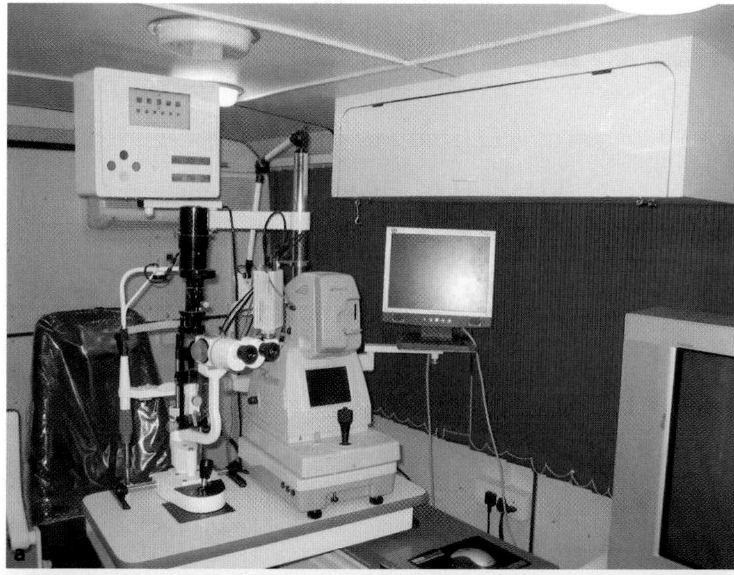

Fig. 18.3. a, b Ophthalmic equipment inside the teleophthalmology bus

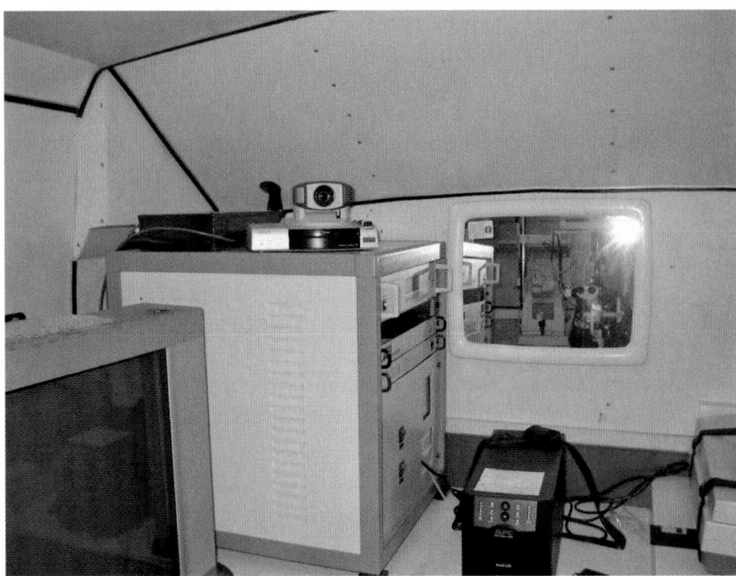

Fig. 18.4. Teleconferencing equipments inside the teleophtalmology bus

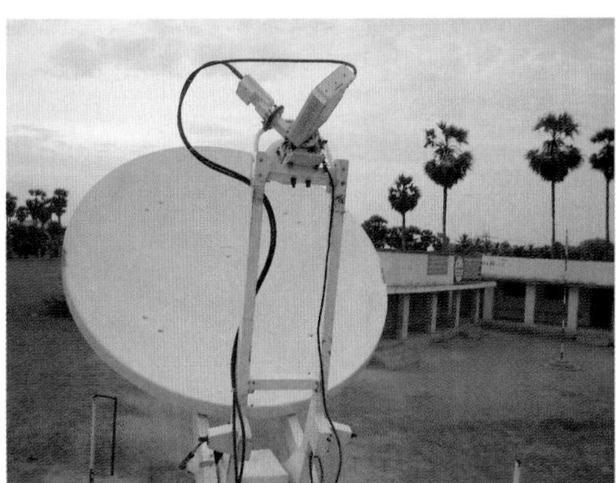

Fig. 18.5. VSAT facility on the top of the mobile bus

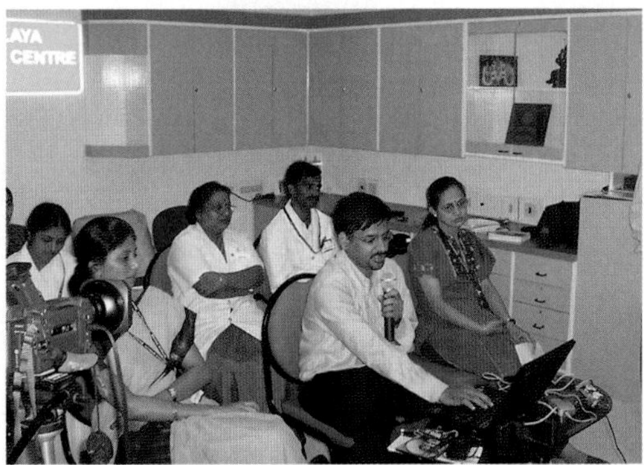

Fig. 18.7. Continuing ophthalmic tele-education between the Sankara Nethralaya team and a team from Tiruvallur general hospital

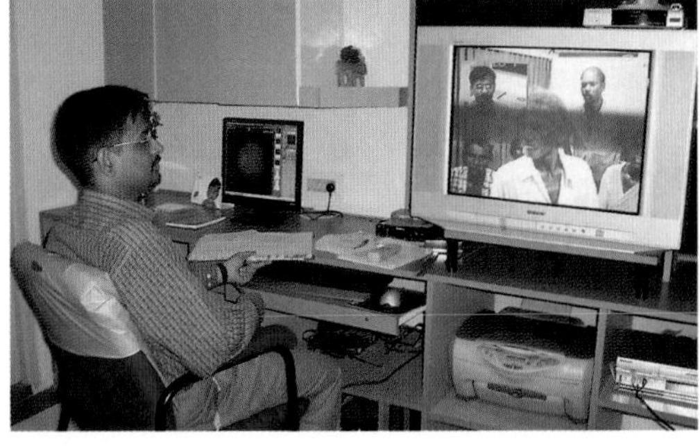

Fig. 18.6. Ophthalmologist during a teleconsultation

were recorded in a register. The control system for the satellite dish antenna malfunctioned due to vibration caused by the generator inside the bus, and the rough terrain of rural roads. There was a loss of continuity in the power supply to the antenna controller. The television used for video conferencing in the bus fell during travel, due to improper anchorage of the device. The rural areas in India usually do not have sealed roads and are very uneven. Proper stationing of the teleophthalmology bus was not possible in many camp sites. Hence, a hydraulic jack was used to provide support for the bus in rough terrains.

18.6 Results

By March 2005, the teleophthalmology bus project had conducted 213 camps in rural areas, and had screened 15,043 patients for eye related disorders. On the day prior to each of the 315 camps, the project also conducted an awareness meeting in the village about common eye diseases, such as cataracts, glaucoma, and diabetic retinopathy. Since corneal blindness is the second most important cause of preventable blindness in India, emphasis was also given to eye care and corneal donation. By interacting with local doctors and directing patients to their clinics for follow-up treatment, the local medical network was strengthened.

Sankara Netralaya teleophthalmology projects were instrumental in screening a large number of patients who were bereft of basic eye care facilities. The patients who were screened by teleophthalmology were segregated into those requiring further tests and opinions from ophthalmologists, and those who required spectacles. A total of 5,852 patients required further opinions from ophthalmologists. About 820 patients were provided with spectacles at cost price.

References

1. Sankara Nethralaya teleophthalmology project (2005) http://www.sankaranethralaya.org/tele_aim.htm. Cited 4 Oct 2005
2. Raman R, Kumari P, Agarwal S, Pradeep, Paul G, Sharma T (2005) Teleophthalmology for mass eye screening in a diabetic population. Poster presented at SERI-ARVO, Singapore 2004

Chapter 19

Teleophthalmology – The Brazilian Experience and Future Directions

19

Cristina Muccioli, Luci Meire P. Silva, Luciano Peixoto Finamor, Rubens Belfort Jr., Daniel Sigulem, Paulo Lopes, Ivan Torres Pisa

This chapter addresses the following

Key Concepts:

- Ophthalmologists are accustomed to diagnosing disease asynchronously from two-dimensional black-and-white and color imagery.
- For teleophthalmology, it is important that examination and diagnosis of the most common eye diseases seen in general practice do not require specialized equipment.
- Teleophthalmology is not yet a basic tool for diagnosis and therapy in Brazil.
- Video consultations using standard, low-cost equipment can be used to connect primary health care personnel and specialists, while providing a reliable method of fulfilling the needs of general practitioners, as well as their diagnostic accuracy.
- Certain practices of asynchronous teleophthalmology can achieve 73.5% accuracy in comparison with traditional consultation.
- Teleophthalmology may never replace traditional hands-on eye examination, but it is a new tool that has the potential of enhancing the practice and distribution of ophthalmology services.

19.1 Introduction

Ophthalmology is a medical speciality with visually intensive dependence, as are other specialties, such as radiology, dermatology, and pathology. Ophthalmologists are trained to interpret images and are accustomed to diagnosing disease asynchronously from two-dimensional black-and-white and color imagery. Therefore, ophthalmology is impacted by new technologies in health informatics, image analysis, and artificial intelligence. The importance of visual information in ophthalmology makes it obvious that telemedicine, supporting the transmission of live or still pictures, offers benefits for ophthalmological consultations.

19.1.1 Communication

Medicine is based on communication between patient and physician, and also between the physician and members of the health care team. Telemedicine maximizes the power of communication in health care.

Digital consultation (e-consultation) in ophthalmology has been able to achieve the following:

- Accurate diagnosis
- Low cost through the use of readily available equipment
- Extended effectiveness of the consultant
- Benefit to patients
- Educational objectives
- Initial acceptance by partner ophthalmologists and their patients
- A format for virtually unlimited expansion after the recruitment of additional partner sites and additional volunteer consultants

Store-and-forward teleophthalmology systems are well suited to sending photographs to specialists for review. Ophthalmologists also work synchronously with real-time systems, diagnosing and managing disease through hands-on patient examination. Teleophthalmology systems with modified traditional ophthalmic peripherals add unique challenges, extra requirements, and increased costs to telemedicine applications, but with numerous possibilities [1].

Most telemedicine being practiced is in the same place it was 10 years ago. It is a formidable tool with relatively few applications to date, but will be increasingly important in the future. Telemedicine is regarded as a way of delivering health care and exchanging health information across distances, however it has not yet become an accepted tool for diagnosis and current therapy in Brazil.

19.1.2 Teleophthalmology Today

Currently, teleophthalmology can be practiced, for example, between primary health care practitioners and specialists, or between ophthalmological units, either in real-time through video conferencing systems, or through store-and-forward processes such as e-mail. Choosing the synchronization model should always be motivated by the needs of the users, reflecting their processes' requirements. Telemedicine is especially suitable for diagnosing and treating eye diseases, since ophthalmologists are well-versed in making diagnoses, prescribing therapy, and designing treatment plans on the basis of visual information obtained from the eyes of patients.

One of the first applications in teleophthalmology was a project done in 1987 to monitor retinal vessels during space flights. A system was developed at the Johnson Space Center in Houston, Texas, in the United States, for real-time transmission of retinal images acquired by a portable video funduscope that was tested on the space shuttle Columbia during mission STS-50 [2, 3].

A survey of teleophthalmology projects in various stages of development reveals innovative applications in ophthalmology [1], including:

- Access to specialists for remote patients
- Linking and sharing diverse medical resources
- Ophthalmic disease screening, monitoring, and management (astigmatism, glaucoma, corneal diseases, and diabetic retinopathy)
- Research and clinical trial collaboration
- Distance learning and continuing education

19.2 Technical Issues

In teleophthalmology, it is important that examination and diagnosis of the most common eye diseases seen in general practice should not require specialized equipment. The diagnoses most often confused by general practitioners (GPs) are related to external eye diseases, for which diagnosis requires no specialized diagnostic equipment. Thus, teleophthlamological equipment requirements are relatively modest. In most cases, a digital video camera that allows for still photography is sufficient. In contrast, eye examinations leading to more complicated diagnoses such as iridocyclitis require specialized instruments and personnel who are trained to use them. These factors limit the applicability of sophisticated teleophthalmology to a certain extent.

Based on our own experience, video consultations using standard low cost equipment can be used in consultations between primary health care personnel and specialists. This type of consultation provides a reliable method of fulfilling the needs of general practitioners and can improve their diagnostic accuracy. However, clinical decisions in teleophthalmology are never 100% accurate, because teleconsultation in general cannot surpass face-to-face examination in terms of accuracy. All new telemedicine systems should be based on open standards where applicable. This is important because today's technology will be old tomorrow, and obsolete the day after.

For example, if a camera system is built around a proprietary camera, replacing the camera with a better one will be very expensive. However, if standard components are used, replacing them is usually less expensive. Using open and clearly defined interfaces between different components will also make upgrading and maintenance easier.

It is a common misconception to think that proprietary systems are safer because they are not publicly known. In practice, a highly secure system has to be based on publicly known and verified security concepts, rather than on what are often unsafe proprietary systems. The use of ordinary office equipment (digital cameras, desktop scanners, standard e-mail programs) should also be encouraged. These may not be reliable enough in critical applications, but the costs savings are very significant in non-emergency use. In addition, the technology used in office equipment is often more up-to-date than that used in proprietary equipment.

19.3 Fundus Imaging and Screening Studies

The importance of screening for diabetic retinopathy has been established, but the best method of doing so has not yet been determined [4]. Telescreening for diabetic retinopathy, using an assessment of two-field 50° non-stereo digital images is a valid screening method [5, 6]. However, detection of CSME by biomicroscopy is superior to detection by digital or standard non-stereo photographs [7]. Viewing digitally reconstructed photographic images of the retina on a video display has caused some doctors to lose confidence in their ability to make a diagnosis [8]. This loss of confidence has also been noted in other specialties, and serves as a safety factor in the process of teleconsultation. Although small pupil cameras can be used, dilating the pupils of patients has a positive effect on the quality of photographs in screenings.

Teleophthalmological consultations have also been performed in photo-refractive surgery [9], corneal transplants [10], glaucoma [11–13], strabismus [14–16], diabetes [17], macula and retinal diseases [17–19], diabetic retinopathy [20, 21], ocular trauma [22], and cytomegalovirus retinitis [23]. The possibility of making computer-assisted diagnoses by using computer vision algorithms may also provide interesting alternatives [24]. There are no published studies on teleophthalmology in Brazil.

19.4 Brazilian Experience

In 2002, the Virtual Diagnostic Center was developed in cooperation with the Ophthalmology Department and Health Informatics Department (DHID) of the Federal University of São Paulo, with the objective of creating a new way to offer ophthalmological evaluation for patients as well as for doctors with practices outside major centers of science and medicine (Fig. 19.1).

19.4.1 Background

After defining the project, the first actions were to develop the group involved in the project (doctors, nurses, and technical support team), to define what equipment to buy, and to determine how to develop the virtual diagnostic center.

An electronic file was created with the objective of receiving all the clinical history of the patients, as well as receive their clinical pictures. Clinical diagnosis and orientation for treatment could be obtained, as well as second opinions in ophthalmology.

19.4.2 The First Study

The first study focused on patients that presented clinical manifestations of Acquired Immunodeficiency Syndrome (AIDS). Teleophthalmology

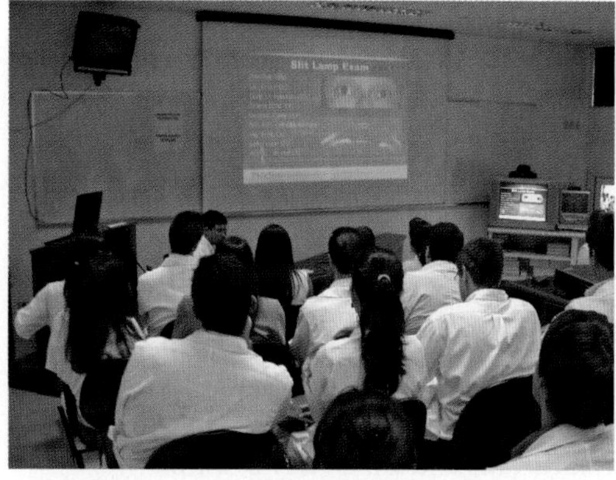

Fig. 19.1. Virtual diagnostic center: cooperation between the Ophthalmology Department and Health Informatics Department of Federal University of São Paulo

has not yet become an accepted tool for diagnosis and current therapy in Brazil. Our experience shows that certain practices of teleophthalmology can achieve 73.5% accuracy in comparison with traditional consultation [25].

This study evaluated the efficacy of teleophthalmology as an auxiliary approach in the diagnosis of infectious and inflammatory ocular diseases, in patients with AIDS and compared to patients with infectious and inflammatory ocular diseases without AIDS. Using an asynchronous method of consultation, this study also evaluated the main problems associated with the conclusion of the consultation, i.e. the inter-observer agreement, as well as standardization and validation of the method.

Two hundred and thirty three 35 mm slides (retinography or biomicroscopy photos) were digitalized and stored on compact disc, to be subsequently viewed and analyzed on a computer monitor by two consultants, both specialists in uveitis and ocular inflammation. The consultants answered a clinical file and a questionnaire, indicating the probable diagnosis and suggestion for treatment for all the analyzed cases. The main difficulties found in the conclusion of the consultation were also assessed by a specific questionnaire.

19.4.3 Results

The kappa statistic, a measure of change-corrected agreement (reproducibility) among the consultants, was calculated. Kappa values of > 0.7 indicate excellent agreement, values between 0.4 and 0.7 indicate fair to good agreement, and values of < 0.4 indicate poor agreement. We found that the agreement between the consultants and the definitive diagnosis was 73.5%. Treatment suggestion or management was not possible in 8% of cases for consultant A, and 10.4% of cases for consultant B.

When addressing the reasons that made diagnosis difficult, high concordance was found among the consultants in relation to a *lack of clinical data* and *low quality of the images*.

19

From this study the authors concluded that teleophthalmology, through asynchronous methods, is an efficient method for the diagnosis of patients with infectious and inflammatory ocular diseases, in patients with or without AIDS.

As observed in this study, the main problems affecting the teleophthalmology consultation were mostly about the lack of detailed clinical data and the low quality of the images. This study will allow the improvement of the consultant form and the establishment of a teleophthalmology service in the Ophthalmology Department of Federal University of São Paulo.

Cyber-ambulatory ophthalmology was created with the mission to offer high quality ophthalmology consultation to doctors in areas where there are few scientific resources and no specialists in ophthalmology.

19.5 Future Directions

The development of modern information and communication technology has occurred with extraordinary rapidity, and is still growing. Health care market information technology (IT) spending is expected to grow at 8% annually between 2003 and 2008, thus offering significant opportunities for hardware, software, and IT service vendors [26]. Telemedicine is part of this picture, involving the health care processes and services in every institution, regardless of size.

Telemedicine holds great potential, especially in rural areas, to greatly improve the quality, access, and affordability of health care. It can reduce the need for travel in rural areas, and provide needed backup and access to specialists for primary care health professionals in these underserved areas. In particular, teleophthalmology is in an experimental phase, and it is one of telemedicine's more challenging applications [1]. The eye's small size and the high degree of training and skills required to provide adequate eye care necessitates a steep learning curve for remote presenters learning to use video ophthalmic peripherals to capture high-quality images. The cost of converting ophthalmic peripherals to digital is also a barrier, particularly for health care units and services with precarious financial support.

Teleophthalmology may never replace the traditional hands-on eye examination. However, it is a new tool that can enhance the practice and distribution of ophthalmology services. Costs and technical barriers will decrease as the technology advances. When that happens, comprehensive teleophthalmology will become a reality, playing a critical role in the lives of health care workers, patients, students, and the public at large [27].

19.6 Health Care Workers

It is likely that in the future more medical interventions will take place at a distance. For some disciplines, such as radiology, this has already occurred to a substantial extent. But ophthalmologists have also become significant consumers of technology, including image peripherals, web systems, and mobile devices. Thus, they are health care professionals with good acceptance, and adaptable skills to include telemedicine applications in their consultation. During these consultations new kinds of information will be available, including three-dimensional eye representations and enhanced computer vision. Mobile devices are well accepted by ophthalmologists, allowing the development of multimodal systems that take into account the union of patient record information, image analysis, second opinion systems, medical decision support systems, telephone services, and internet navigation.

19.7 Patient Care

From the patient's perspective, it should always be possible to receive medical care, whenever and wherever it is requested. Without barriers in the health care system, patients of the future will not be dependent upon their own doctor; instead, they may use their health care agent's assistance to choose the most appropriate health service. In teleophthalmology, there is a lot of information about vision care and related diseases available to the public via the commercial and academic internet. Moreover, it is possible to communicate the vital signals automatically with monitoring centers; patients can then be contacted for further follow-up if necessary.

A simple example of such a monitoring program would be continuous monitoring of the blood sugar concentration of diabetic patients. Based on the results of such monitoring, ophthalmological care can be delivered. In fact, the global availability and better access to health care is likely to result in a complete restructuring of how medical care is delivered. With a shift away from health care being concentrated in health care institutions, toward monitoring and treating individuals in their own environments. This, however, raises questions about how telemedicine services should be funded. In rural areas, border regions and aboriginal communities, there are a lot of doubts about the impact of telemedicine, considering the actual funding model practiced, especially in third-world countries. Teleophthalmology seems to be a medical specialty that presents good results in these cases. However, teleophthalmology application and evaluation in these areas will become more and more a political and financial support decision rather than a technological impossibility.

19.8 Tele-Education

The improvements in information and communications technologies have been influencing education at all levels, and for all groups. The public at large, however, is sometimes forgotten, even though it is the group for whom information is likely to result in the greatest changes in health and how it is delivered. Currently, a substantial proportion of Internet access represents consumer searches for health and medical information.

With regard to health care professionals, tele-education has been radically changing how educational organizations are structured and how information is imparted within these organizations, with more interactive, multimedia-enabled, network-based educational sessions based upon problem-based teaching.

Finally, teleophthalmology will contribute toward the transfer of medical competence from specialists to general practitioners [28]. However, it is important to note that teleophthalmology is not a replacement for traditional eye care. This is because the quality of a telemedicine consultation is intrinsically linked to the remote presenter's expertise and their ability to use digital diagnostic tools. Without the use of every instrument normally available in an ophthalmologist's examination room to directly examine a patient, evaluation of a patient's visual systems is limited. All aspects of telemedicine applied to ophthalmology in its broadest sense (remote assistance, telecare, telehealth, teleconsultation, tele-education, etc.) are likely to be rapidly affected by future developments.

References

1. Li HK (1999) Telemedicine and ophthalmology. Surv Ophthalmol 44:61–71
2. Hunter N, Caputo M, Billica R (1993) Portable dynamic fundus instrument: uses in telemedicine and research. Seventh Annual Workshop on Space Operations Applications and Research (SOAR) 2:555–556
3. Caputo MP (1994) The Application of Digital Satellite Communications in Conducting Telemedicine. Dissertation, University of Houston, Houston, TX, pp 1–94
4. Williamson TH, Keating D (1998) Telemedicine and computers in diabetic retinopathy screening. Brit J Ophthalmol 82:5–6
5. Liesenfeld B, Kohner E, Piehlmeier W, Kluthe S, Aldington S, Porta M, Bek T, Obermaier M, Mayer H, Mann G, Holle R, Hepp KD (2000) A telemedical approach to the screening of diabetic retinopathy: digital fundus photography. Diabetes Care 23:345–348
6. Constable IJ, Yogesan K, Eikelboom R, Barry C, Cuypers M (2000) Fred Hollows lecture: digital screening for eye disease. Clin Exp Ophthalmol 28:129–132
7. Berger JW, Shin DS (1999) Computer-vision-enabled augmented reality fundus biomicroscopy. Ophthalmology 106:1935–1941
8. Briggs R, Bailey JE, Eddy C, Sun I (1998) A methodologic issue for ophthalmic telemedicine: image quality and its effect on diagnostic accuracy and confidence. J Am Optom Assoc 69:601–605
9. Maldonado MJ, Arnau V, Martinez-Costa R, Navea A, Mico FM, Cisneros AL, Menezo JL (1997) Reproducibility of digital image analysis for measuring corneal haze after myopic photorefractive keratectomy. Am J Ophthalmol 123:31–41
10. Shimmura S, Shinozaki N, Fukagawa K, Shimazaki J, Tsubota K (1998) Real time telemedicine in the clinical assessment of the ocular surface. Am J Ophthalmol 125:388–390
11. Beauregard D, Lewis J, Piccolo M, Bedell H (2000) Diagnosis of glaucoma using telemedicine – the effect of compression on the evaluation of optic nerve head cup-disc ratio. J Telemed Telecare 6:123–125
12. Yogesan K, Constable IJ, Barry CJ, Eikelboom RH, Morgan W, Tay-Kearney ML, Jistskaia L (1999) Evaluation of a portable fundus camera for use in the teleophthalmologic diagnosis of glaucoma. J Glaucoma 8:297–301
13. Tang R, Li H, Schiffman J (1997) Screening for open-angle glaucoma through telemedicine in a rural family practice setting. In: American Academy of Ophthalmology Annual Meeting Final Program, p 180
14. Jason C, Cheung M, Dick P, Stephen P, Kraft SP, Yamada J, McArthur C (2000) Strabismus examination by telemedicine. Ophthalmology 107:1999–2005
15. Cheung JC, Dick PT, Kraft SP, Yamada J, McArthur C (2000) Strabismus examination by telemedicine. Ophthalmology 107:1999–2005
16. Helveston EM, Orge FH, Naranjo R, Hernandez L (2001) Telemedicine: Strabismus e-consultation. J AAPOS 5:291–296
17. Teng T, Lefley M, Claremont D (2002) Progress towards automated diabetic ocular screening: a review of image analysis and intelligent systems for diabetic retinopathy. Med Biol Eng Comput 40:2–13
18. Gomez-Ulla, Fernandez MI, Gonzalez F, Rey P, Rodriguez M, Rodriguez-Cid MJ, Casanueva FF, Tome MA, Garcia-Tobio J, Gude F (2002) Digital retinal images and teleophthalmology for detecting and grading diabetic retinopathy. Diabetes Care 25:1384–1389
19. Yogesan K, Cuypers M, Barry CJ, Constable IJ, Jitskaia L (2000) Teleophthalmology screening for retinal and anterior segment diseases. J Telemed Telecare 6:96–98
20. Klein R, Klein BE, Neider MW, Hubbard LD, Meuer SM, Brothers RJ (1985) Diabetic retinopathy as detected using ophthalmoloscopy, a non-mydriatic camera and standard fundus camera. Ophthalmology 92:485–491
21. Garden G, Keating D, Williamson TH, Elliot AT (1996) Automatic detection of diabetic retinopathy using an artificial neural network: screening tool. Brit J Ophthalmol 80: 940–944
22. Simon DP, Thach AB, Bower KS (2003) Teleophthalmology in the evaluation of ocular trauma. Mil Med 168:205–211
23. Li HK, Temprano J, Horna J, Tang R (2000) Diagnosing cytomegalovirus retinitis through teleophthalmology. Internet J Ophthalmol Vis Sci 1(1) http://www.ispub.com/ostia/index.php?xmlPrinter=true&xmlFilePath=journals/ijovs/vol1n1/retinitis.xml. Cited 21 July 2003

24. Madjarov BD, Berger JW (2000) Automated, real time extraction of fundus images from slit-lamp fundus biomicroscope video image sequences. Brit J Ophthalmol 84:645–647
25. Finamor L, Muccioli C, Lopes P, Sigulem D (2005) Teleophthalmology as an auxiliary approach in the diagnosis of infectious and inflammatory ocular diseases. Rev Assoc Med Bras (in press)
26. Claps M (2004) Western Europe, Healthcare Sector, 2003–2008, IT Spending Forecast, p 46
27. Pedersen S (1999) Telemedicine in the future. In: Wootton R, Craig J (eds) Introduction to telemedicine. The Royal Society of Medicine Press, London, UK
28. Craig J (1999) Introduction. In: Wootton R, Craig J (eds) Introduction to Telemedicine. The Royal Society of Medicine Press, London, UK

Chapter 20

Teleophthalmology as a Service Delivery Model – An Experience from a Developing Country

20

R. Kim, R. D. Thulasiraj, K. M. Sasipriya, R. Vasantha Kumar

This chapter addresses the following

Key Concepts:

- Several teleophthalmic modes are available in India, including primary (patient interacting directly with doctor), secondary (ancillary eye care worker interacting with patient and doctor) and tertiary (specialists interacting to gain second opinions or additional information).
- Primary care through affordable Internet connectivity has led to the development of Internet kiosks, facilitating accessibility to information. Kiosk operators are trained to screen for preliminary general examinations, and to take good ocular pictures with webcams, which enable patients to access an eye care provider. A complete treatment is not provided through this approach, but adequate guidance is given regarding further treatment.
- Secondary care through vision centers provide care by trained ophthalmic assistants who can take more appropriate medical details (including pictures), and help patients interact directly with ophthalmic specialists at eye hospitals.
- Outreach screening, which uses a mobile van with appropriate infrastructure to achieve the same level of secondary care in remote areas, is best suited for retinopathy and glaucoma screening, diabetic and creating awareness about eye problems.
- Teleconsultation through both video conferencing and store-and-forward modes allows general ophthalmologists in remote settings to seek opinions from ophthalmic specialists for complicated conditions.

20.1 Introduction

For a country like India, with limited clinical expertise and resources catering to a select population, creating equity and accessibility for the entire population is a major challenge. In India, there are approximately 12,000 trained ophthalmologists, of which a handful are trained to provide super-specialty care (in ophthalmology). The limited number of eye specialists is further aggravated by the uneven distribution of personnel, which is skewed toward urban regions that cater to 10–15% of the population who require such services.

Another major hurdle that further exacerbates the problem is the increase in eye problems that lead to blindness, such as diabetic retinopathy and glaucoma. Clearly, there are not enough well-trained, mid-level ophthalmic personnel who could be entrusted with at least 40% of activities in an ophthalmic setting. Lack of personnel further reduces the productivity of the already scarce ophthalmic professionals.

Comprehensive and sustainable teleophthalmology services may become an alternate, viable approach. Ensuring that quality care crosses geographical borders, time zones, and personnel shortages, and opening doors to economical, widespread screening of diseases, and more accessible clinical service delivery systems. The potential inherent in teleophthalmology suggests that no region of the world is too remote or poor to receive high quality medical care [1].

20.2 Applications of Teleophthalmology in Different Sectors

We have broadly classified teleophthalmology into three levels of eye care, depending on who is accessing it: (1) primary, wherein the patient interacts directly with doctors, (2) secondary – when an eye health care worker is present who interacts with both the patient and the doctor, and (3) tertiary, wherein a doctor interacts with another expert doctor for second opinions.

20.2.1 Primary Care: Creating Access to Primary Eye Care for the Rural Population through Rural Internet Kiosks

Emphasis on primary health care is high on the State agenda, and International organizations such as the World Health Organization (WHO) are also striving to provide such care. The availability of affordable internet connectivity has lead health care organizations and businesses throughout India to invest in setting up internet kiosks that facilitate accessibility to information at the mouse click – be it health care, agriculture, market prices, or interaction with government offices, etc. These kiosks are built on a viable business model that nurtures entrepreneurial skills. Kiosk centers provide primary eye care through teleophthalmology, enabling patients to access an eye care provider in real-time, or through the store-and-forward mode of teleconsultation.

20.2.2 Consultation

Kiosk operators are trained to screen for preliminary or general examinations that identify common problems such as mature cataracts. Training is also provided so operators can take quality ocular pictures using a standard webcam. These pictures are sent to the ophthalmologist in the nearest Aravind Eye Hospital along with a description of the patient's problems, either through voice mail or as text (Fig. 20.1).

Consultations also happen in live mode, where patients interact with trained staff using webcams and voice chat. This happens at a very low bandwidth, using specialized data and video compressing software. The patient is charged a nominal amount by the kiosk operator for the internet usage. Patients are not provided complete treatment through this approach, due to the quality of the images received, but adequate guidance is given regarding further management. This way more patients access a medical doctor, rather than ignoring the problem or using native medicine, which often compounds the problem.

Kiosk centers are becoming an acceptable approach in rural areas as they help patients overcome vital barriers, such as inaccessibility, fear, loss of wages, and lack of support from people who accompany them. These kiosk centers also provide health education, creating awareness through the content developed and uploaded on the web by Aravind. Currently Aravind is working with more than 60 such kiosks that link with Aravind centers. In 2004 alone, 1,170 patients accessed rural kiosks seeking eye care services; of this group, 920 patients were asked to come to a base hospital for further treatment. As a result, sixty-five patients underwent cataract surgery at Aravind Eye Hospital who would not otherwise have done so if such a facility was available.

20.2.3 Business Model

These centers are promoted by n-Logue, a rural Internet service provider who identifies a local person who has the acumen to run this program. Setting up a kiosk requires less than 1,000 USD for connectivity, a desktop computer, and other accessories. These kiosks need to earn between 70 and 80 USD per month to break even, which in a village of about 1,000 people translates roughly to seven or eight cents per person per month. At this price, services are affordable to the rural populace [2].

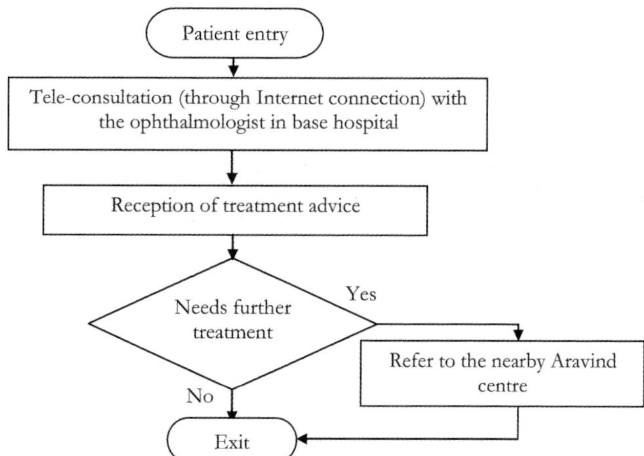

Fig. 20.1. Process at the Internet kiosk center

20.2.4 Secondary Care: Taking Eye Care to the Doorsteps of Rural Populations through Vision Centers

Setting up eye care services in vision centers with Internet connectivity at a low cost is increasingly becoming an option that will better reach the rural and remote population at the right time. This service is further aimed at changing the passive health seeking behavior of the rural population.

The objective of vision centers (Fig. 20.3) is to provide secondary care through well trained ophthalmic assistants. These centers are always connected to an Aravind center through low Internet bandwidth and webcam, which has last mile connectivity by wireless local loop, and provides access to quality eye care for the rural population. The bandwidth available through this technology is around 36.5 kb/s, and the compression software used enables video chat requiring just 14–19 kb/s of bandwidth. Patients interact directly with doctors at the hospitals over video chat, who then give appropriate consultations (Figs. 20a and 20b). Patients are only asked to go to the hospital when interventions such as surgery, or examinations for specialty eye problems are required.

This model is a cost-effective way of providing eye care services in rural areas. It also facilitates easier access to eye care services that otherwise would have required travel and loss of wages to the patient and accompanying persons.

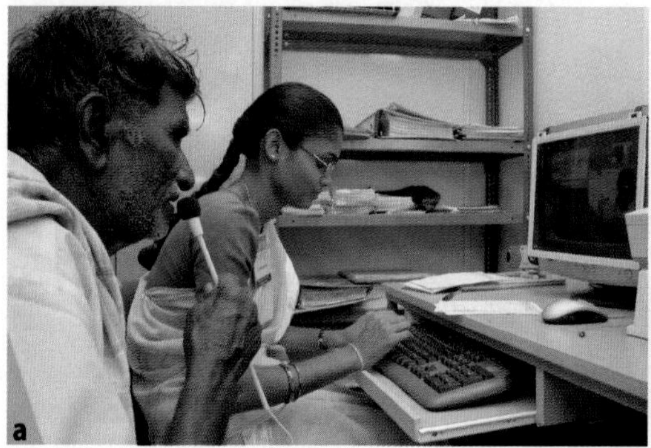

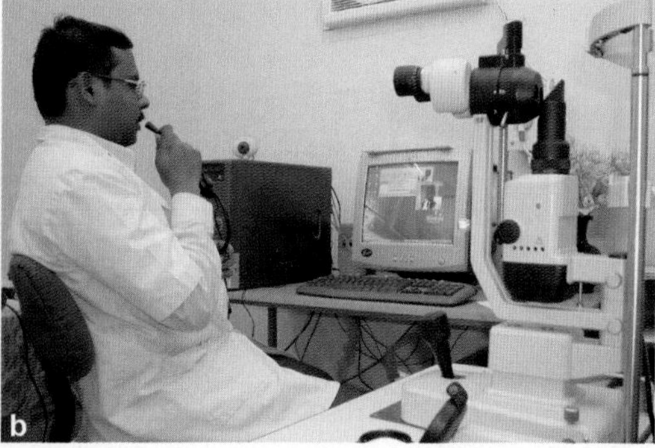

Fig. 20.2. **a** Patient from Vision center Ambasamuthiram village speaking to the **b** Medical Officer, Aravind Eye Hospital

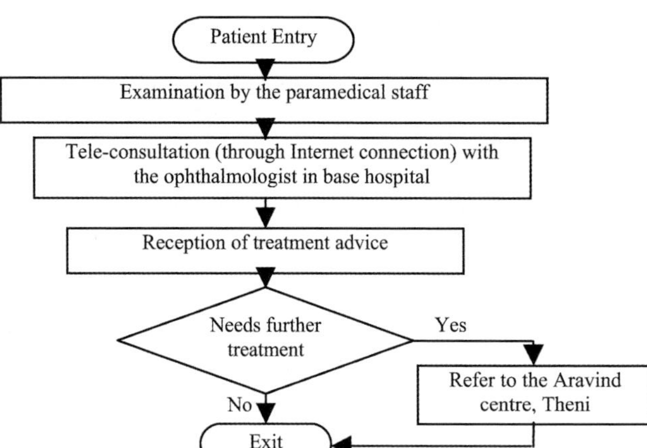

Fig. 20.3. Process at the Vision center

20.2.5 Advanced Screening on a Mobile Unit

Today teleophthalmology applications are not just confined to a specific location, they have become mobile through advances made in space technology. VSATs are increasingly used to connect to health care facilities from a remote location. The ISRO has taken proactive steps to provide free satellite connectivity to health care organizations whose only objective is to reach remote areas. Today remote areas in the northeast, Himalayas, and Island States like Andhaman Nicobar are connected to tertiary care centers through this satellite connectivity using VSAT.

20.2.6 Set-Up

Outreach screening using a mobile van (Figs. 20.4a and 20.4b) with adequate infrastructure (in terms of ophthalmic diagnostic equipment and VSAT connectivity) is best suited for screening and improving awareness of eye problems such as diabetic retinopathy and glaucoma. The mobile van at Aravind is equipped with a Topcon non-mydriatic fundus camera (NW100) and a Topcon SLD7 digital slit lamp. Provisions are made for teleconsultation by video conferencing as well. The mobile van is managed by an ophthalmic technician who handles patients, and a technician who handles VSAT operations.

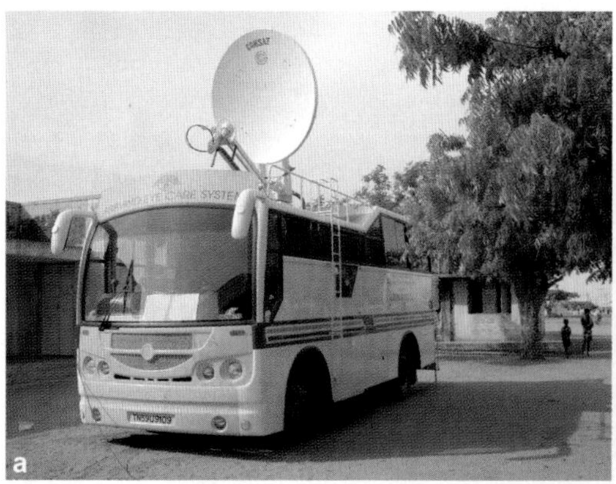

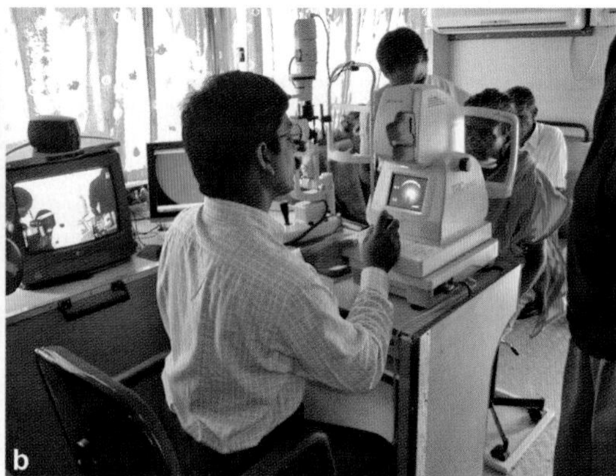

Fig. 20.4. **a** Mobile van for advanced screening **b** Trained ophthalmic technician taking a retinal image in the mobile van

The mobile van, which is currently used to screen for diabetic retinopathy, operates by going to collection points, such as a physician's office. The local diabetologists give appointments to their patients on a particular day when the mobile van is deployed to carry out screening for diabetic retinopathy. The ancillary eye care worker in the van takes digital fundus images using specialized software. These images are sent to the reading center located at the main Aravind Eye Hospital using VSAT connectivity. The size of each still image is around 6 MB and takes 6 full minutes to send to the reading center. Here the severity level is graded and management options are generated by trained graders using specialized software. A report is sent back to the mobile van containing the graded results and suggested treatment protocol within an hour. This report is printed for the patient, who is then counseled about the eye condition. If necessary, teleconsultation can be done through video conferencing, where the doctor can directly interact with the patient.

This system instills confidence both in the referring diabetologists as well as in the patients, who are given comprehensive tertiary care treatment. Between June to December 2004, 1,181 diabetic people were examined, and of these 237 (20.1%) had diabetic retinopathy. In this group, 105 (44.3%) were diagnosed for the first time. The mobile van has made screening for these diseases easier without the need for the specialist to travel.

20.3 Tertiary Care: Extending Tertiary Care to Remote Areas

Teleophthalmology allows a general ophthalmologist in a smaller setting to seek opinions from a specialist for a complicated condition. It also becomes a powerful learning tool to manage similar cases in the future.

The consultations can happen in two modes–live or store-and-forward. In our experience, we find the need to do live consultations is very low. As ophthalmic diagnoses are usually image-based, it is often enough to get the case history bundled with the relevant images and sent to the expert for an opinion.

20.3.1 Live Consultation

The hardware requirement for live consultation increases the cost of this mode. Basically, the equipment needed are:

- Ophthalmic: video slit lamp, fundus camera, and a video indirect ophthalmoscope
- Communications: video conferencing equipment, ISDN lines, and a computer

It is very important to have a minimum of 384 kb/s of bandwidth to view the ophthalmic images (moving) clearly in this mode. Here again, the consultants have the option of storing an image and viewing it and the resolution is not lost. The advantage of this mode is that the experts can directly interact with the patients and the referring doctors, to clarify any doubts instantaneously.

Disadvantages include (1) coordinating the appointment between the two sides, (2) expense, (3) time consumption, and (4) dependency on bandwidth availability, which may not be available in all locations.

20.3.2 Store and Foreward Consultations

The store-and-forward mode is more useful because it is easily accessible, does not depend on bandwidth, both parties can view, send in their own time and it is less expensive. Since in ophthalmology emergency situations rarely arise, this mode becomes more practical.

There are many Web-based programs available for store-and-forward teleconsultation. Aravind has developed and deployed software called *eyesTalk* that is Microsoft Dot-Net based, making it easier to use. Since the software resides locally in the respective servers, Internet connectivity is required only while sending or receiving the electronic case sheets.

Entering the data and images to the case sheet can be done off-line, unlike Web-based programs where data entry can only be done on-line. It is designed so that a referring doctor (called the *client*) can send data to a hospital (called the *provider*) after a licensing process is given by the provider. The doctor can send data directly

Table 20.1. Details about the requirements of different sectors

Sector	Human resource	Equipment		Software	Connectivity
		Ophthalmic	Non-ophthalmic		
Primary care	Referral end Internet kiosk operator Specialist end General ophthalmologist	Nil	Computer with multimedia and a webcam	OOPS Isee proprietary (compression software)	– Wireless local loop @ 36.5 kb/s – Dial-up Internet connection
Secondary care *Vision centers*	Referral end – Ophthalmic assistant Specialist end General ophthalmologist	– Stand alone slit lamp – anterior segment examination – Trial set to check for refractive errors – Streak retinoscope – Glucometer	– Computer with multimedia – Digital still camera (replacing web cam for better resolution)	OOPS Isee proprietary (software that compress the video file)	– Wireless local loop @ 36.5 kb/s – Dial-up Internet connection
Advanced screening on a mobile van	Referral end – Trained ophthalmic technician – Hardware technician to take care of connectivity Specialist end Specialist ophthalmologist	– Digital video slit lamp – Non-mydriatic camera	– Computer (laptop) and laser printer – Videoconferencing unit television monitor – 14 inches	Store and forward software (DRAGON) to capture retinal images and patient details (in-house development)	– VSAT (1.8 diameters antenna) – Bandwidth – 384 kb/s
Tertiary care	Referral end Ophthalmologist Specialist end – Specialist ophthalmologist – Hardware technician (optional) – Teleophthalmology program in charge	– Digital video slit lamp – Mydriatic camera – Video in-direct ophthalmoscope	Computer Videoconferencing unit Television – 14 inches	Store-and-forward software (eyesTalk) to capture images and patient details (in-house development)	– ISDN Lines (384 kb/s for video-conferencing) – Internet connectivity of minimum 56 kb/s for store-and-forward consultation

to any department (retina, uvea, etc.). Once the case sheet is received at the specialist's end, in the specific department required, an alert is given to the specialist for consultation. This almost acts as an electronic medical record, and has provisions to seek opinions or transfer the case sheet to other sub-specialties in the system. If required, an external opinion can also be obtained from other centers without having to deploy the software externally.

20.4 Setting up Teleophthalmology in Developing Countries

Today many health care organizations across the world are developing telemedicine systems that meet their needs. Much should be attributed to the rapid strides witnessed in the technology, both in health care and in information technology (IT). However a careful analysis for a sustainable solution is required while proceeding toward a structured teleconsultation process. Teleophthalmology may in fact have a more profound impact in developing countries than developed countries, if implemented appropriately.

20.4.1 Considerations

The following subsections address some issues that need to be considered when setting up a teleophthalmology unit.

20.4.1.1 Choosing the Technology

The availability of the communication network very often determines the technology used. In teleophthalmology, the diagnosis is dependent on the quality of the images, so it is very important to have enough bandwidth when in live mode. It is necessary to have a minimum of 384 kb/s of bandwidth to view a good quality video image. In store-and-forward mode it is enough to have reliable Internet access, which is now becoming readily available in all countries. The store-and-forward mode of teleconsultation is the best mode to seek consultations. It requires less bandwidth and hence a lower investment.

20.4.1.2 Imaging in Ophthalmology

With the advent of digital imaging systems, it has become easier and cheaper to acquire ocular images. Currently a range of imaging equipment, both low-end and high-end in terms of cost and quality, is readily available. The user can choose based on the available budget. Work is continuing to further reduce the cost of equipment, making it more accessible. It is important to know if the equipment complies with the standards set for image transmission such as Digital Imaging and Communications in Medicine (DICOM).

20.4.2 Protocols and Systems

Considering the paradigm shift occurring in the way eye care is provided, developing and implementing appropriate protocols is important to ensure effective utilization of this technology. This applies to any level of teleconsultation, be it primary care or tertiary care. We have developed structured protocols and systems for each level of care. This help to maintain and track the system. The protocols helps to define the responsibility of all involved, and the systems define the process. For example, in primary care it is helpful to have a structured questionnaire to capture relevant patient information.

20.4.2.1 Security

It is very important to safeguard the security of patient information, particularly as the information is sent over the Internet. At present, there are no appropriate laws in developing countries such as India to facilitate this process. Regardless, it is possible to comply by following equivalent laws, such as those delineated in the Health Insurance Policy and Accountability Act (HIPAA) in the United States.

20.4.2.2 Sustainability

The idea to seek consultations through teleophthalmology is relatively new. A considerable investment has been made to provide teleconsultations in terms of equipment, manpower, and other resources. At present, we are still developing this concept as an acceptable mode. But like any other service, teleophthalmology services should eventually become sustainable for both the clients who seek services and for the service providers who offer such services. It will be necessary to develop appropriate payment protocols.

20.5 Conclusion

In view of a developing country's immense need to deliver quality eye care service, teleophthalmology clearly emerges as an alternate service delivery model, that will ensure accessibility to quality eye care for rural and remote populations. To ensure the successful adaptation of this technology, sustainable and affordable models should be developed. The immediate challenges of costs, security and protocols should be addressed by policy makers to ensure effective adaptability of the technology.

References

1. Li HK (1999) Telemedicine and Ophthalmology. Surv Ophthalmol 44(1):61
2. Ashok J, et al. (2004) The story of a Rural Service Provider in India. Commun Info Res Net 1:1:32–40

Chapter 21

An Overview of Telemedicine Technology in the Russian Countries

21

Nikica Gabrić, Petar Raštegorac

This chapter addresses the following

Key Concepts:

- Russian telemedicine has been shaped by the space program, and is largely driven by problems with access to medical expertise in rural areas.
- The Russian Republic and all of the former Soviet states have weak telecommunications infrastructures, and do not have the capital resources to improve this situation, although several new networks are under development.
- Development of telecommunications infrastructure is crucial for the advancement of telemedicine.
- The two major factors determining growth over the next few years are whether the federal government truly decides to commit to health care as a national priority, and whether the telecommunications infrastructure is developed enough so that it can adequately support reliable, timely transfer of large amounts of medical data.

21.1 Background Information

Telemedicine began in the 1960s when the National Aeronautics and Space Administration (NASA) studied the physiological changes of astronauts during their space journeys. NASA scientists demonstrated successfully that physicians on earth could monitor physiological functions, such as blood pressure, heart rate, and body temperature of astronauts in space. Other early experiments also demonstrated that it was possible to undertake remote diagnosis through transmission of medical data [1].

21.2 Existing Teleophthalmology Technology and Digital Imaging in Russian Countries

There are some interesting similarities between Russian and United States (US) telemedicine. Both have grown up with and been shaped by the space program, and both are to a great extent driven by serious problems about access for medical consumers to medical expertise in rural areas.

The technology developed for transmitting medical information from space stations and spaceships to earth was used extensively after the Armenian earthquake of 1988, and after the Ufa gas pipeline explosion in 1989, in which many people were injured. Currently the Russian Center for Space Biomedicine (which is in fact a telemedicine center), Moscow State University, and the Institute of Medical Biological Investigation are collaborating with NASA through an agreement by the Gore–Chernomyrdin Commission. Among other things, this collaboration includes the creation of several Silicon Graphics workstations for medically related video sessions between hospitals in Russia and the US.

21.2.2 Infrastructure

The Russian Republic and all of the former Soviet states have weak telecommunications infrastructures, and do not have the capital resources to improve this situation. In 1992, an American financier donated 100 million USD to support science in the countries of the former Soviet Union. One of the outcomes of this has been the development of a university-based Internet project, charged with creating a new generation of Internet users. The first University Center opened in June 1996 in Yaroslavl, the second will open soon in Novosibirsk. In all, 32 regional universities will be linked.

21.2.3 South Moscow Supportive Network

The South Moscow Supportive Network (SMSN) is also being upgraded to fiberoptics, and will support 100 Mb/s transmission. The SMSN is essentially a Wide Area Network (WAN) that provides Internet access and computer networking for leading medical, scientific, and educational institutions in Moscow and St. Petersburg.

The SMSN is currently a hybrid network consisting of four data channels. Two of these operate via satellite, which allows very high throughput but suffers problems with dependability and delay in signal passage; the other channels are land based.

Access to the SMSN trunk is via regular phone lines or via ISDN lines for higher-end users. Another network under development is the Russian University Network, financed by the Ministry of Science, that will presumably link with and extend the SMSN [2].

21.3 Low- and High-End Applications

The Russian telemedical community feels strongly that development of telecommunications infrastructure is crucial for the advancement of telemedicine. Not only does it support *low-end* telemedicine applications such a Web-based medical education, still image archiving, and distribution for modalities (such as telepathology, and transmission of medical records), it also (1) raises professional and public awareness of the potential contribution of telecommunications to patient care, and (2) opens the gates to perceiving the potential of *high-end* applications such as interactive teleconsultations. Many Russian telemedicine applications are now POTS-based, but even that is hampered by the fact that the quality of many of these lines is poor, and cannot reliably support high speed, unbroken modem data links.

21.4 Satellite-Mediated Applications

Satellite-mediated applications that have been piloted in Russia include international case conferences via the International Telebridge. These have typically run at 128 Kb/s, and have linked the Department of Medical Science at Moscow State University to Baylor College of Medicine (Houston, TX) in the US, and to the University Hospital of TromsŻ in Norway. Other links have been to telemedicine centers in Moscow, Novosibirsk, and Ekaterinburg.

21.4.1 Challenges

While screen resolution for these conferences was high, the low bandwidth made for poor motion handling, and satellite transmission delays of up to 3 seconds made true interactivity a challenge. The screen resolution of transmitted radiographs and pathology slides appears to be adequate, at least for teaching purposes.

Elsewhere throughout the countries of the former Soviet Union, telecommunications and telemedicine infrastructure is being supported by the American International Health Alliance, which has the mission of improving ties between medical systems in the US and in the newly independent states. For example, in the past year there have been eight teleconferences between the Boston University School of Medicine in the US, and hospitals in Yerevan, Armenia, using Winrad technology and VTEL (VideoTelecom) equipment.

21.4.2 Local and International Links

A regular link that has been established between Arkangelsk Medical Academy in northwestern

Russia and Tromsö Regional Hospital in northern Norway, uses regular phone lines and modems, as well as periodic higher-bandwidth digital links. This has been used both for patient care and for teaching. Telemedicine in this extremely northern part of Russia is seen as a high priority, because of the high costs of transporting patients for specialty care, especially in winter.

On a more local level, the Moscow office of Paragraph International is developing a new kind of cardiac monitor which enables electrocardiogram transmission over regular phone lines directly from patient homes, using palmtop computers.

21.5 Significance of Telemedicine

An indicator of the perceived importance of telemedicine in Russia is the development of a new curriculum and specialization in telemedicine at the Arkangelsk Medical Academy.

Russian telemedicine is at an important crossroads. The need is clear, and professional enthusiasm is high. There are two major factors determining growth over the next few years: first, whether the federal government truly decides to commit to health care as a national priority; and second, whether the telecommunications infrastructure is developed to the point where it can adequately support reliable, timely transfer of large amounts of medical data.

References

1. Perednia DA, Allen A (1995) Telemedicine technology and clinical applications. JAMA 273(6):483–488
2. Grigsby J, Barton PL, Kaehny MM, Schlenker RE, Shaughnessy PW (1994) Telemedicine policy: quality assurance, utilization review, and coverage. Center for Health Policy Research, Denver, CO

Chapter 22

Teleophthalmology in Lithuania

22

Alvydas Paunksnis, Valerijus Barzdžiukas, Skaidra Kurapkienė

This chapter addresses the following

Key Concepts:

- A telemedicine center was established at Kaunas University of Medicine in 2002, to initiate and guide telemedicine developments in the university and across the country.
- Infrastructure is oriented toward teleconsultations and second opinions for clinical practice, distance education of medical staff and the general population, creation of international medical databases, and research.
- An Internet web site and Internet-based distance education course have been created to facilitate training of medical students and general practitioners.
- The telemedicine center took part in a massive casualty training exercise, responding in conjunction with civil and multinational military medical personnel to a simulated train crash.
- Diagnostic information systems and decision strategies are being developed for clinical decision support.

22.1 Introduction

Modern technologies are widely used for the early diagnosis and prevention of disease. The resolution of the minister-level conference and exhibition held in Brussels, European Union (22–23 May 2003) urges the consolidation of all information technology (IT) of experts and professionals, to assure the availability of the highest quality telemedicine health care to all European Union (EU) residents [1].

Information technologies give an opportunity for early diagnosis, treatment, and permanent patient follow-up (home care). The mission of the information society is to serve the people, to make life easier and, of course, the highest priority is meeting peoples' vital needs. Human health is not only a vital need, it affects national wealth as well [2].

22.1.1 Teleophthalmology as Priority

Teleophthalmology takes priority in this field: ophthalmological diagnosis is usually based on evaluation of anterior eye segment and fundus images. Digital fundus image processing is very helpful for the early diagnosis of diabetic retinopathy, hypertensive retinopathy, atherosclerosis, and in laser ocular surgery.

The main ophthalmic services in Lithuania are predominantly concentrated in the two biggest cities: Vilnius and Kaunas in particular, where the Hospital of Kaunas University of Medicine and the Kaunas University of Technology are located. These institutions carry most of the human and technical resources and provide the widest and most sophisticated services in Lithuania. In rural areas eye care is limited to the basic diagnostic and therapeutic levels due to a lack of appropriate equipment and experience of local personnel.

22.1.2 Challenges

The increase in mean life duration increases the number of visually impaired and blind people. Patients, predominantly the elderly, are sometimes forced to travel long distances to centers of ophthalmology, due to minor problems with their eyes.

In addition, the costs of medical services increase rapidly, diagnostic possibilities lag behind West Europe, and Lithuanian medical reform has just begun.

22.1.3 Collaborative Effort

Teleophthalmology in Lithuania started through a collaboration between Kaunas University of Medicine and St. Erik Eye Hospital in Stockholm (Sweden) in 1997. A video conference between the Eye Clinic of Kaunas University of Medicine and the International Telemedicine Conference in Visby, Sweden, was held in 1998. The first Lithuanian–Swedish telemedicine project, Litmed 1, connecting the medical societies of Sweden and Lithuania, was founded in 2000 after these presentations.

The Litmed 1 project started in three cities: Kaunas, Lund and Stockholm, and which included two medical specialities: ophthalmology and otorhynolaryngology. The participants involved in this project were: St. Erik Eye Hospital (Stockholm, Sweden), Lund University Hospital (Lund, Sweden), Tieto Enator AB (Sweden), Euromed Networks AB (Stockholm, Sweden), Kaunas Medical University Hospital (Lithuania) (Fig. 22.1), and Kaunas University of Technology (Lithuania) [3, 4].

The infrastructure for common Swedish–Lithuanian networking has been established under the framework of this project.

22.2 Telemedicine Center

Telemedical infrastructure has been utilized for the creation of high quality medical image databases, and the development of clinical routines, teleconsultations, second opinions, distant education and clinical decision support (Fig. 22.3). As a result of our telemedicine activities, a Telemedicine Center of Kaunas University of Medicine (Fig. 22.1) was established (tmc.kmu.lt) in 2002 [4, 5].

22.2.1 Goals

The aim of the telemedicine center are to initiate, guide and introduce the politics of telemedicine development in the University and across the country, and to prepare relevant recommendations for health care institutions and government institutions.

These include the following:

- To provide methodical leadership for the application of telemedicine technologies for medical diagnostics, consultation, monitoring, and scientific investigations in all stages of the undergraduate and postgraduate studies, and to coordinate them
- To search for programs and sources of finance that stimulate the development of telemedicine
- To organize sessions and conferences on telemedicine
- To organize and participate in national and international telemedicine and e-health projects

22.2.2 Patient-Oriented IT Solutions

Analysis of the problem showed the novelty of these ideas in a world-wide context. All available teleophthalmological experience was generalized in the NetLit project and realized by the Telemedicine Center of Kaunas University of Medicine and Kaunas University of Technology.

22.3 Infrastructure

The organizational and technical infrastructure for e-health in Lithuania, and for networking with foreign countries, was prepared in the Kaunas Medical University Hospital. Initial connections were made using ISDN between Kaunas Medical University Hospital, St. Erik Eye

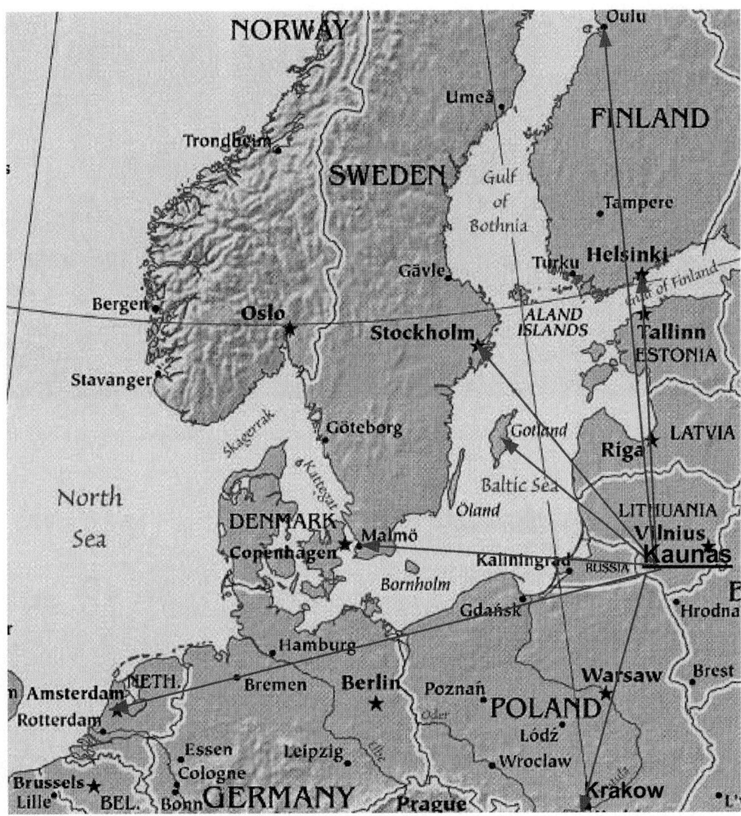

Fig. 22.1. Location of Telemedicine Center of Kaunas University of Medicine

Hospital, Lund University Hospital, and Uppsala University in Sweden.

The infrastructure created was oriented toward:

- Teleconsultations and second opinion for clinical practice
- Distant education of medical staff and the general population in Lithuania, using the existing distance education facilities of the telemedicine center
- Research and creation of international medical databases, and information exchange on both medical and technological fronts

The Telemedicine Center of Kaunas University of Medicine has rooms available for small (~10 people) and big (~140 people) video conferences (Fig. 22.2)

The teleophthalmology service infrastructure (Fig. 22.3) consists of the following items:

- Computer net (one server, six computers)
- Telemedicine workstation Eurotel I with Zydacron video conferencing board: codec Z360 and ISDN communications Z280, two Sony EVI-D3 robot video cameras, framegrabber, video switcher
- Slit lamp Topcon SL8Z with Sony 3 Charge Coupled Device (CCD) camera attached
- Digital fundus camera Canon C60UVi (6.3 megapixels)
- Ultrasound diagnostic equipment (Mentor Advent AB system)
- Video connection by three ISDN lines (384 kb/s) or IP

The infrastructure includes software for:

- Video conferencing – Zydacron OnWan
- Image and database management – Olympus Migra (Euromed AB, Sweden). Migra is a software client with high-resolution picture grabbing, live picture/voice (30 frames/s),

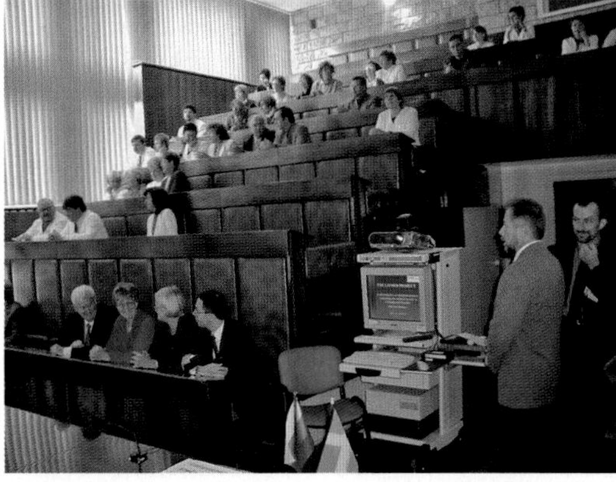

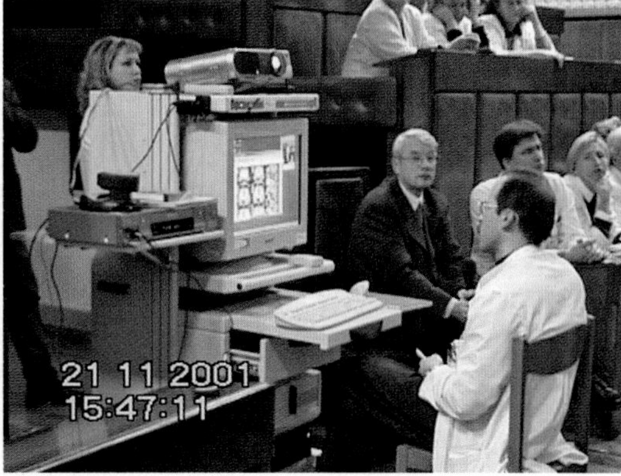

Fig. 22.2. A Swedish–Lithuanian telemeeting and a distant multispeciality consultation from the Kaunas Eye Clinic

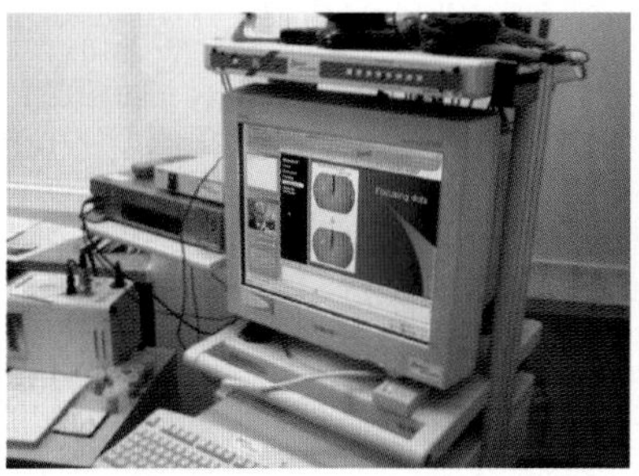

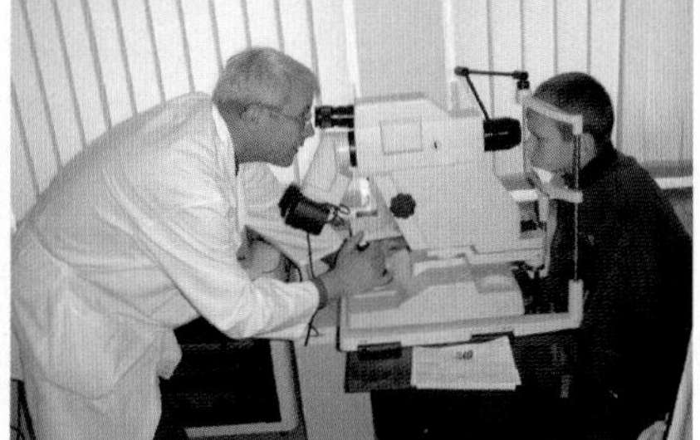

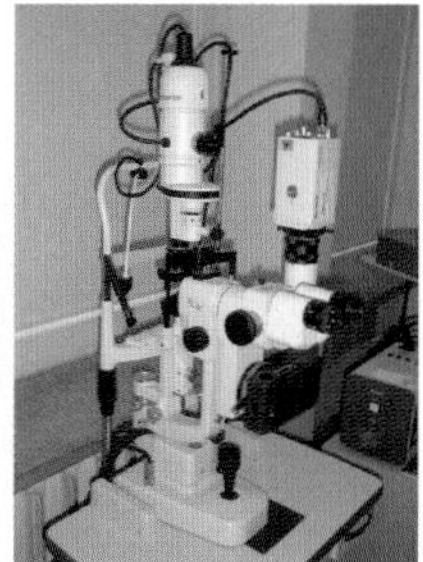

Fig. 22.3. The system for teleophthalmology service

e-mail with compression functions, microscope measurement *White Board* (live pointing and writing in the same picture) and database storage (Open DataBase Connectivity). Transmission of pictures during a video conference session is possible (dynamic bandwidth)

- Image management, processing and video conferencing – MediPas. Medipas is MS Windows Multiple Document Interface based software for image management and on-line telemedicine applications. It contains a module for image acquisition including a standard interface and Matrox Meteor framegrabber. Images can be opened from multiple picture formats or grabbed from analog and digital sources into a temporal high speed buffer, into a workspace or directly into a database. The database module is for storage of images and related text information. There are two database management systems supported: local database (MS Access based) and a central database (MS SQL server). The data entry forms and user interface are easily customizable by users. The high performance hardware videocodec Zydacron 360 is integrated in Medipas to achieve the best video and audio quality in on-line telemedicine applications. When video conferencing hardware is not available, the integrated software based video codec can be used. The video conferencing session allows sending and receiving of images, synchronization of desktops, drawing on the image and adding the drawings into the database [8, 9]

This system is connected with the databases via LAN, ISDN and IP for international networking (Fig. 22.4).

The technical possibilities for storing, processing, and accessibility (data exchange) of ophthalmological information, and for the creation of multi-objective analyses based on clinical decision support strategies have been established.

22.4 Distance Education

Distance education in ophthalmology started with live lectures between St. Erik Eye Hospital in Stockholm and Kaunas Medical University Hospital in Lithuania in 2002. This experience allowed us to develop new distance educational programs in ophthalmology.

As a first step, the web site titled *Digital Ophthalmology – Information System for General Practitioners* (Fig. 22.5) in English and Lithuanian, sponsored by the Open Society Fund Lithuania (bmii-www.tef.ktu.lt:8081/unrs/akys), was created. The web site has been created in order to promote and facilitate consulting and training of medical students and general practitioners. The web site contains a diagnostics-focused database built on differential diagnostic tables with comprehensive visual information (biomicroscopic and ophthalmoscopic images). All visual materials are original and are stored in the telemedicine center of Kaunas University of Medicine and the Institute of Biomedical Engineering of Kaunas University of Technology. The internet application for this site is based on Java Servlet technology, using the Velocity template engine and Tomcat Servlet container [10, 11].

An internet-based distant education course for general practitioners, including a dictionary and films on *Eye Diseases for General Practitioners* (72 h) was prepared in Lithuanian in 2004 (Fig. 22.6). It consists of the following topics:

- Acute painless visual loss (18 h)
- Red eye (18 h)
- Eye and systemic diseases (18 h)
- Eye trauma (180 h)

The program has been approved by the Lithuanian Ministry of Health as a continuing medical education (CME) program.

Each course, which is held two times per year, is available for 15–20 general practitioners; and

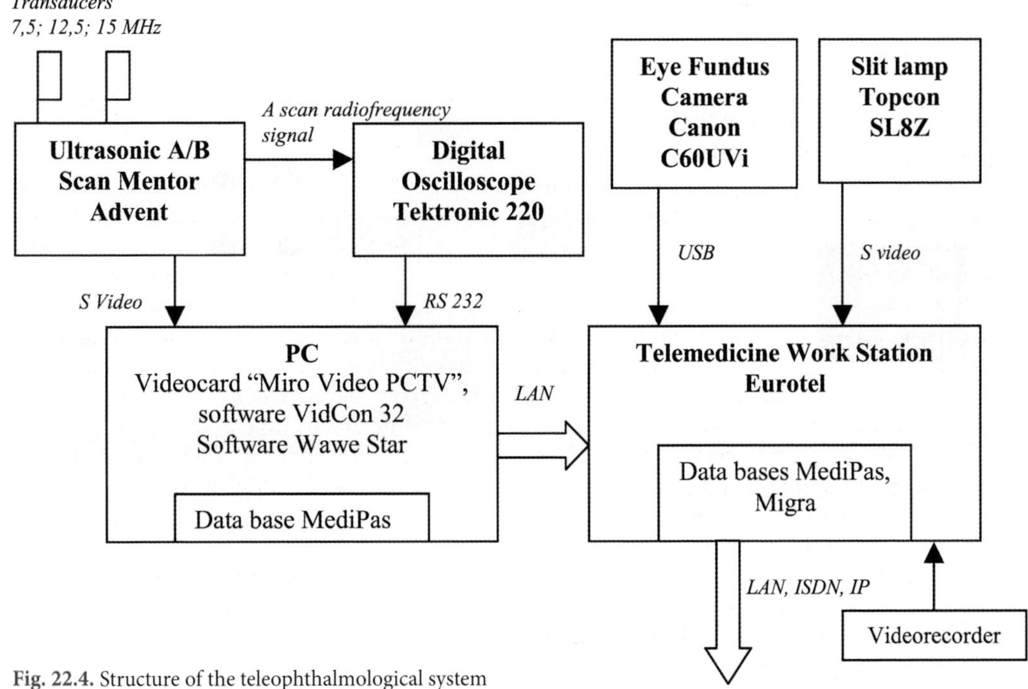

Fig. 22.4. Structure of the teleophthalmological system

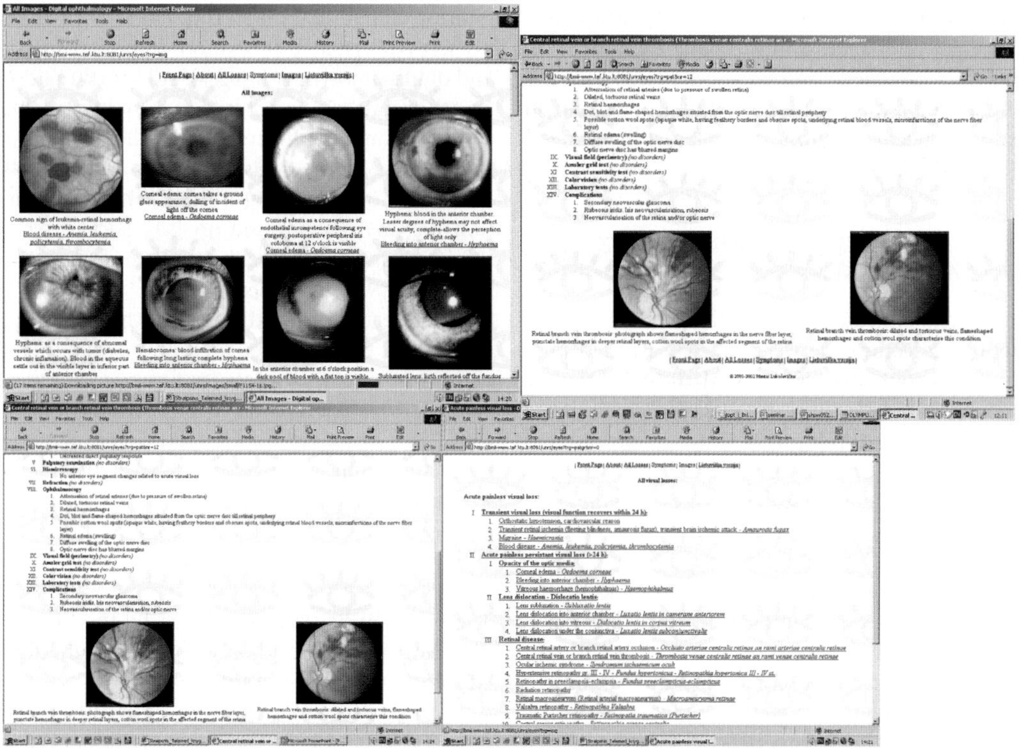

Fig. 22.5. Windows of the web site *Digital Ophthalmology*

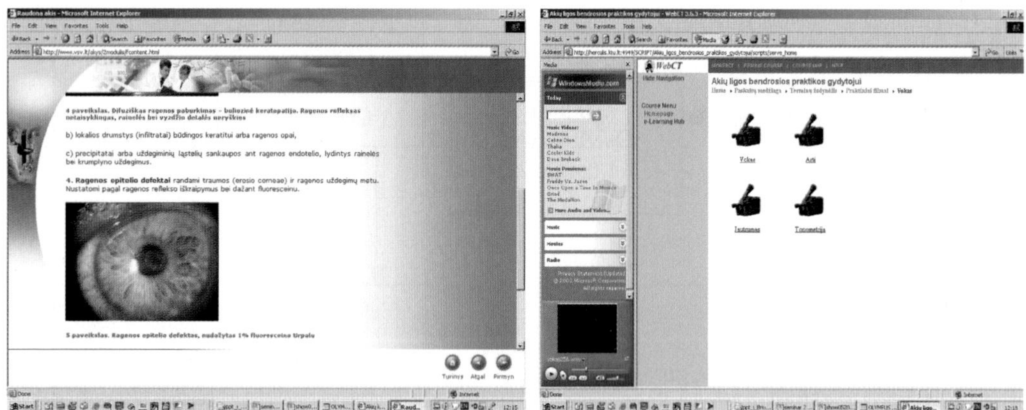

Fig. 22.6. Internet-based distant education courses for general practitioners

about 20 cities are connected (multipoint) to this source.

22.5 Teleconsultation and Second Opinions

International consultations started in 2002. The main ophthalmological pathologies include eye trauma, ophthalmic oncology, ophthalmic pathology, pediatric ophthalmology and rare diseases.

The use of existing infrastructure in the telemedicine center allows live (on-line) and delayed (off-line) international distance ophthalmological consultations. Live consultations, are more expensive and used for urgent situations only. Use three ISDN lines (384 kb/s), with direct transmission of images from a slit lamp Topcon SL8Z to the consulting site.Off-line consultations are more frequent, using anterior segment or eye fundus images transmission via the Internet.

22.5.1 Possibilities re Telemedicine Use in Massive Casualties Situations

The facilities at the telemedicine center of Kaunas University of Medicine (tmc.kmu.lt) allow for live (on-line) distant consultations from high-level medical specialists to rural areas. In order to expand the use of distant consultation facilities, telemedicine can be applied to mass casualty events, decreasing the geographical isolation of a casualty location.

22.5.1.1 RESCUER/MEDCEUR Project

On 23–28 July 2004, the Telemedicine Center took part in a RESCUER/MEDCEUR project exercise. RESCUER/MEDCEUR 2004 is a United States Army and Europe-led exercised called *In the Spirit of Partnership for Peace*; it was designed to train US, NATO, and Partner nations, to respond to a disaster relief/mass casualty situation. Three hundred and twenty soldiers from 12 countries, namely Lithuania, Armenia, Azerbaijan, Bulgaria, Estonia, Georgia, United States of America, Croatia, Latvia, Moldova, Romania, and Ukraine, took part in the RESCUER/MEDCEUR 2004 exercises, alongside six observers from the Netherlands, Poland, Luxemburg, and Germany.

The telemedicine center used appropriate telecommunication devices (Satellite, ISDN, IP) to help coordinate the joint activities of civil and multinational military services in critical situations, such as mass casualty events. ISDN lines and IP radio connections (Fig. 22.7) were used.

22.5.1.2 Simulated Emergencies

On 28 July, the final and most intensive day of the anti-terrorism drills, the multinational force of medics at the Kairiu Training Range in Lithuania reacted to a large mass casualty event – treating hundreds of victims from a simulated train crash. The Telemedicine Center arranged live, direct, high-level medical multispecialist teleconsultations between Kaunas Medical University Hospital and the crash location. The most complicated initiated cases of eye trauma, neurosurgical trauma, maxilloface trauma and traumatic amputation of limbs were evaluated and selected by Kaunas Medical University Hospital specialists at the event location using telemedicine facilities. All those cases were then transported to Kaunas and Vilnius Universities' Hospitals by helicopter (200 and 300 km from the event location) [12].

The use of existing telemedicine infrastructure highlights the military medical personnels' capability to provide medical services for casualties, as well as their ability to cooperate with civil institutions during rescue operations. These results show that the existing telemedicine infrastructure needs further development into an International Integrated e-Health Network for very fast international exchange of medical information, remote consultations of specialists from the world's best civil and military medical centers in emergent, large mass-casualty events and distant education.

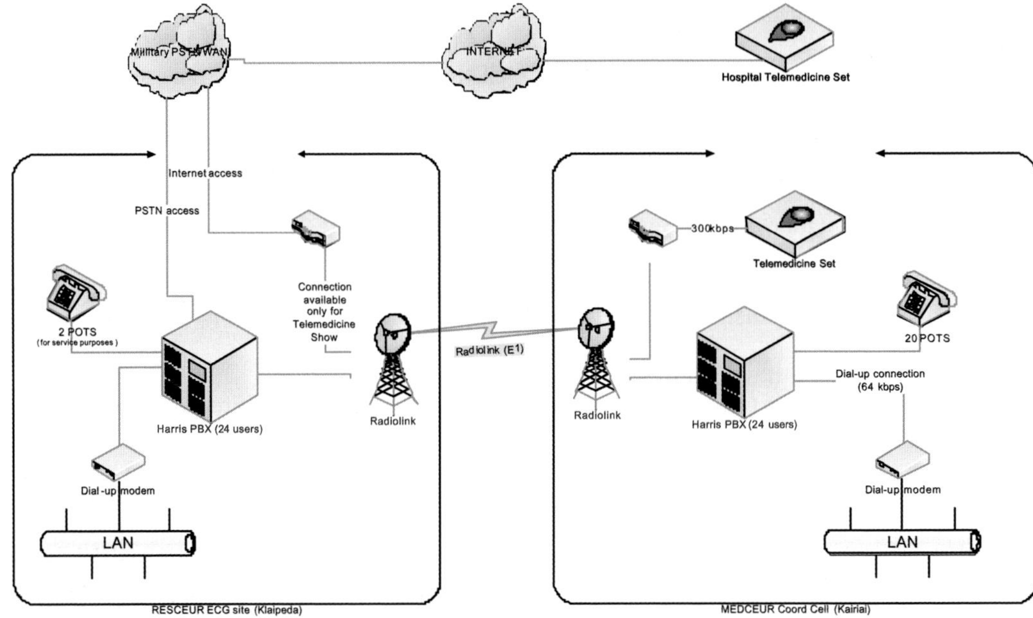

Fig. 22.7. Radio link connectivity

22.6 Clinical Decision Support

The program titled, *Information Technologies for Human Health: Clinical Decision Support* (IT Health), which is supported by the Lithuanian State Science and Studies Foundation, started in 2003. Participants included the Kaunas University of Medicine, Kaunas University of Technology, and the Vilnius Mathematics and Informatics Institute. The proposed project aims are to combine the efforts of experts and researchers from both areas to improve health care quality, by focusing attention directly on the needs of the patient and the physician in supporting them for individual patient diagnostic decisions.

The objectives and tasks of the project are oriented into two interrelated clusters:

1. Development of clinical decision support strategies, based on multi-objective analysis methods using pilot databases of medical images and signals, and telemedicine networks.
2. Development and evaluation of information systems for making preventive clinical decisions to decrease the risks of disability-causing diseases

One of the most important tasks is to evaluate the qualitative and quantitative informative parameters for clinical decision support, using analog and digital analysis of nonlinear complex systems, parameterization of ophthalmological findings and images [13, 14].

Pilot databases of medical images and signals, and telemedicine networks serve this purpose (Fig. 22.8).

Development of IT technologies makes the processing and systematization of large amounts of different information, and assessment of the subsequent data, possible.

The storing of ophthalmological images in databases with integration to international telemedicine networks has been undertaken. The data is used for parameterization (classification) and training of the decision support algorithms. Initially, ophthalmological image classification by digital parameters and expert assessment methods are developed.

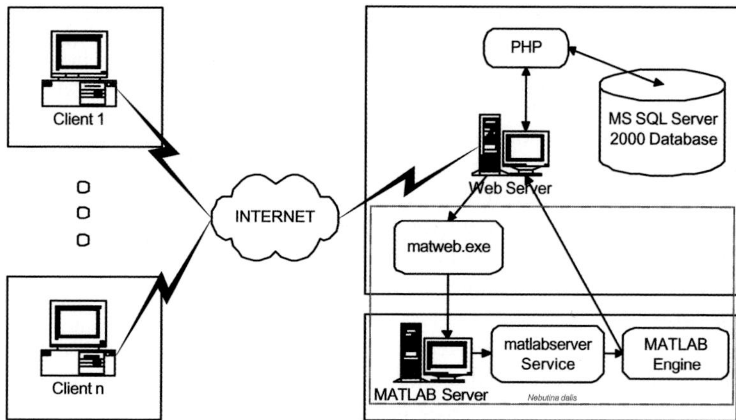

Fig. 22.8. Structure of distant automated medical data analysis

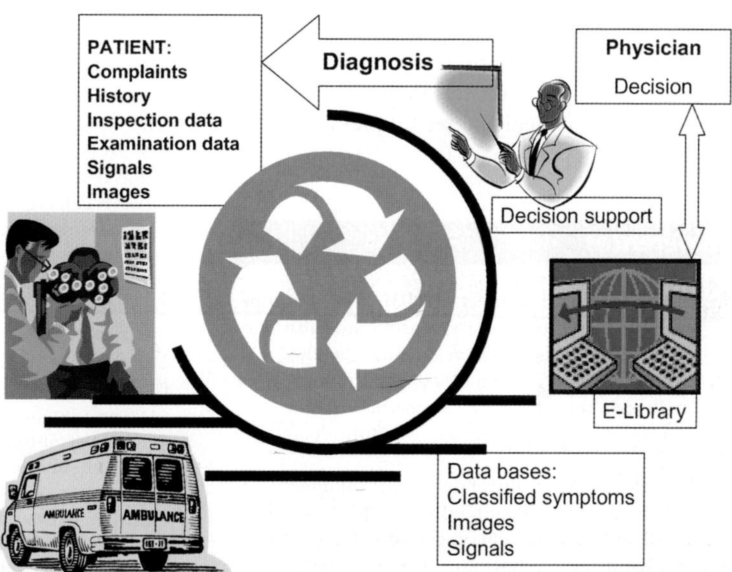

Fig. 22.9. The ophthalmologist (user and expert) diagnostic–information system for clinical decision support

The sequence of eye fundus image parameterization, following the logical eye fundus examination assessment, established:

1. Parameterization of the optic nerve head
2. Parameterization of the retinal focuses (derivatives)
3. Parameterization of the retinal blood vessels

22.7 Future Development

The direction for future development and advancement of IT methods (mathematical methods, algorithms, computer network decisions) helping in the formation of preventive and clinical decisions were also developed (Fig. 22.9) [14–17].

The connection between the ophthalmologist (user and expert) and the diagnostic information system for clinical decision support is based on the storage of patient data in a high capacity ophthalmic and cardiologic data and digital image base. After classification processing and parameterization, the clinical and experimental data will be stored and used for the creation of new multi-criteria decision strategies for analyzing patient-population data and the creation of ophthalmological clinical decision support, with links to internet information (e-library). The ophthalmologist then makes a final diagnostic decision.

According to our experience in developing the infrastructure in Lithuania, a world-wide teleophthalmology network could be created. Development of telemedicine services in Lithuania has great importance for the Lithuanian health care system, as there is great potential to reduce preventable disease, improve the quality of health care and increase the professionalism of doctors by using distant training, consultations with modern telemedicine techniques and clinical decision support.

References

1. EU Information Society (2003) http:://europa.eu.int/information_society/eeurope/e-health/conference/2003/index_en.htm. Cited 4 Oct 2005
2. Ingram D (2004) The journey of health informatics. In: Proceedings of the 2nd International Conference E-health in Common Europe, Krakow, Poland, pp 3–18
3. Paunksnis A, Calissendorff B, Blomdahl S, Lukoševičius A, Barzdžiukas V, Kurapkienė S, Gricius R, Almquist LO, Varnauskas E (2001) Teleophthalmology: cooperation between Sweden and Lithuania. Int J Health Care Eng 9(4):367
4. Paunksnis A, Barzdžiukas V, Lukoševičius A, Blomdahl S, Kurapkienė S, Jurkonis R, Jegelevičius D, Almquist LO (2002) Teleophthalmology: impact for Lithuania. In: Abstracts of 7th International Conference on the Medical Aspects of Telemedicine Integration of Health Telematics into Medical Practise. Eur J Med Res, Regensburg, Germany, pp 60–61
5. Paunksnis A, Lukoševičius A, Kurapkienė S, Barzdžiukas V, Jurkonis R, Almquist LO, Severgardh P, Uloza V (2003) Achievements of telemedicine in Lithuania. In: Proceedings of Advanced Learning Technologies and Applications, ALTA'03, pp 55–56
6. Paunksnis A, Barzdžiukas V, Kurapkienė S, Severgardh P (2004) Trends of telemedicine development in Lithuania. In: Abstracts in International E-Health Exhibition and Conference "Med-e-Tel", Luxembourg, pp 71–72
7. Paunksnis A (2003) Integrated E-health network in Lithuania for clinical practise, education and research. Ministerial Conference and Exhibition E-health: the contribution of ICT to Health, Brussels, pp 10–11
8. Marozas V, Gelžinis A, Lukoševičius A, Severgardh P, Kurapkienė S, Paunksnis A (2002) The method to achieve online telemedicine capabilities using general purpose videoconferencing software. In: Abstracts of 7th Intenational Conference on the Medical Aspects of Telemedicine Integration of Health Telematics into Medical Practise, Eur J Med Res, Regensburg, Germany, p 47
9. Marozas V, Jurkonis R, Kazla A, Lukoševičius M, Lukosevičius A, Gelžinis A, Jegelevičius D (2004) Development of teleconsultations systems for e-health. In: Duplaga M, Zielinsky K, Ingram D (eds) Transformation of Healthcare with Information Technologies series Studies in Health Technology, IOS Press 105:337–348
10. Lukoševičius M, Paunksnis A, Barzdžiukas V, Lukoševičius A, Kurapkienė S (2002) Model based ophthalmologic knowledge structuring and presenting via Internet. In: Biomedicininė inžinerija proceedings. Kaunas University of Technology, pp 143–146
11. Lukoševičius M, Paunksnis A, Barzdžiukas V, Lukoševičius A, Kurapkienė S (2002) Digital ophthalmology, acute visual loss: the informational diagnosis focused ophthalmological web site for general practitioners and medical students. In: Abstracts of 7th International Conference on the Medical Aspects of Telemedicine Integration of Health Telematics into Medical Practise, Eur J Med Res, Regensburg, Germany, p 47
12. Kurapkienė S, Paunksnis A, Barzdžiukas V, Vaičaitienė R, Sereika V (2005) An assessment of telemedicine possibilities in massive casualties situations. In: Euroregional Conference on Building Information Society in the Healthcare in Euroregion Niemen Abstracts, p 62
13. Kurapkienė S, Paunksnis A, Lukoševičius M, Barzdžiukas V, Almquist LO, Severgardh P (2004) An experience of virtual clinical practise, education and research in medicine. In: Abstracts in the 5th International Telemedicine Congress "Telemedum", Umea, Sweden, pp 20–21
14. Šaltenis V (2004) Outlier detection based on the distribution of distances between data points. Informatica 15(3):399–410
15. Barzdžiukas V, Paunksnis A, Lukoševičius M, Kurapkienė S, Almquist LO, Severgardh P (2003)

Teleophthalmology for second opinion and clinical decision support. In: Proceedings in the 2nd international conference "E-health in Common Europe", Krakow, Poland, p 61

16. Barzdžiukas V, Paunksnis A, Kurapkienė S (2005) The use of teleophthalmology for the second opinion and clinical decision support. In: Abstract in Euroregional Conference on Building Information Society in the Healthcare in Euroregion Niemen, Bialystok, Poland, p 61
17. Paunksnis A, Barzdžiukas V, Kurapkienė S, Almquist LO, Severgardh P (2004) Networking for consultations and education: experience of telemedicine center. In: Proceedings of the 2nd international conference "E-health in Common Europe", Krakow, Poland, p 30

Chapter 23

Teleophthalmology in Japan

23

Akitoshi Yoshida

This chapter addresses the following

Key Concepts:

- Asahikawa Medical College has developed new standards in highly compressed, high quality, three-dimensional streaming video transmission to meet the demands of ophthalmological medical treatment.
- International telemedicine conferences have been developed between Asahikawa Medical College and Harvard University, and lectures have been broadcast between Asahikawa Medical College and the Affiliated Hospital of Nanking University.
- These and other teleophthalmology developments are discussed in detail.

23.1 Introduction

As the only telemedicine medical center in Japan, Asahikawa Medical College is presently developing a revolutionary and innovative form of medical practice. The following summary of our efforts span the past 12 years, during which time we have attempted to define telemedicine research in the field of ophthalmology.

In 1994, Asahikawa Medical College Department of Ophthalmology was the first in Japan to successfully transmit moving images through the transmission of video footage. A system was constructed between the ophthalmology unit at the Yoichi Association Hospital and the Department of Ophthalmology at Asahikawa Medical College by incorporating transmission signals over a distance of 200 km. Color video sequences were transmitted via a single InterNet communication Settings (INS) Net 64 ISDN line.

The following year, with the cooperation of Panasonic Corporation, our present system of telemedicine, using an INS Net 1500 ISDN optical fiber line, began delivering full-speed, full quality, 30 frames per second streaming video. The system transmits via Nippon Telephone and Telegraph's INS Net 1500 line (1.5 Mb/s) and then the images are converted via a codec device. Utilization of this telemedicine system in the field of ophthalmology has made it possible to support remote diagnosis and operations. Following our efforts in Yoichi, Kushiro, Sapporo and other cities, the telemedicine system has continued to expand (Figs. 23.1 and 23.2).

In 1996, the first practical use of an international network was achieved when communications were set up between the Department of Ophthalmology at Asahikawa Medical College

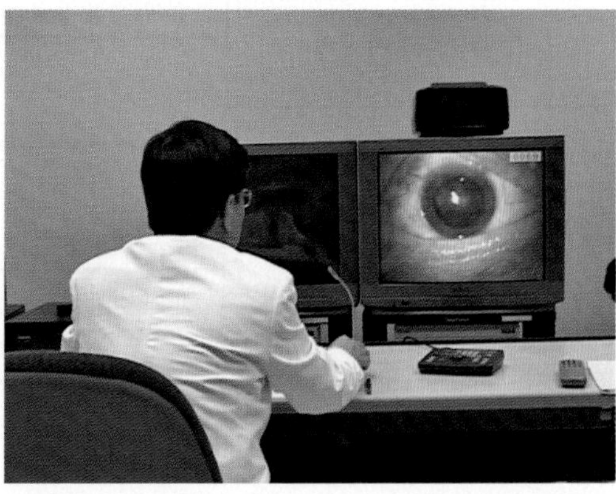

Fig. 23.1. Asahikawa Medical College's Department of Ophthalmological Medicine

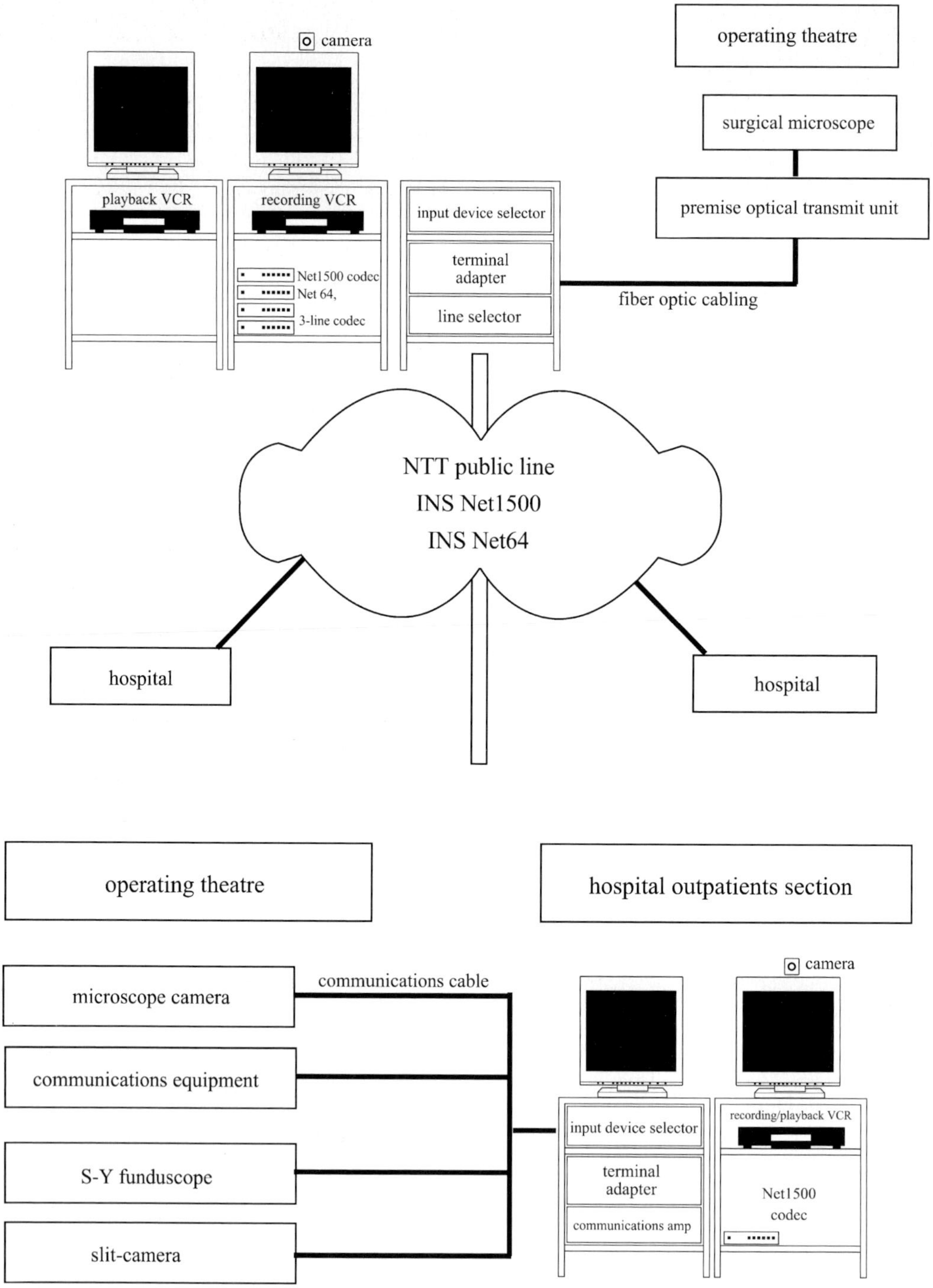

Fig. 23.2. Structural diagram of communication system at Asahikawa Medical College's Ophthalmology department

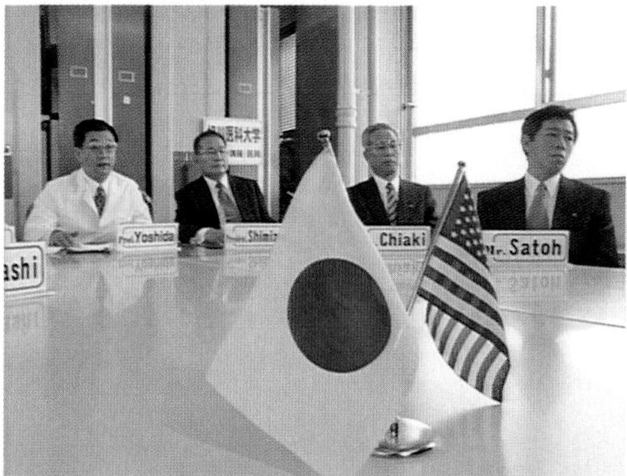

Fig. 23.3. First real practical demonstration of on-line visual transmission

and the Stephens Eye Research Institute at Harvard University's Faculty of Medicine (Figs. 23.3 and 23.4).

During the conferences, discussions regarding diagnosis and treatment methods were discussed, as well as live surgery in real-time for both participants. For the innovation of this system, we were awarded the Governor's award by Governor William F. Weld of the State of Massachusetts, as well as the Global Interoperability for Broadband Network award, which was chosen during a G7 Summit Meeting in 1994 (Fig. 23.5).

23.2 Recent Activities

Between 1997 and 2002, we established a research laboratory, and built a collaborative research, manufacturing, and administrative project team. We also developed high standards in technological advancement that were aided by the transmission of highly realistic, solid, three-dimensional images to meet the demands of ophthalmological medical treatment (Fig. 23.6).

Using an ophthalmic surgical microscope and our imaging techology, high-resolution images have been acquired, stored, compressed, and transmitted to distant sites. The result is a new, highly-compressed, high quality, three-dimensional, ophthalmological streaming video transmission, based on a new compressed algorithm concept. A fixed quantity method was used to deal with block distortion caused by compression in the doctor's "Region of Interest" (ROI), which is an important feature of the compression algorithms. These high definition images have opened up areas that could not previously have been reliably done with telemedicine, such as endoscopic surgery, receiving more medically accurate diagnostic images, and medical treatment and decision support.

In 1997, the international telemedicine achievements for Tertiary Telemedicine (Asahi-

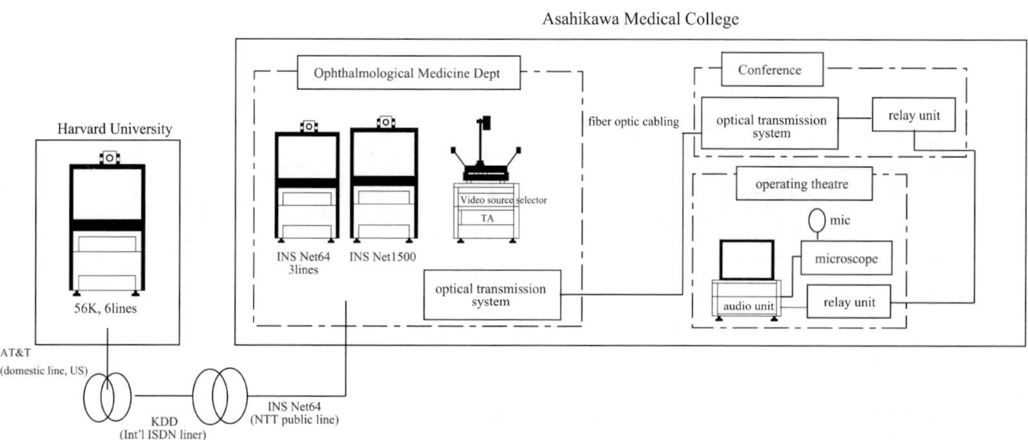

Fig. 23.4. Regional ophthalmological telemedicine network system

23

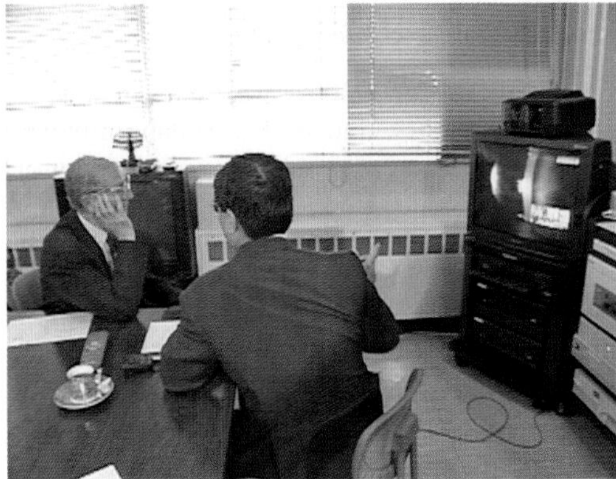

Fig. 23.5. Charles Schepens inspecting and testing the telemedicine system at Asahikawa Medical College

Fig. 23.7. History and practice of telemedicine at Asahikawa Medical College's Department of Ophthalmology

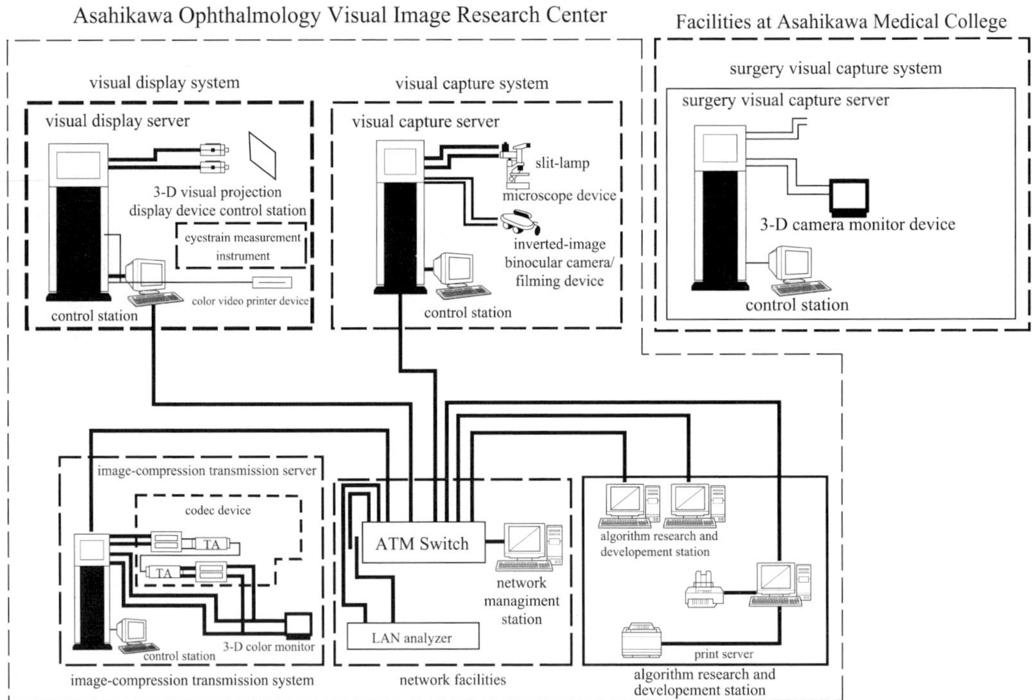

Fig. 23.6. Structure diagram of research and development facilities

kawa Medical College/Harvard University/Nanking Hospital) was launched.

Conferences that were set up have aided all participants in comparing and learning the latest treatment techniques, and in undertaking research on retinal diseases, particularly macular disorders. Through these conferences, it is possible to hold discussions about the rapidly increasing occurrence of eye diseases in Japan and to provide an avenue for sharing ideas and the latest information regarding ophthalmic conditions (Fig. 23.7).

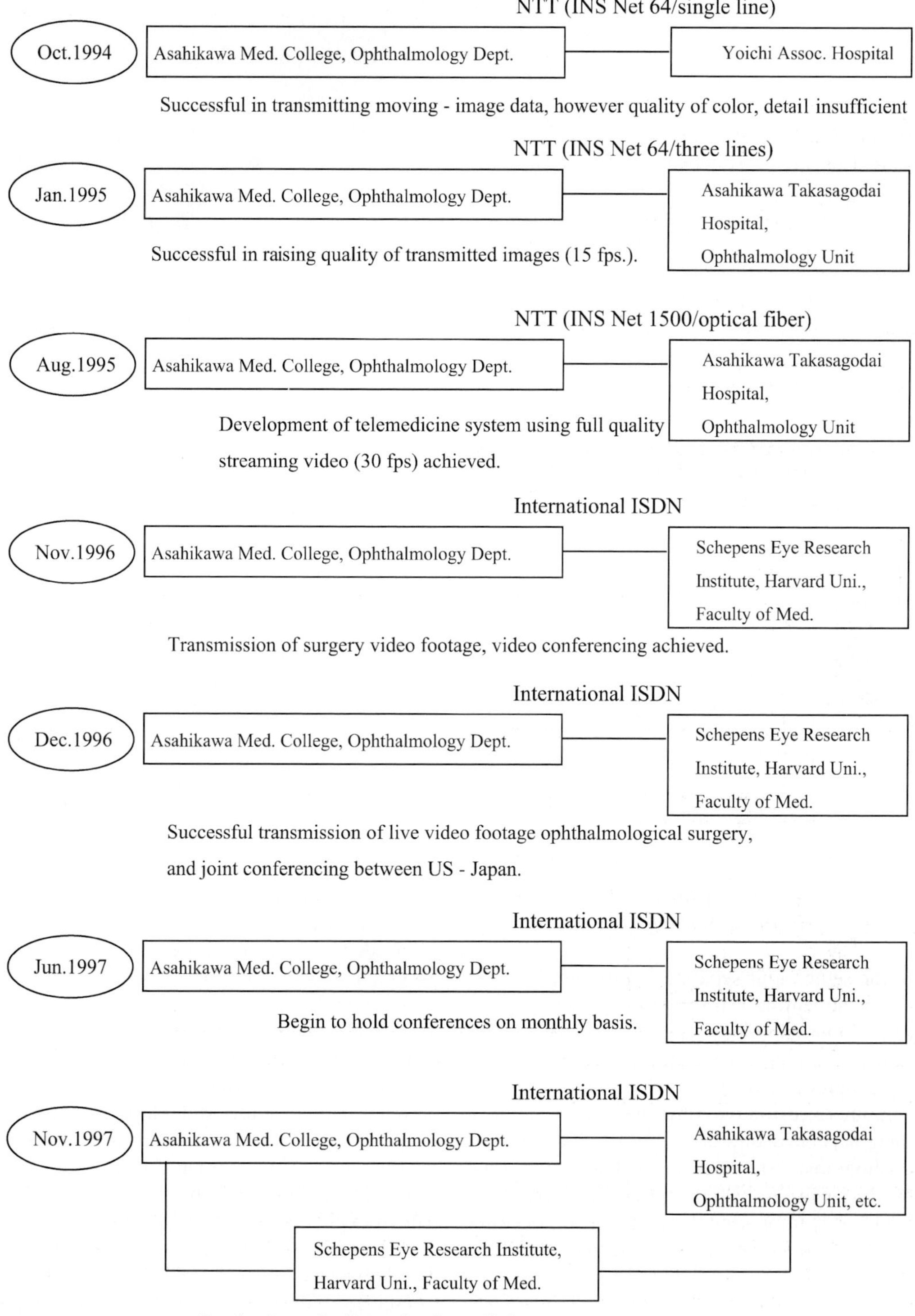
NTT (INS Net 64/single line)
Oct.1994
Asahikawa Med. College, Ophthalmology Dept.
Yoichi Assoc. Hospital
Successful in transmitting moving - image data, however quality of color, detail insufficient
NTT (INS Net 64/three lines)
Jan.1995
Asahikawa Med. College, Ophthalmology Dept.
Asahikawa Takasagodai Hospital, Ophthalmology Unit
Successful in raising quality of transmitted images (15 fps.).
NTT (INS Net 1500/optical fiber)
Aug.1995
Asahikawa Med. College, Ophthalmology Dept.
Asahikawa Takasagodai Hospital, Ophthalmology Unit
Development of telemedicine system using full quality streaming video (30 fps) achieved.
International ISDN
Nov.1996
Asahikawa Med. College, Ophthalmology Dept.
Schepens Eye Research Institute, Harvard Uni., Faculty of Med.
Transmission of surgery video footage, video conferencing achieved.
International ISDN
Dec.1996
Asahikawa Med. College, Ophthalmology Dept.
Schepens Eye Research Institute, Harvard Uni., Faculty of Med.
Successful transmission of live video footage ophthalmological surgery, and joint conferencing between US - Japan.
International ISDN
Jun.1997
Asahikawa Med. College, Ophthalmology Dept.
Schepens Eye Research Institute, Harvard Uni., Faculty of Med.
Begin to hold conferences on monthly basis.
International ISDN
Nov.1997
Asahikawa Med. College, Ophthalmology Dept.
Asahikawa Takasagodai Hospital, Ophthalmology Unit, etc.
Schepens Eye Research Institute, Harvard Uni., Faculty of Med.
Beginning of trilateral telemedicine

23

23.3 Time Savings

With the advent of the international telemedicine system, the burdens of time and cost have been greatly reduced for both health provider and patient. In 1998, international telemedicine visual transmissions between Asahikawa Medical College's Department of Ophthalmology, and the Affiliated Hospital of Nanking University of Traditional Chinese Medicine were initiated. Transmissions and lectures on vitreous surgery and refractive surgeries have been broadcasted from Japan. The use of the excimer laser, with many examples of operations for correcting myopia, has been transmitted from China.

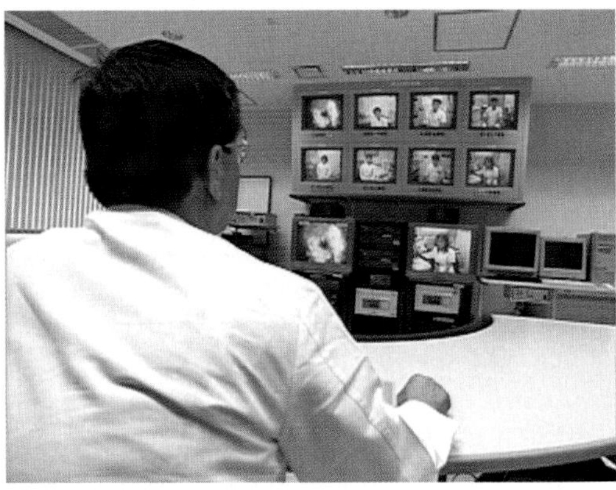

Fig. 23.8. Asahikawa Medical College Telemedicine Center

23.4 Telemedicine Center and New Models for Cooperation

In 1999, to further promote international telemedicine, the Starr Center for Scientific Communications was opened at the Schepens Eye Research Institute at Harvard University. Presently this center, along with Asahikawa Medical College, is networking between city hospitals in countries world-wide. Asahikawa Medical College's telemedicine center is also linked to 34 facilities within Japan and two facilities outside Japan. It is a base working at full capacity on both national and international levels (Fig. 23.8).

23.4.1 Inside Japan's Telemedicine Center

In the center, four separate rooms have been set up for streaming transmissions for sensory organs (ophthalmology, ears/nose/throat), diagnosis, streaming video transmissions for pathology diagnosis, streaming video transmissions of computerized tomography, magnetic resonance imaging, endoscopy, ultrasound images, electrocardiograms, and electroencephalograms, each of which can also be transmitted. Telemedicine is continually improving the transmission of close-grained detailed images and streamlined videos.

23.4.2 A Growing Network

In 2000, a network was set up that linked all diagnoses, procedures, and treatment rooms between Asahikawa Medical College and Nemuro City Hospital by the telemedicine center. In 2001, using a fiberoptic line at 64Mb/s between the Asahikawa Medical College operating rooms and Sapporo-Kosei General Hospital, for the first time ever in real-time, a three-dimensional ophthalmology operation was transmitted. Furthermore, a completely new educational method for teaching surgical techniques was verified when both hospitals simultaneously used virtual reality technology (a vitreous surgery simulator) to conduct a simulated operation.

In 2002, a peer-to-peer style information correspondence network for research was initiated. Research is being conducted with the peer-to-peer network, particularly for medical images for three-dimensional (high definition) image compression transmission algorithms and three-dimensional vision. This aims to integrate data between telemedicine and electronic medical records, which is the first such medical system for the world. This national project is presently receiving attention from the governmental U-Japan strategic initiative. In addition, in 2005, the Asia Broadband framework also began. Asahikawa Medical College and Singapore National Eye Center are trying to initiate three-dimensional, high definition international telemedicine between the two sites.

23.5 Goals

Asahikawa Medical College aims to become the key center for telemedicine practice with research and electronic medical records. We propose to provide all people, no matter where they live, the chance to enjoy the world's highest standard of medical treatment. Our goal is to make telemedicine ubiquitous and for it to spread throughout all countries, allowing it to function smoothly. In this regard, Asahikawa Medical College is working as an information center, and is being actively progressive in thinking of new medical treatment strategies for the future.

References

1. Akitoshi Yoshida, Yoshihiko Kamehata (2000) Telemedicine. Kogyo Chosakai, Tokyo, Japan
2. AkitoshiYoshida (2000) http://www.pr-yoshida.com. Cited 10 June 2000
3. Asahikawa Medical College Department of Ophthalmology (2003) http://www.asahikawa-med.ac.jp/dept/mc/ophtha. Cited 9 May 2003
4. Asahikawa Medical College Telemedcine Center (2003) http://www.asahikawa-med.ac.jp/hospital/astec. Cited 4 Oct 2005

Chapter 24

ORBIS Telemedicine: Cyber-Sight

24

Eugene M. Helveston, Mohan J. Thazhathu, Lynda M. Smallwood

This chapter addresses the following

Key Concepts:

- A DC10 flying eye hospital conducts programs of two to three weeks duration in developing countries.
- Hospital-based programs are carried out in countries that are visited by the plane.
- Digital images and the Internet are used to maintain contact between partners and ORBIS doctors when the plane leaves or when the hospital-based program concludes.
- Teleconsultations are answered in hours or days.
- A variety of teaching programs are available on the ORBIS web site.
- Cyber-Sight intends to reach those ophthalmologists and eye health care workers with the biggest job and the fewest assets.

24.1 Introduction

ORBIS is an international non-governmental blindness fighting organization with a history of more than 25 years working in the field. Its programs are best known for their used of a Flying Eye Hospital (FEH), the first used a DC8 and since 1994, a DC10 aircraft fully equipped with classroom, operating room, procedure room, recovery room, and appropriate support areas, including a fully functional audio-visual studio.

Recognizing the need for more program continuity, in the past several years ORBIS has sponsored *in country* hospital-based programs (HBP) in addition to the FEH. These HBPs have provided ORBIS the ability to reach many partners and patients who are in need but who, because of a variety of conditions, are out of reach of a traditional FEH program.

24.2 FEH and HBP Programs

FEH programs, which usually last three weeks, consist of three one-week sessions. HBPs usually last one week. Each are conducted by one or several ORBIS volunteer faculty (VF) who carry out patient evaluations while providing clinical teaching, performing surgery (mostly for demonstration and teaching purposes), delivering formal lectures, and providing other services requested by their partners as long as they fit within the guidelines of ORBIS programs.

Both FEH programs and HBPS have over the years delivered the ORBIS message effectively. This message stresses teaching doctors, and to some extent those they serve, about methods for both treating and preventing avoidable blindness. At the individual level, ORBIS programs strive to meet the unique needs of each partner, helping that person to be the best health care provider they can be.

24

24.2.1 Communication Challenges

These initial efforts notwithstanding, and in spite of attempts to stay connected, some ORBIS programs have been frustrated by the lack of ongoing communication between partners and ORBIS mentors. The challenge to continuity is apparent: an ORBIS VF works with the FEH or arrives in a small group at a hospital or clinic (HBP), carries out an intense program for three weeks (FEH) or one week (HBP) and then departs. The time spent by ORBIS VF working with partners is effective in most cases, enhancing the professional development of partner doctors. At the same time, ORBIS VFs experience the satisfaction of giving. But no student can learn everything there is to know in one week, and no teacher can teach everything he or she knows in one week. In addition, new techniques and understanding are always on the horizon. It became apparent something should be added to in ORBIS programs. This something was effective communication between VF and partners dealing with a variety of issues both carried over from the ORBIS visit and newly arising.

24.2.2 IT: Communication Rx

This started to change during the 1990s with the advent of effective communication that became widely available through information technology (IT). Thanks to digitization, text and images can be transferred by wire and through space via satellite, effectively joining partner and VF in the practice of medicine and linking teacher and student in the quest for knowledge.

24.3 ORBIS' Program Development

The first ORBIS effort in what is now universally referred to as telemedicine started in Havana Cuba in 1998. During a one week HBP it became clear that a week was woefully inadequate to launch an effective pediatric ophthalmology program at the Ramon Pando Ferrer Eye Hospital. This was so in spite of an intelligent and eager young staff serving a varied and challenging patient population. To overcome the obstacle of having a pediatric ophthalmology/strabismus clinic in Cuba and a teacher in the United States, a connection was established using e-mail and attached images. This technique immediately proved effective. Several hundred consultations, mainly dealing with strabismus, were carried out successfully. The concept was tested initially for accuracy of diagnosis. This validation began with 10 experts agreeing on the diagnosis of a dozen patients presented through e-mail consultation.

24.3.1 Cyber-Sight

In addition a mentor visiting the Cuban clinic demonstrated that the *in-person* evaluation of 15 previously examined patients matched the on-line consultation. After this, the program expanded to Bucharest Romania, Tirana Albania, Kakinada India and Santo Domingo in the Dominican Republic.

Based on the success of the e-mail based consultation program and recognizing the limitations of using e-mail as the method of communication, a corporate partner was sought. ORBIS, the most logical partner, adopted the program fully and the unique brand of ORBIS telemedicine, Cyber-Sight was established. This program now utilizes a server based in Flushing, New York. This server supports a unique format for managing the patient consultation process and also provides the framework for an extensive educational program.

24.3.1.1 The Teaching Modules: E-Consultation

Cyber-Sight is located on the World-Wide Web at www.orbis.org. Once there, the home page is accessed by clicking on *ORBIS telemedicine*. From there, three main choices are available. These are E-Resource, E-Consultation, and E-Learning. Two of these are teaching modules available to anyone accessing the site. E-Consultation, available only to qualified partners, will be described first.

E-consultation is the patient care link of Cyber-Sight. It is offered free of charge to qualified partners anywhere in the world. Most partners are selected after personal contact has been established by means of an ORBIS FEH program or HBP. This personal contact can occur as a result of a partner application or it can occur during a FEH or HBP encounter. Once selected, partners are given a digital camera, and when needed, a computer. Some partners are also helped in obtaining an Internet connection. The digital camera for external imaging is simple.

At this time we are employing the Nikon 2200 camera because it is low cost and has a suitable macro lens (but many cameras can meet the needs of the program). This Nikon camera can be employed with a standard slit lamp by holding it against an ocular. A better solution is the use of a hand held slit lamp with a specially fashioned camera adaptor. Posterior segment imaging is more difficult to obtain, but a picture of a picture can be useful. A digital fundus camera is ideal but is very costly. Magnetic Resonance Imaging and Computerized Tomography images can be sent without difficulty. A sample of images sent via Cyber-Sight are shown in Fig. 24.1.

Partner doctors, after training in the program, are given a user name and password allowing them to access a page that is suitable for uploading patient information (Fig. 24.2). When partners are accepted and given a username and password they are also assigned to a mentor team. This mentor team consists of ophthalmologists who include all of the sub-specialties in ophthalmology, with one or more experts in retina, glaucoma, oculo-plastics, pediatric ophthalmology/strabismus, uveitis, retinopathy of prematurity, ophthalmic genetics, retinoblastoma, cataracts, and other disciplines.

When a partner doctor sends a patient for consultation, a request is first made for timing of the response – either routine, or one of two classes of expedited response (24 h or 12 h). Then a *drop-down* box is used to select the appropriate sub-specialty. For each mentor team a specific doctor(s) will receive notification via e-mail that a consultation request has been sent.

Upon receiving notification that this consultation request is made, the mentor signs in with a unique user name and password to gain access to the patient information. The consult is answered and submitted, at which time the partner is notified by e-mail. The partner looks at the mentor's response, acknowledges or asks for more information and sends the case back.

Before a partner submits a case, the partner must click on a response stating that the patient has given consent for the consultation and that the pictures can be used for ethical teaching purposes. Partners agree to download the consent form, have the patient sign the form and keep it on file. Mentors likewise acknowledge the disclaimer that they are taking responsibility for sending a response to the partner. However, in these combined forms it is clearly stated that the responsibility for care of the patient rests *solely* with the partner.

24.3.1.2 The Process

Several things are important in this process. Some are mundane and technical and some are far-reaching and philosophical. Digital images should be obtained with the camera on the *lowest* setting available, i.e., 640×480 pixels. However, the latest compression techniques enable capture of high-resolution images, lessening the problem of bandwidth. If it is anticipated that a print of this picture will be made, especially with an enlargement, a second picture at higher resolution can be taken. High-resolution images are of *no* value in the Cyber-Sight process, and only result in delayed or even failed transmission.

The second, more philosophical, point is that the Cyber-Sight consultation process is mostly a teaching/learning experience/exercise. While information about individual patient management is imparted, the thrust of the program is *teaching*. A large part of the dialogue tends to include questions such as, "Have you done this test?" What do you think of this option? Have you looked at that piece of information?

24.3.1.3 Completed Consultation

A completed consultation contains the patient information, digital images imparting the necessary clinical information, the partner's tentative diagnosis, tentative treatment plans and any other questions or comments by the partner. Upon

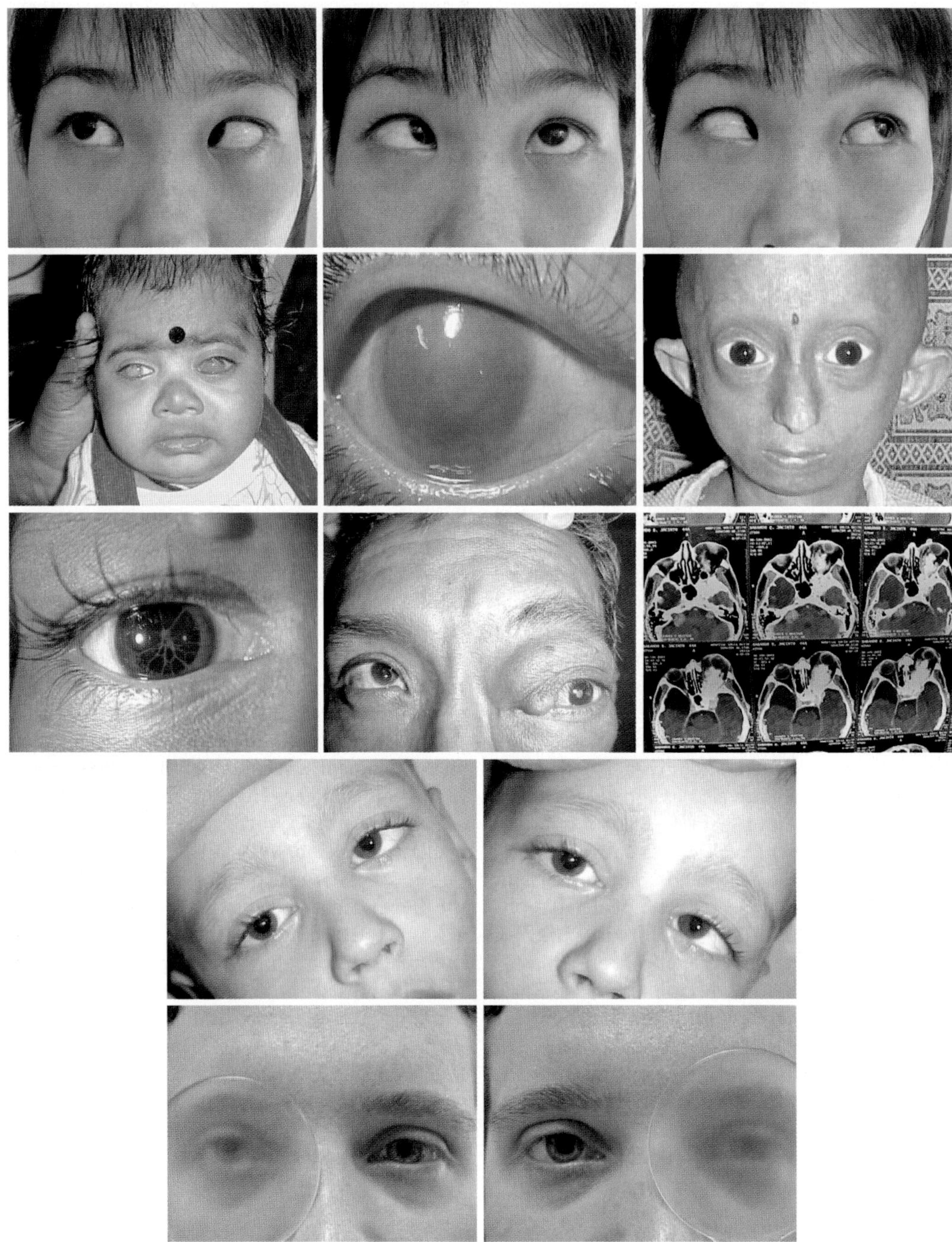

Fig. 24.1. The variety of images seen on e-consultation. *Top row:* strabismus. *Second row:* congenital glaucoma, uveitis, Hallerman-Strief. *Third row:* persistent supillary membrane, proptosis, MRI. *Fourth row:* strabismus. *Bottom row:* alignment with translucent occluder

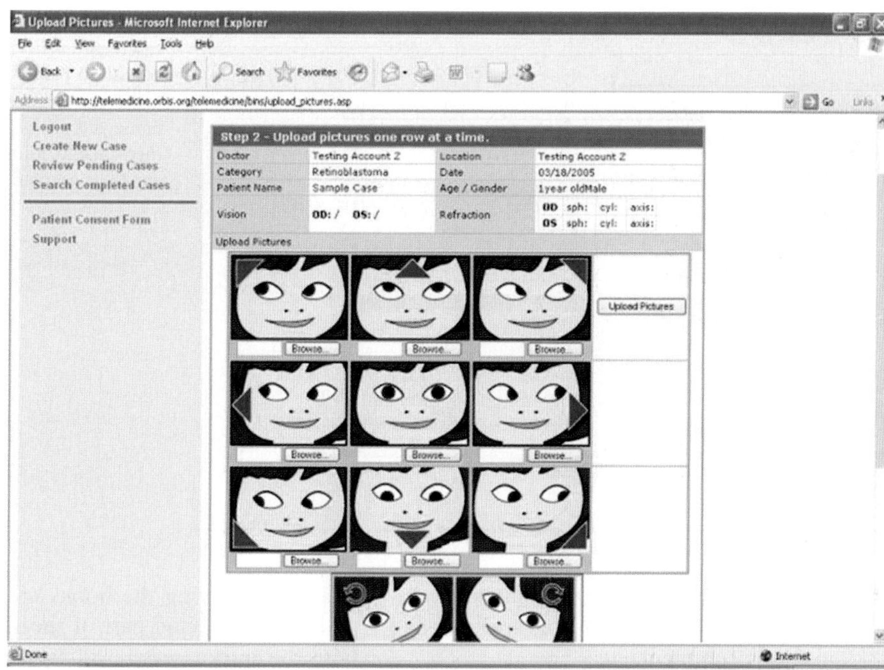

Fig. 24.2. Template for submitting a patient consultation

receiving this information/request, the mentor studies the case and submits a response.

At this point the partner can accept the advice and close the case or can ask another question. This dialogue continues until the partner is satisfied and closes the case. All cases are archived and are periodically monitored.

As of 2005, more than 2,000 case studies and approximately 6,000 communications have been recorded in the Cyber-Sight program and reside on the server. In addition, the archived material has provided data for two scientific papers on the process and a presentation on the clinical characteristics and classification of Duane syndrome [1, 2].

24.3.1.4 Teaching Modules: Education Components

In addition to the E-consultation part of the Cyber-Sight Web site, two other parts make up the educational component of the teaching modules: E-Resource and E-Learning.

E-Resource includes a few components. *Question of the Week* is a weekly quiz dealing with a new subject each week. The format is that of a case presented with images and history, and multiple-choice question are posed. One week later answers are given along with an explanation. This feature has been in place since 20 January 2004. The *Ophthalmology Minute* is a series of short lectures specially designed to be read on the Internet. Sub-specialties with *minutes* include strabismus, ophthalmic nursing, neuro-ophthalmology, and retinopathy of prematurity. The aim is to eventually cover all ophthalmic sub-specialties. A book section has an algorithm-based text book *Strabismus: A Decision making Approach* with the addition of several illustrations not present in the book form. In the future other printed material especially suited for the Internet will be included.

On the *E-Consultation* segment a section includes featured cases. These are made up of a series of images followed by a listing of the medical findings. Then one or more experts comment on the case, imparting their own clinical experience.

24

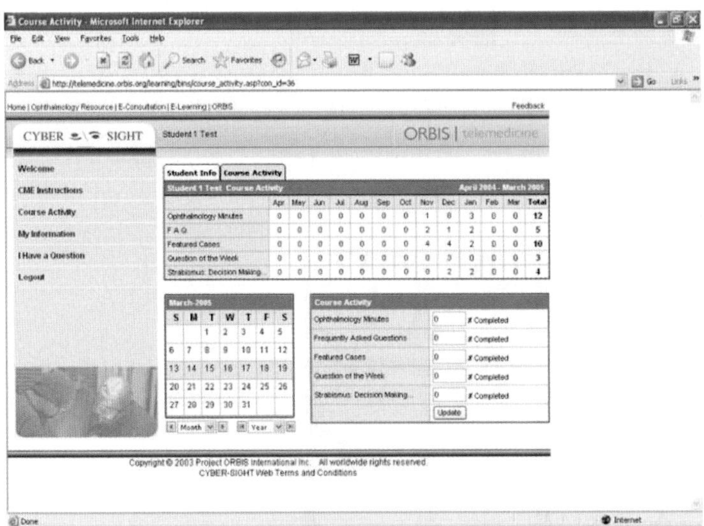

Fig. 24.3. Student visiting the site can record visits to the various education pages. First students must register to obtain a user-name and password. Continuing medical education credit (attendance) is granted for this

A series of *Frequently Asked Questions* is also included. Throughout the site visitors are invited to ask questions, comment, etc.

The *E- Learning* section provides the opportunity for students to enroll, for the purpose of recording the amount of time spent studying on the site. For example; if a student visits the site and answers a question of the week or reads an ophthalmology minute, the student can go to the *course activity* page and record this activity. The guide and the course activity recording site are shown in Fig. 24.3. Students will also be awarded one hour of credit for each consultation submitted. Study of the material on the site, which is free to all, earns Continuing Medical Education *attendance* credit granted by the Indiana University of Indianapolis Indiana, USA. A certificate suitable for framing is given with the Continuing Medical Education award.

Selected students are enrolled in a restricted part of *E-Learning* which uses the American Academy of Ophthalmology Basic and Clinical Science Course book set as a text. This 14 volume, approximately 5,000 page work covers all of the recognized sub-specialties in ophthalmology, in addition to featuring a volume on general medical principles. Under an agreement with the American Academy of Ophthalmology, ORBIS purchases book sets and gives them to students who would otherwise be unable to purchase and/or have free access to this material. Students receiving the books are enrolled in a password-protected part of the site which contains the approximately 900 work questions and answers found at the end of each Basic and Clinical Science Course volume. The tests taken and successfully completed on-line are automatically recorded. Upon completion of the tests, students receive category I Continuing Medical Education credit.

24.4 The ORBIS Philosophy

The philosophy supporting ORBIS Telemedicine, Cyber-Sight is one of sharing. By our best estimates there are 160,000 ophthalmologists in the world who are at the front line meeting patients and attending to their needs in support of better vision, including the fight against preventable blindness. It is estimated that half or 80,000 of these ophthalmologists who are the best trained and the best equipped care for between 5 and 10% of the world's blind or potentially blind.

This leaves the daunting task of caring for up to 90% of the world's blind to the other 80,000, who happen to have the least training and are the poorest equipped. Such gross inequity can be met in a variety of ways. This is being attempted by several organizations world-wide. The special role of ORBIS Telemedicine, Cyber-Sight is to find ways to empower our partners through capacity building so that those we assist can grow in their capabilities to both help those in need and teach other caregivers. An important part of capacity building is teaching, and that is what Cyber-Sight is all about.

References

1. Helveston EM, Orge F, Naranjo R, Hernandez L (2001) Telemedicine: Strabismus e-consultation. J AAPOS 5(5):291–296
2. Helveston EM, Kopecky G, Smallwood LM (2004) Cyber Sight – ORBIS Telemedicine. Insight 29(3):15-18

Chapter 25

Teleophthalmology in Spain

25

Francisco Gonzalez, Adrian F. Castro

This chapter addresses the following

Key Concepts:

- An increasing number of telemedical techniques applied to ophthalmology are being used in Spain, with virtually all of them aimed at detecting diabetic retinopathy or retinal diseases.
- The authors present a short analysis and results of a teleophthalmology link between two primary care centers and a tertiary hospital.
- A bibliographic search on publication output in teleophthalmology in Spain shows that most teleophthalmology projects were not published in scientific publications.

25.1 Introduction

The Spanish National Health System is a public health care insurance system with universal coverage for the population of 41 million people. The country is politically and administratively divided into 17 autonomous communities and the cities of Ceuta and Melilla (Fig. 25.1), with autonomous regional governments that are responsible for their own public health systems, and which are largely independent of each other. However, they are coordinated by the national government and fully financed by the general tax fund.

Virtually all hospitals and primary health care centers (PCCs) belong to this system and are publicly owned. All the autonomous communities have at least one university, and most universities have agreements with the local public health systems to share their resources for teaching and research purposes. It is within this framework that most telemedical projects take place in Spain.

A recent study of publication output in telemedicine in Spain shows that, as in many other countries, telemedicine activity evolved along with the proliferation of the Internet [1]. If we assume that publication output is related to telemedical activity, this study shows that telemedicine in Spain started in 1988, with a sudden increase from 1995 caused by the massive expansion of the Internet. The time course of research activity in telemedicine in Spain is similar to that reported by Moser et al. [2] world-wide, and is in accordance with the previously reported rapid growth in telemedicine during the 1990s [3].

In the Spanish National Health System, general practitioners (GPs) at the PCCs play a critical role in reducing waiting lists to access specialized care because they act as gatekeepers. Therefore every effort to help GPs select patients who actually need to be referred to a specialist is supported by the public administration. In ophthalmology, image inspection is a key factor for diagnosis; therefore, sending ocular images from PCCs that would be inspected by an ophthalmologist to hospitals, would certainly reduce the number of referrals [4]. In such an environment, ophthalmology teleconsultation techniques are helpful for this purpose. In this chapter, we report on the results obtained after performing a search for activity in teleophthalmology in Spain.

25.2 Search Methods

To assess the activity in teleophthalmology in Spain, we performed a search that included the Medline database, Internet search engines, and direct contact with key people or institutions by e-mail, regular mail or phone calls.

25.2.1 Medline Search

We used several combinations of words related to telemedicine and ophthalmology (i.e., teleophthalmology, telecare, teleconsultation) together with the word *Spain* linked by means of the *and* logical operator. The results were examined to exclude those documents not related to teleophthalmology.

25.2.2 Internet Search

We also performed a search using the *Google* search engine on the Internet by using several queries that included similar words as those used for searching in the Medline database, but in this case in Spanish. The hits were examined to detect those web pages that genuinely provided information about teleophthalmology projects or activities.

25.2.3 Direct Request of Information

To gain a more detailed account on activity in teleophthalmology in Spain that could not be identified by the previous search, we requested information by means of regular mail or e-mail from the Departments of Health of every community, and from the ophthalmology services of 50 major hospitals and eye-care related institutions in all the communities and autonomous cities. Some additional information was also gathered by direct phone calls to key individuals whom we expected to have direct or indirect relationships with this activity.

25.3 Search Results

The search in the Medline database showed five studies addressed teleophthalmology activity [4–8]. Most of these documents focused their attention on retinal images taken with non-mydriatic funduscopic cameras. However it is possible that more studies have been reported that were not found in Medline, either because of an inadequate query, or because they had been published in journals that are or were not indexed in the database at the moment of publication. This is the case, for instance, for two articles reporting on the potential use of telemedicine in ophthalmology [9] and on a teleconsultation system for ophthalmology [10] published in journals not indexed in Medline.

From direct requests made by e-mail, regular mail and phone calls, we obtained a total of 12 answers reporting either activity or no activity on teleophthalmology.

25.4 Community Activity

We derived the information in this section from the hits found in our search on the Internet. Here, we summarize all the information gathered on teleophthalmology activity in Spain, grouped by communities (Fig. 25.1).

25.4.1 Andalusia (Andalucia)

The Hospital Regional Universitario Carlos Haya of Malaga began a project at the beginning of 2005, designed to obtain eye fundus images with a non-mydriatic camera in three PCCs, and to send them to a hospital where an ophthalmologist could make a diagnosis (personal communication).

Currently the project is in an initial phase, in which several technicians are learning how the images can be obtained. It is predominantly aimed at detecting diabetic retinopathy, but data about visual acuity and IOP is also included in the transmission.

In Sevilla and Huelva several pilot projects have recently started by which seven hospitals

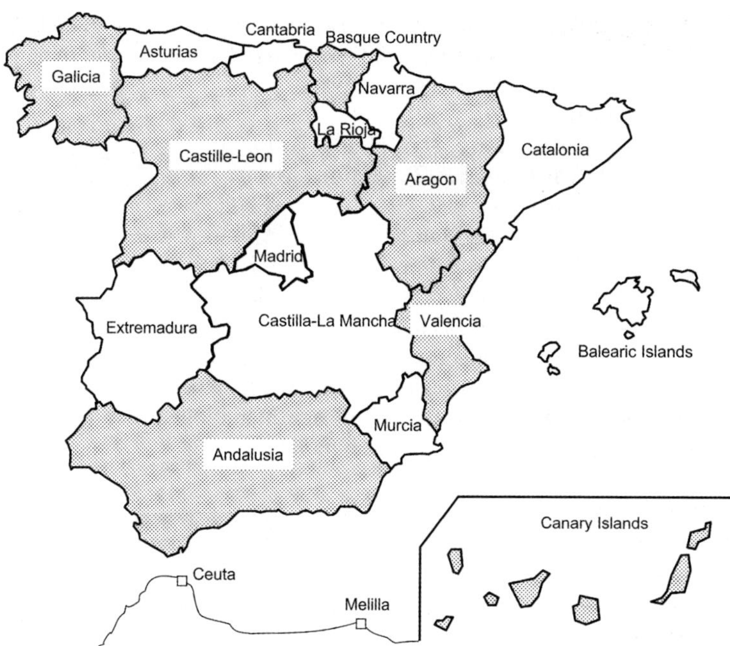

Fig. 25.1. Map showing the autonomous communities (*dotted*) where we were able to find activity in teleophthalmology

and the PCCs of eleven districts are to be connected by a teleophthalmology system (personal communication). The main purpose of these projects is the early detection of diabetic retinopathy.

25.4.2 Aragon

In 2000, the Fundacion para la Diabetes and the Hospital Universitario in Zaragoza started a pilot project for diabetic retinopathy screening using a non-mydriatic funduscopic camera in an endocrinology out-patient clinic [11, 12].

25.4.3 Basque Country (Pais Vasco)

The Hospital de Cruces, in Barakaldo, started a teleconsultation link with two PCCs in 2004 (personal communication). Digital eye fundus images are taken with a non-mydriatic funduscopic camera at the primary health care center (PCC) by a technician and sent via Internet to the hospital where they are examined by an ophthalmologist. This system is predominantly intended to detect diabetic retinopathy.

25.4.4 Canary Islands

In 1998, Ferrer-Roca et al. [5] reported a study on telemedicine using regular telephone calls in several medical specialties in the Canary Islands. In ophthalmology, 84 calls from patients were registered in 24 days. The call failed to solve the problem in 36% of cases, which required face-to-face consultation.

A paper published in 1999 [10] reported the results of a system for teleconsultation in ophthalmology running from August 1997 to January 1999. Teleconsultations could be freely requested by any person by means of a web page. The response was given via e-mail. Within this period of time 71 consultations were made, most of them related to refractive surgery and retinal diseases. Consultations originated predominantly in Spain, but teleconsultations from Central and South America were also made.

Since 1999, the Hospital de la Candelaria in Tenerife has used two funduscopic cameras located in two PCCs to collect digital retinographies to be inspected by an ophthalmologist at the hospital (personal communication). The cameras are moved periodically to different PCCs to access a larger population.

25.4.5 Castille-Leon (Castilla-Leon)

The possibility of making computer-assisted diagnoses by using computer vision algorithms may provide interesting alternatives in teleophthalmology [13–15]. In Spain, the Instituto Universitario de Oftalmobiologia Aplicada (IOBA) in Valladolid has developed a software tool that is able to detect lesions associated with diabetic retinopathy in digital retinal images. The program was tested with 20 images and showed a sensitivity of 79.6% with a mean three false positives per image [8]. Seven hundred copies of this software were freely distributed among general practitioners.

In 1999 the same institution started a pilot project for diabetic retinopathy screening in rural areas of Spain to improve the ability of GPs to detect diabetic retinopathy [16, 17]. For this, the GPs were trained to obtain mydriatic fundus photographs in diabetic patients and send them in real-time or store-and-forward mode through a private ISDN network using standard e-mail software to be reviewed by an ophthalmologist at the IOBA.

A teleophthalmology project linking the IOBA and the Instituto Oftalmologico Nacional of Angola has been announced in the web page of this institution (last updated about four years ago). However, we were unable to find further published information on this project.

25.4.6 Galicia

Since 1999 in Galicia, there has been a direct teleophthalmology link between the Complejo Hospitalario Universitario in Santiago de Compostela and a PCC where a non-mydriatic fuduscopic camera is used to capture retinal images. A second PCC was included in 2002. The images are sent via intranet to the hospital to be inspected by an ophthalmologist, who sends back the diagnosis to the general practitioner at the PCC [4, 6]. This experience is reported in more detail below. A similar system has recently been used between the Instituto Gallego de Oftalmologia in Santiago de Compostela and a PCC located in the northern part of Galicia. In addition, a project to validate teleophthalmology for diabetic retinopathy screening was carried out in 2002 at the Complejo Hospitalario Universitario in Santiago de Compostela [7].

25.4.7 Valencia

The Fundacion Jorge Alio in Alicante developed a screening program for ocular diseases including anterior and posterior segments using digital image techniques. The images were stored for later analysis. However, the images of those cases which were considered to have a severe problem were sent to an ophthalmologist for inspection using regular e-mail [18].

25.5 Teleophthalmology Between a Primary Care Center and a Reference Hospital

Since 1999 there has been a teleophthalmology link between a PCC (Centro de Salud de Vite) and a reference hospital (Complejo Hospitalario Universitario de Santiago de Compostela) in the Community of Galicia [6]. Three years later a second PCC (Centro de Salud de Muros) was also linked to the hospital. In the Centro de Salud de Vite, located in a suburban area, five GPs delivering medical care to a population of about 9,000 adults (older than 14) participated in the program. In the Centro de Salud de Muros, located in a rural area, six GPs delivering medical care to about 7,500 adults participated in the program.

25.5.1 Diabetes and Hypertension

Eye fundus images are obtained with a non-mydriatic fundus camera, compressed as JPEG files and sent for diagnosis to an ophthalmologist at the hospital using a store-and-forward mode. For this, specific software was built by the Computing Department of the local public health system (SERGAS) of the Community of Galicia (Fig. 25.2).

In 2004, 391 teleconsultations were made involving 346 patients. The reasons for requesting a teleconsultation were focused on reaching

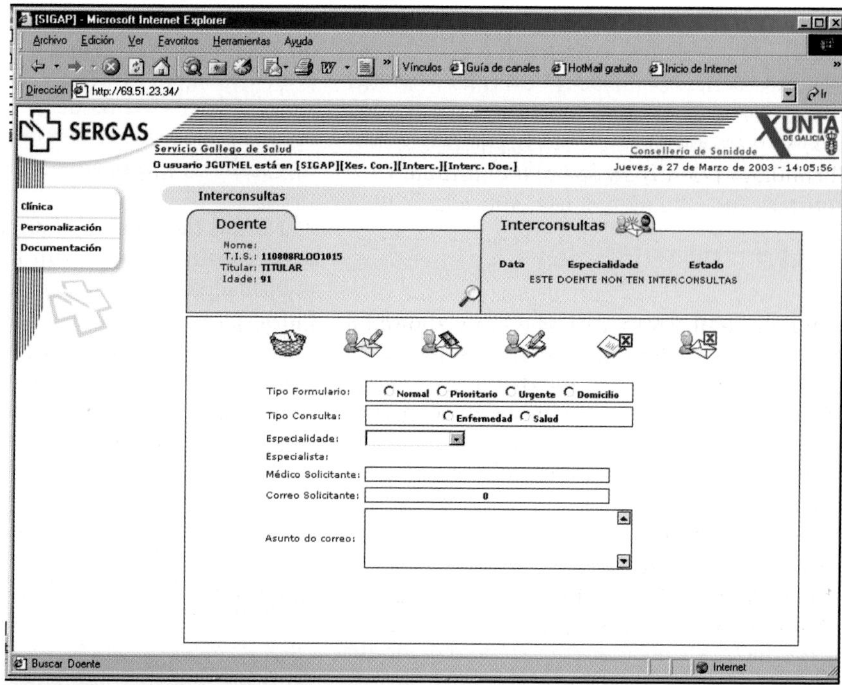

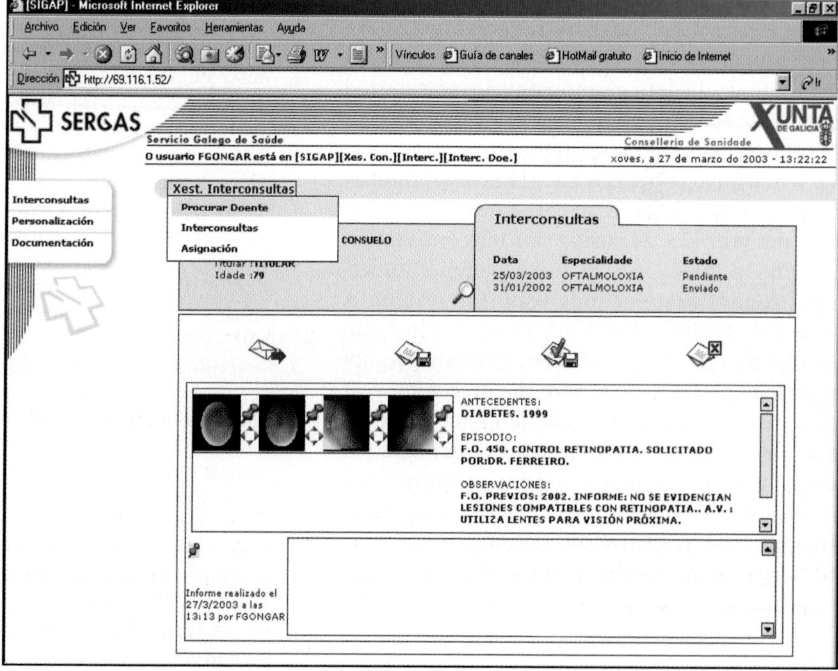

Fig. 25.2. Computer window available for teleconsultation in ophthalmology as seen by the general practitioner who requests the consultation (*top*) and the ophthalmologist (*bottom*). This software uses a store-and-forward mode of transference and automatically controls the transferring of information between the appropriate doctors. It also meets the legal requirements for preserving the confidentiality of the data. The system is being used by several specialties

diabetics with concurrent systemic hypertension (31%), only systemic hypertension (41%), only diabetes (25%), and other reasons (3%). The large number of patients with systemic hypertension occurred because a study on hypertensive retinopathy was also being carried out.

25.5.2 Diabetic Patients

The estimated direct cost of diabetes in 2002 ranged from 2.4–2.67 billion EUR in Spain [19]. Since screening for diabetic retinopathy is one of the most cost-effective health interventions [20], this system was predominantly intended to assess this condition. The reliability of teleophthalmology for detecting and grading diabetic retinopathy has been demonstrated in a recent study [7].

The prevalence of known diabetic patients in the population served by the two PCCs is 6%, which is similar to that reported for the adult population in Spain by the 1997 Spanish National Health Survey [19, 21]. About 55% of diabetic patients do not have retinopathy [22]. In the Spanish National Health System the patients with known diabetic retinopathy are transferred directly to an ophthalmologist [4] who schedules the subsequent follow-up appointments.

We targeted patients without known retinopathy should have at least one eye fundus examination per year [23, 24] using our teleconsultation system. In 2004, 36% of these patients underwent fundus examinations with our system. A recent study showed that in a rural area in Spain similar to ours, 73% of diabetic patients had not received ophthalmology care the preceding year [25]. Therefore our teleophthalmology system was able to increase the number of diabetic patients who received eye fundus examinations. We expect that in the near future teleophthalmology systems such as ours could provide a full coverage for eye fundus examination in diabetic patients.

25.6 Conclusions

Telemedical techniques in ophthalmology are currently being used in Spain. Our search shows that virtually all projects and settings are based on non-mydriatic cameras that obtain digital retinal images, which are then transmitted in store-and-forward mode to be examined by an ophthalmologist. The aim in most cases is to detect diabetic retinopathy in known diabetic patients.

Despite the number of projects carried out on teleophthalmology in Spain, there are still too few published studies to reach general conclusions. However, we believe that teleophthalmology is a useful and feasible technique, at least for diabetic retinopathy screening. In Spain, as in many other countries, this disease fuels the implementation of teleophthalmology as a tool to manage ocular diseases. Unfortunately, although early treatment of diabetic retinopathy is of proven value in reversing or preventing visual loss, the infrastructure to detect appropriate patients for treatment is not yet universally available.

References

1. Gonzalez F, Castro AF (2005) Publication output in telemedicine in Spain. J Telemed Telecare (in press)
2. Moser PL, Hauffe H, Lorenz IH, Hager M, Tiefenthaler W, Lorenz HM, Mikuz G, Soegner P, Kolbitsch C (2004) Publication output in telemedicine during the period January 1964 to July 2003. J Telemed Telecare 10:72–77
3. Perednia DA, Allen A (1995) Telemedicine technology and clinical applications. JAMA 273:483–488
4. Gonzalez F, Iglesias R, Gomez-Ulla F, Fernandez MI (2003) Telemedicine reduces referral of diabetic patients to ophthalmologists. J Telemed Telecare 9:307–308
5. Ferrer-Roca O, Estevez M, Gomez E (1998) The environment for telemedicine in the Canary Islands. J Telemed Telecare 4:161–167
6. Gonzalez F, Iglesias R, Suarez A, Gomez-Ulla F, Perez R (2001) Teleophthalmology link between a primary care centre and a reference hospital. Med Inform Internet Med 26:251–263
7. Gomez-Ulla F, Fernandez MI, Gonzalez F, Rey P, Rodriguez M, Rodriguez-Cid MJ, Casanueva FF, Tome MA, Garcia-Tobio J, Gude F (2002) Digital retinal images and teleophthalmology for detecting and grading diabetic retinopathy. Diabetes Care 25:1384–1389
8. Sanchez Gutierrez CI, Lopez Galvez MI, Hornero Sanchez R, Poza Crespo J (2004) Retinal image

analysis to detect lesions associated with diabetic retinopathy. Arch Soc Esp Oftalmol 79:623–628
9. Grande Baos C (1998) Teleophthalmology: telemedicine in ophthalmology. Arch Soc Esp Oftalmol 73:99–102
10. Abreu Gonzalez R, Abreu Reyes JA, Ferrer-Roca O (1999) Ophthalmologic advice on Internet. Arch Soc Can Oftalmol 10:125–130
11. Faure E, Marcuello C, Mateo A (2002) Estudio epidemiologico de la retinopatía diabetica en la ciudad de Zaragoza mediante retinografo no midriatico digital. Avances en Diabetología 18(1):30
12. Faure E, Mateo A, Marcuello C, Roche MJ, Cristóbal JA (2004) Proyecto RetinDiab2. Utilidad del retinografo TRC-NW65 en la clasificacion y seguimiento de la retinopatía diabetica. Sociedad Española de Endocrinología y Nutrición 51(1):15
13. Gardner GG, Keating D, Williamson TH, Elliott AT (1996) Automatic detection of diabetic retinopathy using an artificial neural network: a screening tool. Brit J Ophthalmol 80:940–944
14. Madjarov BD, Berger JW (2000) Automated, real time extraction of fundus images from slit-lamp fundus biomicroscope video image sequences. Brit J Ophthalmol 84:645–647
15. Teng T, Lefley M, Claremont D (2002) Progress towards automated diabetic ocular screening: a review of image analysis and intelligent systems for diabetic retinopathy. Med Biol Eng Comput 40:2–13
16. Lopez M, Velilla S, Diez A, Sanchez P, Pastor JC (2000) A pilot study of telemedicine in diabetic retinopathy screening. ARVO 2000 Meeting, IOVS (S647) Abstract 3436-B534
17. Lopez-Galvez MI, Hornero R, Acebes-Garcia M, Calonge T (2003) Teleophthalmology for diabetic retinopathy screening in a rural area of Spain. In: American Telemedicine Association 8th Annual Meeting, Abstract 33
18. Alio JL, Rodriguez Prats JL, Ayala Espinosa MJ, Schimchack Ugartemendia P, Galal A, Khalil H, Pacheco JJ (2005) Campaña para la prevención de ceguera en la 3ª edad. Poster 1263, XXV Pan-American Congress of Ophthalmology, Santiago, Chile
19. Oliva J, Lobo F, Molina B, Monereo S (2004) Direct health care costs of diabetic patients in Spain. Diabetes Care 27:2616–2621
20. Javitt JC, Aiello LP (1996) Cost-effectiveness of detecting and treating diabetic retinopathy. Ann Intern Med 124:164–169
21. Encuesta Nacional de Salud (1997) Centro de Investigaciones Sociologicas. Madrid
22. Fernandez-Vigo J, Sanchez Macho J, Diaz Rey A, Barros J, Tome M, Bueno J (1993) The prevalence of retinopathy in northwest Spain: an epidemiological study of diabetic retinopathy in Galicia. Acta Ophthalmol Scand 71:22–26
23. American Diabetes Association (1998) Diabetic retinopathy. Diabetes Care 21:157–159
24. Kohner EM, Porta M (1991) Protocols for screening and treatment of diabetic retinopathy in Europe. Eur J Ophthalmol 1:45–54
25. Lopez IM, Diez A, Velilla S, Rueda A, Alvarez A, Pastor CJ (2002) Prevalence of diabetic retinopathy and eye care in a rural area of Spain. Ophthalmic Epidemiol 9:205–214

Chapter 26

Telemedicine to Improve the Quality and Cost Efficiency of Providing Eye Care

26

Vladimir Kazinov

The following key concepts about just-in-time telemedicine and physicians interaction and communication are covered in the chapter:

This chapter addresses the following

Key Concepts:

- Every physician in charge of treatment, diagnosis, or decision making and surgery should receive relevant medical consultation in the workplace, and on an as needed basis.
- Physicians can consult with and train distant colleagues.
- Medical data is available in a form that is quite similar to that derived from face-to-face interaction with the patient, or with the medical equipment.
- A simple user interface, high usability rate, and ease of learning, is available.
- It is possible to receive relevant data from diverse equipment and transmit it over varied communication channels.
- An entirely new level of interaction can be established between physicians of various specialities.

26.1 Introduction

Public health reforms aimed at improving the quality and cost-efficiency of disease prophylaxis, diagnosis, treatment, and surgery are underway in almost every country. In developing countries, these efforts are noted by a focus on financial expenditure for public health in the budget. Improved health care in such countries is ultimately the result of high standards of medical care combined with rational and well conceived financing of the public health service. The growing percentage of middle-aged and aged citizens whose health care needs are greater than those of the younger generation should also be taken into consideration.

Public demand for improvement in the quality and timeliness of medical aid can present an insurmountable obstacle for the budgets of developing countries with limited ability to finance the public health service. Without changing the structure of which services the health budget currently covers, further increases are impractical. *Just-in-time* telemedicine may be an effective tool for improving the quality, timeliness, and cost-efficiency of medical care.

26.2 Telemedicine Just-in-Time

The major principles of telemedicine just-in-time operation include the following ideas:

1. Every physician in charge of treatment, diagnosis, or decision making and surgery should obtain relevant medical consultation, at the workplace, in the just-in-time format. This means that the information should come neither before nor after it is required, but rather, when it is needed, in the required amount, and at an appropriate quality. Only under those conditions will the effectiveness of those providing medical care be maximized, without adding unnecessary labor for physicians and other care providers. Additional

efforts of physicians to obtain or provide telemedicine consultations would unnecessarily increase their labor.

2. The expert physician should consult and train distant colleagues, making use of the availability of acquired medical data. Medical data should be available in a form that is as similar as possible to that gained in face-to-face interaction with the patient or the medical equipment. Even slight deviations in the quality or quantity of transferred medical data may dramatically increase the workload of expert medical consultants.
3. The cost of telemedicine systems used by physicians and consultants should not exceed 10% of the cost of medical instrumentation at diagnostic centers or surgical suites.
4. Telemedicine systems to be used by physicians, specialty consultants, and public health service managers should offer a simple user interface, high usability rate, and ease of learning. If a system is designed correctly, health care providers will realize that telemedicine does not need to add to their workload. Rather, it can ease their patient-care duties, and should be as familiar as ordinary medical equipment.
5. Every medical institution should be equipped with local telemedicine networks linking doctors' workplaces. Local telemedicine networks should be set up in a staged program, with a gradual increase in the number and variety of workplaces. A local telemedicine network should become a symbol of progress in hospital-based medical information systems. The process of setting up telemedicine networks at clinics must be accompanied by adaptation of the telemedicine systems to individual doctors and management requirements at specific medical institutions.
6. Telemedicine systems should be structured so they are capable of receiving relevant data from diverse medical equipment, and transmitting it with appropriate quality over varied communication channels.
7. Every local telemedicine network should have the capacity to access global telemedicine networks using appropriate communication channels. The global telemedicine network should be constructed based on the telecommunication and information infrastructure established by leading communication providers.
8. Telemedicine centers at local and regional clinics should perform mainly dispatching and technical functions within the telemedicine operation. They should also be responsible for record keeping of telemedicine sessions. Data on telemedicine consultations and other events using telemedicine technologies should be easily available to insurance or other public health companies or agencies that finance public health services.
9. Insurance companies and agencies that administrate or financially support clinics should undertake continuous financial analysis of the telemedicine clinic network operation. Such oversight is necessary in order to inform decisions for further development of the telemedicine system.

26.3 Telemedicine Just-in-Time in Ophthalmology

Local telemedicine networks at ophthalmology clinics should be available at the workplace of various subspecialties. This allows the construction of an entirely new system of interaction among such medical staff.

26.3.1 System of Interaction

In order to assess the advantages of this system of physician interaction, the existing system in most ophthalmologic clinics should be analyzed. The current system of interaction between physicians and patients in a clinic implies a succession of non-intersecting (or minimally intersecting) actions made by physicians of various specialties. This succession of actions with the patient implies that the patient moves sequentially in time from one physician to another.

The case history, accompanied by relevant and accumulating data, produces the base of interaction between each physician and the patient. The interaction begins with the registration office, moves through time from one analysis to another, and from one treatment method or surgical operation to another. Ultimately, the patient should arrive at the last action, i.e., discharge from the clinic.

26.3.2 Colleague Consultation

Normally, every physician performing a given action with the patient is guided by the results of their own interaction with the patient, as well as occasionally by the results of interactions with previous doctors. Prior to formulating their results, however, ophthalmologists of various specializations sometimes consult with other doctors who have previously had interaction with the patient. For instance, prior to performing surgery, a physician may consult with the person who performed an ultrasonic examination of the eye. However, these consultations are suspended, in that they are held after the ultrasonic diagnostic physician has performed all the tests with the patient and formulated a conclusion; typically, this opinion is given without a repeated ultrasonic test or lengthy re-examination of results. Similarly, a pathologist consults with the surgeon who performed a tumor removal, but the consultation is usually held after completion of the operation, and often nothing can be changed without additional surgery.

26.3.3 New Level of Interaction

If the ophthalmologic clinic is equipped with a telemedicine network (Fig. 26.1), an entirely new level of interaction is established among physicians of various specialities. This provides an opportunity to establish a system of direct mutual consultations of physicians, during their interaction with the patient. This can be done without any movement of physicians from their workplace. For example, while conducting a relevant ultrasound test, the physician should be able to contact another doctor through the telemedicine terminal and network of the clinic. They could show these diagnostic results to the operating surgeon in real time.

Although watching the diagnostic study from another workplace, the surgeon is still directly involved in the session, and can record, store images and sequences of interest, and exchange opinions with the ultrasound technician or ophthalmologist. Thus the surgeon can affect and understand the results prior to surgery. If the patient is later directed to the specialist surgeon, that person has already encountered the ultrasonic diagnostics, and has more accurate and jointly developed information for the forthcoming surgery. Likewise, similar interactions with the ophthalmic surgeon and pathologist can be arranged for conducting intraoperative histological or cytological consultations.

26.3.4 Provider-Patient Interaction

The illustration in Fig. 26.1 presents the existing scheme of interaction among physicians in an ophthalmologic clinic when every physician performs actions with the patient (blue line illustrates the actions of each doctor) and formulates the results of their actions (red line shows the result of each performing physician's action). The second scheme shows that within the telemedicine network of an ophthalmologic clinic an opportunity may arise, and in some cases a real necessity, to consult other physicians in the just-in-time mode. In this latter scheme, the result of the physician–patient interaction is generated with the participation of other physicians. The results of such interaction are made available at an earlier stage to those physicians to whom the patient will be directed at a later time.

26.4 DiViSy Telemedicine Systems for Providing Just-in-Time Consultations

DiViSy TM21 (manufacturer DiViSy Group – www.divisy.com) (Figs. 26.3 and 26.4) telemedicine systems belong to a third generation of telemedicine systems.

Their capabilities and characteristics take into account the operating experience of the two previous generations, DiViSy PM1 and DiViSy TM2000. The newest system offers the following features:

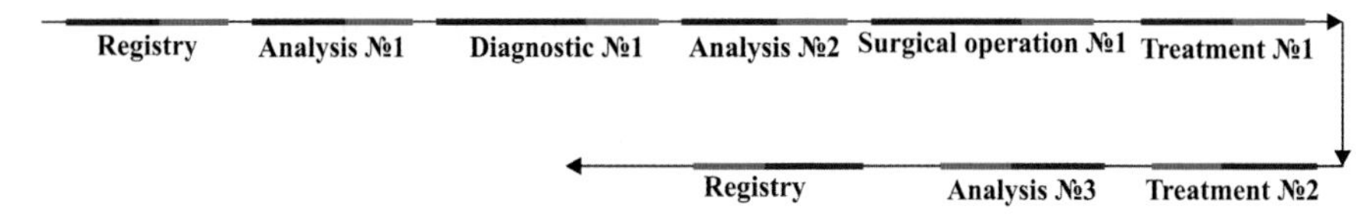

Diagnostic and treatment of patient in hospitals
Existing process of diagnostic and treatment in hospital

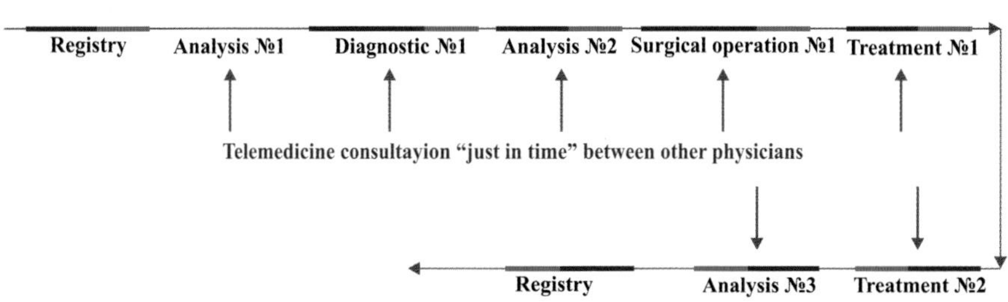

26

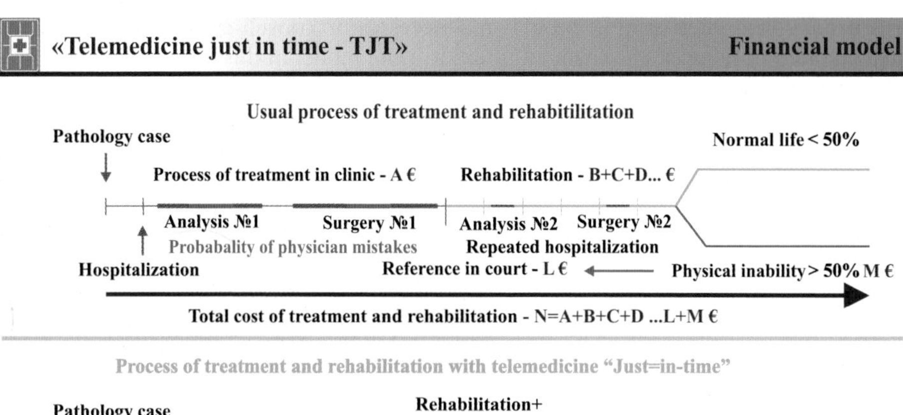

Fig. 26.1. Scheme of interaction among doctors in an ophthalmologic clinic

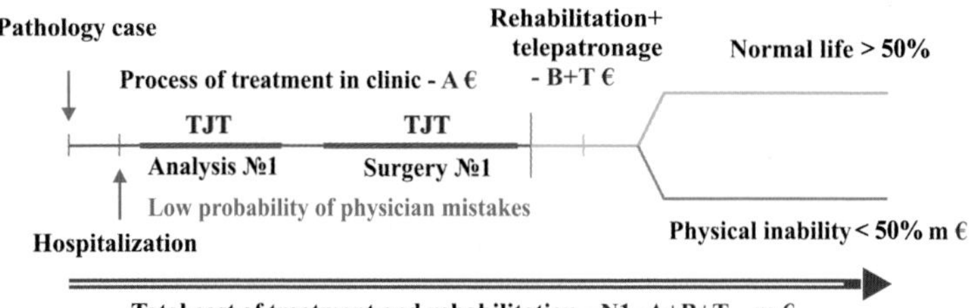

Fig. 26.2. Financial model of just-in-time telemedicine operation

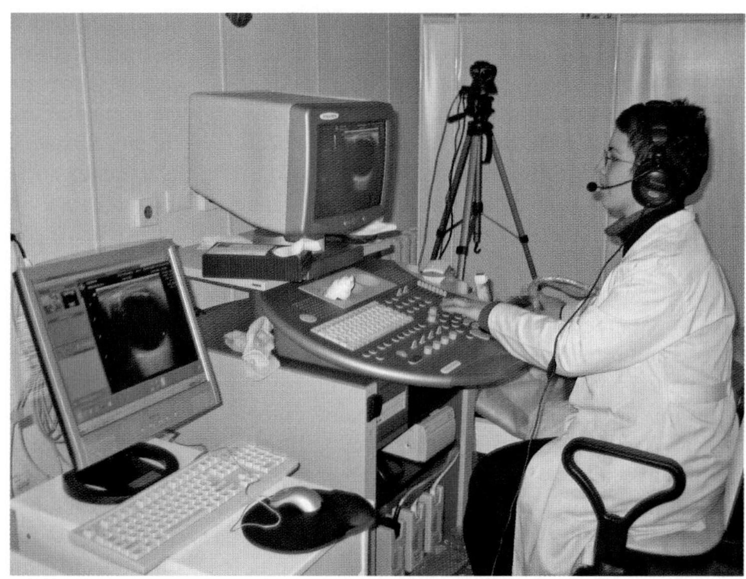

Fig. 26.3. Telemedicine system DiViSy TM21 in ultrasound diagnostic room. All medical information is transferred to the local telemedicine network for consultations and distance medical education

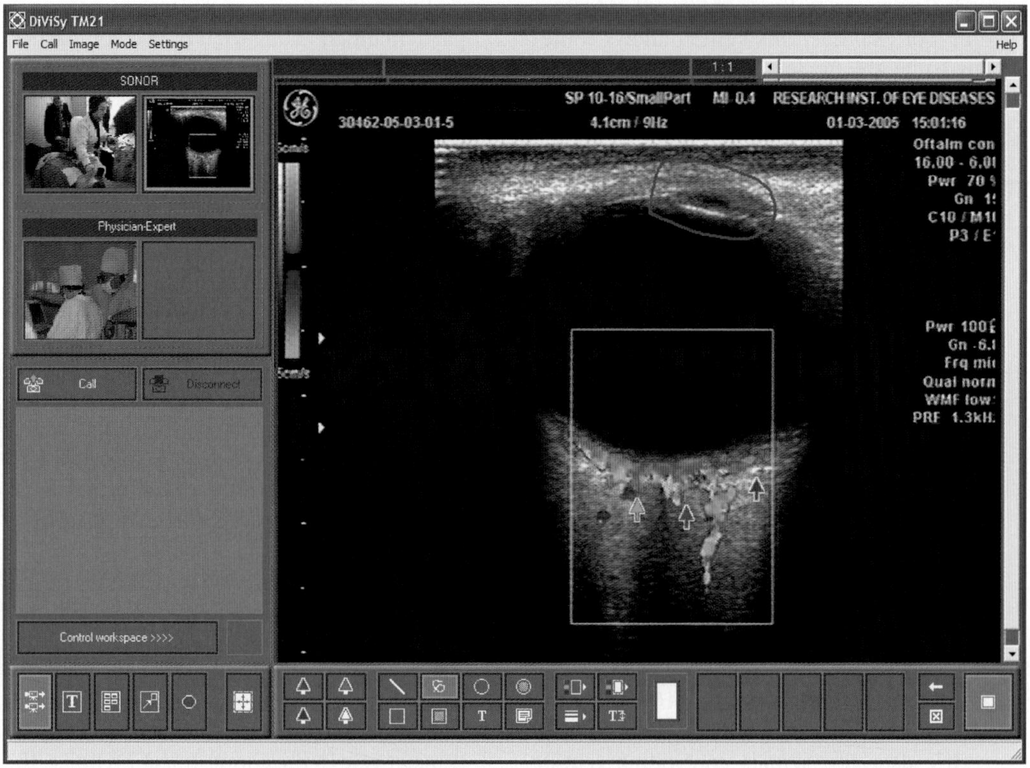

Fig. 26.4. Interface of telemedicine system DiViSy TM21 during a telemedicine consultation between physicians in an ophthalmology clinic. Ultrasound scanning of an eyeball and an orbit. A grey scale mode in combination with color Doppler. A color image of vascular system of an eyeball

26

1. Medical data communication via five channels simultaneously – two parallel channels for medical video information, one channel for communicating medical telemetry data and signals from local and remote medical instruments, a duplex audio channel, and a channel for text data communication. The number of data transmission channels can be optionally increased. The channels themselves have the following characteristics (a–d):

a. Two channels for medical video data transmission provide entry, digitization and transmission of medical video images having resolution up to 768×576 bits (for analog video cameras), and up to the maximum resolution of digital video and photo cameras (see Fig. 26.2). Two parallel channels for medical video data transmission and display are required. This allows the remote consulting physician or trainee in the remote medical learning system to simultaneously see the main image, as well as additional information. For example, this system allows someone to be able to see not only the image of the surgical field, but also the image of the operating room and actions of the surgical team as well. Similarly, while conducting an ultrasonic investigation, such a technological framework makes it possible for the remote physician to not only see the image transmitted from the ultrasonic scanning device, but also an image showing the layout of the ultrasonic sensor on the patient's body. This effectively allows the consulting physician to not only provide consultation, but also to modify the diagnostic process to provide the most useful information. From an engineering viewpoint, both channels are equivalent and provide medical imaging data from 768×576 bits resolution (for analog sources of medical video images) to the maximum possible resolution of digital sources of medical video images. Video codecs for medical images can be selected from a menu of formats including MJPEG, H.263, MPEG4, and MPEG2.

b. The channel for communicating medical telemetric data and signals controlling remote medical instruments is capable of connecting medical equipment having digital outputs for telemetric data. It can also be used for the administration of local and remote medical instrumentation (controlled through video cameras, robotic microscopes for pathological consultation, and in the future, robotic remote surgery).

c. The duplex audio channel is intended for audio exchange among remote participants of telemedicine consultancy or remote learning. High quality audio is provided by the addition of audio compression rates 8, 16, 32, 64, 128 KB/sec such as G.711, G.728, and G.723 into the telemedicine systems.

d. The channel for text data communication is intended for real-time text dialog between participants of telemedicine sessions.

2. The DiViSy TM21 telemedicine system offers a desktop feature through which joint analysis and medical image processing can be done. At the discretion of any participant of the telemedicine session, the image currently of most interest is placed on the desktop. Using digital pointers, with each participant choosing their own color, participants of a telemedicine session can illustrate specific areas on the image of greatest interest. Using such integrated digital features, the consultant doctor can show the boundaries of a tumor, or the curve along which a resection is needed. A record of images with all the pointers can be stored by each participant of a telemedicine session.

3. The DiViSy TM21 telemedicine system allows consulting and remote medical learning not only for a single remote doctor or patient, but also for many, performed in video conferencing mode. To that end, there is a DiViSy TM21VS telemedicine server. The telemedicine server controls data flow during the sessions, and runs video conferencing sessions among several remote users.

4. Telemedicine systems such as DiViSy TM21 are intended for operation with virtually any communication link, including telephone, radio, cellular, fiberoptic, satellite, and incorporate data encryption. The medical data transmission rate is limited to the data transfer rate in the communication links. The minimum rate at which data is transmitted through the DiViSy TM21 telemedicine system during tests is 9,600 bit/s (Global System

for Mobile Communication (GSM) cellular channels), with the maximum rate being 20 Mbit/s. The system offers some operational settings to select the quality of video and audio information, depending on the real data transfer rate through the channel.

26.5 Financial Model of Just-in-Time Telemedicine Operating at Ophthalmology Clinics

Figure 26.2 represents a financial model of the just-in-time telemedicine operation at an ophthalmologic clinic or a hospital.

The upper part of the figure presents the existing model of diagnostics, treatment, surgery and rehabilitation of the hospitalized patient. This model depicts the existing system not using modern telemedicine technology.

26.5.1 Description of the Model of Existing Treatment Process

The following describes stages of the existing treatment process:

1. First stage: primary inspection and appointment for hospitalization
2. econd stage: laboratory and clinical analyses, and making a diagnosis. This procedure is prone to medical errors for various reasons (complex disease, atypical for the given region, outdated medical instrumentation, poor quality of consumables, breakdown in the procedure of running analyses and diagnostic processes, etc.). When a medical error arises or is suspected, an inadequate treatment plan is constructed or incorrect data is sent to the surgeon, ensuring an inadequate surgical plan.
3. Third stage: treatment or surgical operation. With inadequate data analysis and oversight, the probability of undertaking optimal treatment or surgical operation is quite low. Indeed, the probable need for conducting repeated analyses or surgical operations increases.
4. Fourth stage: remedial action, during which these analyses or surgical operations will be conducted, either at the same or another medical institution. Real costs therefore increase.
5. Fifth stage: making a decision of disability, the probability of which in the case of medical errors is rather high.
6. Sixth stage: rehabilitation process under disability
7. Seventh stage: legal action and defrayal

Based on the above stages, the costs for treatment and rehabilitation would be as follows:

N = A (cost of analyses, including the cost of surgical operation) + B (cost of repeated analyses and repeated treatment, including repeated surgical operation) + C (cost of analyses at the diagnostics center) + M (invalidity benefit) + L (cost of legal action). The number of components in this formula can only increase.

The lower part of the Fig. 26.2 presents a financial model of diagnosis, treatment, surgical operation, and rehabilitation of the patient with the use of DiViSy just-in-time telemedicine systems.

26.5.2 Description of the Model of Treatment Process Making Use of Telemedicine

The following describes stages of the treatment process using telemedicine:

1. First stage: primary inspection and appointment for hospitalization to the admission office
2. Second stage: laboratory and clinical analyses, making a diagnosis. Within the procedure, necessary telemedicine consultations increase the probability of making the correct diagnosis.
3. Third stage: treatment or surgical operation. With adequate data analysis, the probability of undertaking the optimal treatment or surgical operation is very high. In the course of treatment or consideration of surgery, telemedicine consultations are also held, which further increase the probability of a favorable outcome.
4. Fourth stage: normal process of rehabilitation

5. Fifth stage: discharge of the patient, with the disability minimized
6. Sixth stage: missing
7. Seventh stage: missing

Based on the above stages, the costs for treatment and rehabilitation would be as follows:

N1 = A + a (cost of analyses and treatment, including the cost of surgical operation, where *a* is the cost of telemedicine consultations, which is significantly lower than the cost of *A*) + C (cost of scheduled rehabilitation) + T (cost of in-house monitoring to accelerate the process of final rehabilitation).

26.6 Findings

Comparative analysis of the two models shows that N1 is significantly lower than N. In addition, the duration of a patient's stay at the medical institution is shorter, and the rate of bed turnover in the hospital increases. The costs for sick-list payment also goes down; the patient also achieves a better clinical result sooner, and returns to the workplace within the shortest possible time.

Even at ophthalmology clinics using advanced medical technologies, the difference between N1 and N can be at least 15% of the clinic's total budget.

References

1. Kazinov V, Danilov A (1996) Facilities of DiViSy technology for telepatology seminar for microscopy of Carl Zeiss in medicine, Moscow
2. Kazinov V (1997) Computer systems for digital video - DiViSy. Facilities of applications in Russian telemedicine projects Computer Technology in Medicine No 1, Moscow
3. Kazinov V (1998) Moscow information network of teleoncology base DiViSy Technology. In: 11th International Symposium of Space Biology and Medicine, Moscow, June 1998
4. Kazinov V (1998) Teleoncology in Moscow symposium days of Bavaria in Moscow Medical Technical, Moscow, October 1998
5. Kazinov V (1998) Show of facilities DiViSy technology for telemedicine fair at 17th International Cancer Congress, Rio-de-Janeiro, Brazil, August 1998
6. Kazinov V (1998) Show of facilities DiViSy technology for Telemedicine Fair Health Care, Moscow, December 1998
7. Kazinov V, Danilov A, Pokrovski K (1998) DiViSy telemedicine technology in Moscow clinical practice II, International Telemedicine Symposium, Moscow, 1998
8. Kazinov V, Chissov PV, Danilov A, Sokolov V, Frank G (1999) Perfect DiViSy technology for video network in medicine: the impact of telemedicine on health care management. IOS Press, Amsterdam
9. Kazinov V, Danilov A, Fedorov V, Pokrovski K (1999) DiViSy telemedicine technology and equipment for diagnostic, treatment and surgery. In: Symposium in Frame of Days of Moscow, Bavaria, 1999
10. Kazinov V, Danilov A, Fedorov V, Pokrovski K (2000)General aspects of transmission of medical images in real time telemedicine consulting. In: Proceedings of the III International Moscow Telemedicine Symposium 2000, Moscow
11. Kazinov V (2000) Medical VideoNetwork in Clinical practice, Medical Herald in Moscow, 2000
12. Kazinov V, Danilov A, Fedorov V, Pokrovski K (2000) Implementation of DiViSy technology in clinical practice ITU, SUB-Regional seminar on telemedicine, Geneva, 2000
13. Kazinov V, Shapiro N, Mistcheriakova T, et al. (2002) Computer technology in cytology laboratory in Central Railway Clinic, Live issue in railway medicine, 2000, Moscow
14. Kazinov V (2001) Telemedicine systems in surgery and neurosurgery. In: Symposium: Days of Bavaria in Moscow, Moscow, July 2001
15. Kazinov V, Timin E, Volinsky U (2001) Facilities and limitation in telemedicine. IST, Moscow, 2001
16. Kazinov V, Venedictov D (2001) General facilities of telemedicine in Russia Telemedicine conference. Vladikavkaz, November 2001
17. Kazinov V (2001) Actual problems of preparing and transmission of medical images in real time: first scientific virtual conference on telemedicine in clinical informatics.
Donetsk, Ukraine, 2001
18. Kazinov V (2001) New video technology for education, science and business. In: Proceedings of the III International congress of concentrations in CIS, Moscow, 2001
19. Kazinov V (2001) Distance education in medicine: information technology in health care, 2001
20. Kazinov V, Polyakov S (2003) Telemedicine network of Moscow health department base DiViSy telemedicine systems. In: The 2nd European Congress: Achievements in Space Medicine into Health Care Practice and Industry. Berlin, Germany, 2003
21. Kazinov V, Serebriakov V, Kulagin M, Ilushin G (2005) Telemedicine project Beslan-Moscow: scien-

tific seminar of Russian Academy of Science. Moscow, 2005
22. Kazinov V (2005) DiViSy telemedicine systems for oncology. In: Proceedings of the International Oncology Conference, Kazan, Russia, 2005
23. Kazinov V (2005) DiViSy telemedicine systems for remote medical consultation and education. In:The 6th International conference, Contemporary condition and perspectives for development of the Internet in Russia, September 2005, Moscow
24. Kazinov V (2005) DiViSy telemedicine systems of the fourth generation as the tool for improvement of quality and financial efficiency of healthcare services. In: The Third European Congress, Achievements in Space Medicine into Health Care Practice and Industry. Berlin, Germany, 2005

Chapter 27

Cataract and Refractive Surgery Post-operative Care: Teleophthalmology's Challenge in Argentina

27

Giselle Ricur, Roberto Zaldivar, Maria Gabriela Batiz

This chapter addresses the following

Key Concepts:

- Post-operative follow-up care is as crucial and decisive as the surgery itself.
- In many countries where access to health care, cost inflation, and uneven geographic distribution of quality care are common problems, adequate post-operative care is becoming an issue.
- A teleophthalmology service was set up at Instituto Zaldivar, an ophthalmic ambulatory surgical center, to enhance its outreach to patients who had difficulty visiting the Institute for post-operative eye care.
- A video conference system was established with a remote branch to evaluate the efficiency of post-operative follow-up care through teleconsultation.
- Teleconsultation service was subsequently expanded to include first consultations, pre-operative screening, and regular eye care follow-up visits.
- Camera resolution and high speed connections were crucial factors in assessing adequate post-operative control.

27.1 Introduction

Post-operative follow-up care in any medical discipline is as crucial and decisive as the surgical act in itself; if this were not so, successful surgeries may result in undesired and complicated outcomes. To ensure quality care, follow-up to surgery requires programmed visits, strict follow-up protocols, and ad hoc medication, as well as experienced examining physicians [1].

In many countries where access to health care for large segments of the population, cost inflation, and uneven geographic distribution of quality care and physicians, are common facts, adequate post-operative care is becoming an issue. Most patients make an effort to reach high-end or sophisticated surgical centers in search of treatment for their afflictions, but rarely comply with short- and mid-term follow-up visits, much less for the long-term. How often have we heard patients complain or say: I feel great, so why do I have to go back? It's too far and I don't have time to go by your office; I can't leave work again. It's too expensive to travel back for follow-up, etc.

Effective follow-up is probably one of the major challenges that telemedicine has to overcome. As Rashid L Bashsur clearly described in one of his editorial comments in the American Telemedicine Association's official journal, "access to care has been a direct effect of telemedicine. In fact, to date the presumed increase in access to care for remote population has been the cornerstone of telemedicine development" [2]. Consequently, the use of electronic information and telecommunication technologies to provide or support long-distance clinical health care has been rapidly extending.

While not all of the medical specialties have found their place in this new field, Ophthalmology greatly benefits from it, due to its high volume of diagnostic and follow-up digital imagery [3–5]. Telemedicine offers almost endless possibilities for transmitting imagery, whether still or real-time, depending on the network and communication infrastructure available.

Many reports have been published concerning teleophthalmology models that focus mostly on posterior segment assessments with asynchronous, or store-and-forward, models for diabetic retinopathy or glaucoma screening. Little has been written, however, about synchronous, or real-time consultations, especially in cataract and refractive surgery [6–16].

At the Instituto Zaldivar, an ophthalmic ambulatory surgical center located in Mendoza, Argentina, a teleophthalmology service (focused mainly on phaco-refractive patients) was established in 2001. The initial objective was to enhance its outreach to patients, who, due to the economic and social crisis of the time, had difficulty visiting the Institute for proper post-operative eye care.

27.2 Teleophthalmology Models in Cataract and Refractive Surgery

At first, an asynchronous (store-and-forward) model was implemented by means of an institutional web site (www.institutozaldivar.com) where patients could access standard on-line platforms for booking post-operative follow-up visits. Afterward, the system was upgraded to allow for routine appointments, second opinions, and the possibility of sending ophthalmic images (JPEG, TIFF, etc.) over the Internet. Patients could also access and print educational resources concerning comprehensive eye health care.

The second phase of the telemedicine project contemplated the use of a synchronous (real-time) model, via a video conferencing system over a VPN set up between the Institute in Mendoza and its branch in Buenos Aires.

At first, the purpose of this project was to evaluate the efficiency of short-term laser-assisted in situ keratomileusis (LASIK) post-operative follow-up care through video conference consultations or teleconsultations with real-time imagery transmission. Two main issues were emphasized:

- Physicians' concern regarding imagery resolution and the high-speed connections as crucial factors in assessing adequate post-operative controls
- Physician-patient satisfaction in a non-traditional *virtual* environment

Due to the acceptance of this new consultation modality by both the attending physicians and patients, the service was expanded shortly afterward to include initial consultations, pre-operative screening, and regular eye care follow-up visits, all by means of a hybrid model, i.e., real-time video conferencing was complemented by still imagery and diagnostic images sent previously by e-mail (Fig. 27.1).

27.2.1 Sites

The central hub and spoke sites were established in Mendoza and Buenos Aires, Argentina, respectively, in September 2001. The central hub, Instituto Zaldivar, is the ambulatory surgical eye center, and is located in the city of Mendoza in the central west part of Argentina. The peripheral examining office or remote site lies 1,100 km away on the east coast of the country, in the city of Buenos Aires (Figs. 27.2 and 27.3).

27.2.2 Telecommunication and Information Network

Both sites have their own private information technology (IT) network (intranet) with LAN-based (Local Area Network) workstations (100 Mb/s) that are currently linked to the VPN by six ISDN lines (Integrated System Digital Network: digital telephone lines) supplied by Telefónica Argentina, the local telecommunications company. There are also analog telephone lines (POTS) for voice and fax, and auxiliary communications are carried by a private radio frequency tracking network, called Movilink (a BellSouth mobile communication service).

A scheduler, clinical file and follow-up charts were developed in-house, based on pre-existing

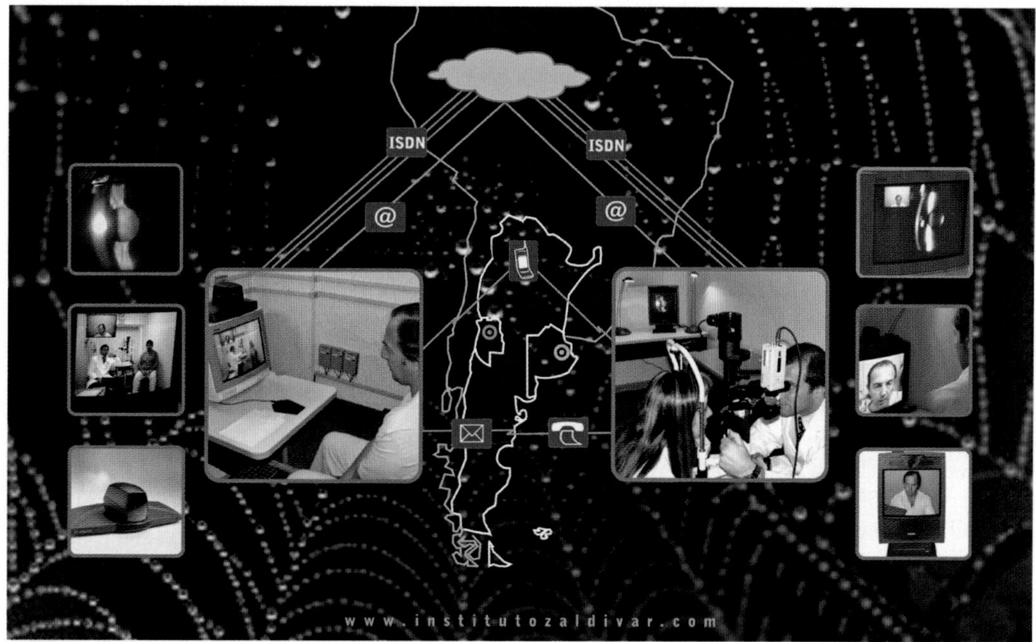

Fig. 27.1. Teleophthalmology hybrid model: the hub in Mendoza (*left*), and the remote site in Buenos Aires (*right*). ISDN: three digital telephone lines (384 kb/s), point-to-point IP connectivity (512 kb/s), private radio frequency tracking network, facsimile, private courier

ones. Although all these touch-screen electronic medical records have their databases on-line, by means of workflow applications software called *Netpack 5.0* (Symbolic System SRL, Buenos Aires, Argentina), they are also stored as a hard copy, due to local regulations requiring that all medical files be kept on paper and signed-in by hand (Fig. 27.4). Therefore, patients' records can travel back and forth from the sites through four different channels:

- On-line access (VPN – intranet)
- E-mail (scanned or forwarded)
- Shipped by private courier in order to comply with federal regulations
- Faxed, for backup reasons or non-programmed emergency consults

27.2.3 Teleconsultation Examining Rooms

The examining and consultant's offices were intentionally designed in the following ways:

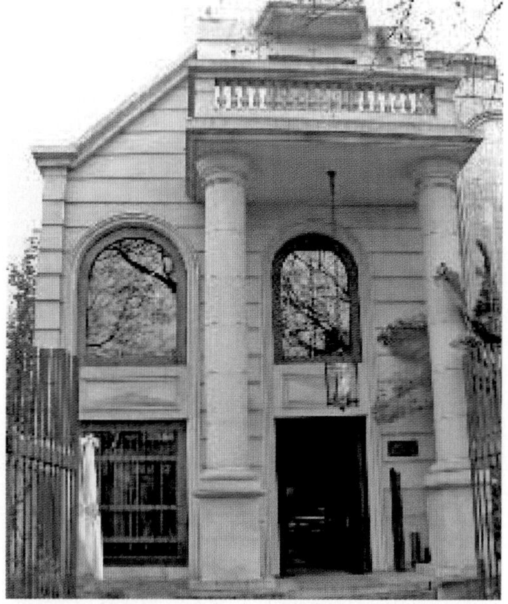

Fig. 27.2. Instituto Zaldivar central hub: Instituto Zaldivar SA. Mendoza, Argentina. Ophthalmic Surgical Ambulatory Center

- The examining room in Buenos Aires was furnished with all the necessary equipment for routine eye examinations (visual acuity chart and projectors, slit lamp and accessories, etc.). A workstation with access to phone and fax lines, two digital video cameras (one for the slit lamp and the second on the wall for recording the surrounding environment), and finally, a Tandberg 1000 video conference system were also installed. Environmental illumination was assured with overhead fluorescent tube lights and pale office walls, and in order to ensure quality audio and privacy, the walls were sound-proofed.
- In Instituto Zaldivar, the consultant's office was equipped with a LAN-based workstation, a Tandberg 500 video conference system, and analog phone and fax lines. The consultant can easily access phone and fax lines as well as the workstation while seated in front of the reading station's monitor. The background wall was painted blue-gray, while the others are pale. Since the consultant's image is always viewed by the patient on the monitor at the spoke site, the background wall was darkened in order to avoid an overexposed image due to the colors of the physician's lab coat or surgical scrubs (Fig. 27.5).

27.2.4 Project Team and Protocols

Specialized staff personnel were selected and trained to take part in this pilot project: two coordinators, one at each site, the intervening physicians, and support staff that included a full-time IT engineer and video production consultant[1]. Standard operating procedures with each team member's duties are described in Table 27.1.

Protocols were designed ad hoc to make them quick and easy to comply with and were given out as surveys, together with the consent forms

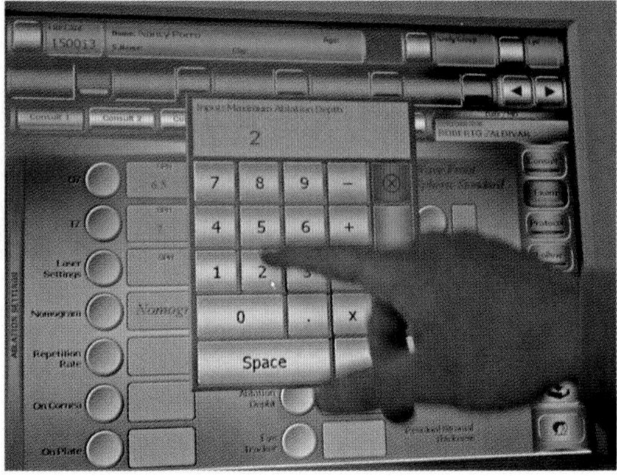

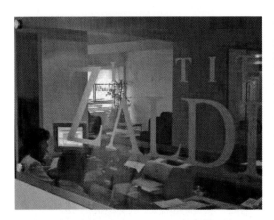

Fig. 27.4. Electronic medical record system, with touch-screen technology, based on workflow applications

Fig. 27.3. Buenos Aires spoke site: Instituto Zaldivar SA. Buenos Aires, Argentina. External Clinic

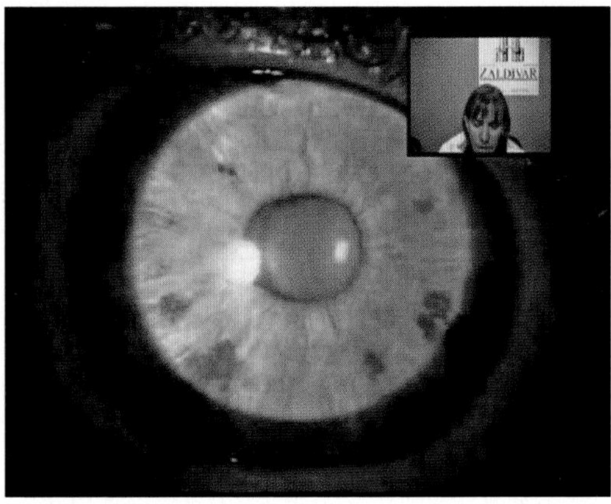

Fig. 27.5. Anterior segment video-captured image with the Tanberg 500 video conference system. Both the patient's eye and the consultant's site can be visualized simultaneously on the monitor. The color of the wall behind the consultant was darkened in order to enhance contrast

(Figs. 27.6 and 27.7). Their objectives were to structure the teleconsultations and gather as much data (feedback) as possible for future revision. From the physicians' point of view, the slip lamp's digital camera resolution and the high-speed connections were crucial factors in assessing adequate post-operative control, so the protocols included questions regarding both factors. A patient satisfaction survey was designed to essentially probe their feelings concerning this new virtual modality of physician/patient relationship.

27.3 Results and Discussion

Large-scale access to health care is scarce worldwide. Argentina, affected by a prolonged political and economic crisis, has suffered over the past years a profound impact on its health care system. Not only have costs, salaries, reimbursements, and import restrictions become crucial issues in medicine, so, too, have health care insurance coverage, transportation, and communication costs, as well as patient access to health care systems.

With 36 million people living in Argentina, an uneven geographic distribution of its patient and medical population have only made things worse. While the World Health Organization (WHO) states that there should be one ophthalmologist per 15,000 inhabitants, in Argentina, estimates drawn from the latest survey performed in March 2001 calculate that Argentina has 4,000 ophthalmologists, 1,700 more than required [17]. The distribution is unequal, with a ratio of ophthalmologist per patient in the urban areas much greater than in rural areas.

Avant garde technology in ophthalmic surgery is also only available on a small scale. High-end ambulatory surgical centers can only be found in the larger metropolitan cities, and health insurance coverage usually falls short of covering these services. For this reason, the Instituto Zaldivar designed a teleophthalmology program to benefit its patients.

Prior to launching the on-line consultation service, ophthalmic consults – other than regular office visits – were limited, and made by regular mail, fax, or by a cost-free telephone. Through the on-line consult or booking service, the response was overwhelming, with a significant increase in the number of consultations, i.e., 4,860 new consultations were performed between December 2001 to December 2004 (Fig. 27.8).

Since the implementation of the real-time model in December 2001, 349 patients have been examined under the video conference or teleconsultation model, of which 79.9% were refractive and cataract surgery patients (Fig. 27.9). All patients originally attended at Instituto Zaldivar for surgery, and had their follow-up visits at the Buenos Aires spoke site.

When relying on non-traditional methods or techniques to evaluate or diagnose a medical condition (and in this case, based almost entirely on patient imagery), image resolution and fidelity must be of the highest order. Some of the drawbacks encountered in telemedicine deal with these issues. Many physicians argue that face-to-face assessments simply can not be replaced by a remote consultation.[2] Many detractors base their claims on the lack of direct interaction with the eye and poor image qualities for properly diagnosing or assessing the patient's eye condition, as well as the lack of direct physical contact with the patient, and consequently dissatisfaction of one or both intervening parties. Another critical issue under the spotlight is the sustainability of current telemedicine programs.

27.3.1 Image Quality

Adequate image resolution is crucial when it comes to diagnosing or assessing any condition, whether at a clinical, surgical or post-operative stage. DICOM is the global standard for exchanging biomedical imaging and image information and efforts are being made jointly by the American Academy of Ophthalmology (DICOM Working Group 9) and the ophthalmic vendor community in search of standards-based approaches to facilitate the use of digital imaging in ophthalmology, an essential factor for teleophthalmology [18, 19].

In this particular study, we analyzed the quality of real-time imagery of the external and anterior segment of the eye, particularly the cornea, under slit lamp examination, and transmitted via

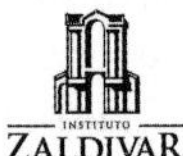

VIRTUAL CONSULT

CONSULT

Date [ ] **Time** [ ] **Medical Record** [ ]

VC Duration [ ]

Patient [ ]

Referring Physician [ ]

Consulting Physician [ ]

MOTIVE

[ ]

OBSERVATIONS

	Good	Regular	Inadequate
SPOKE SITE			
Transmission	[ ]	[ ]	[ ]
Audio	[ ]	[ ]	[ ]
Images	[ ]	[ ]	[ ]
Others	[ ]	[ ]	[ ]
HUB			
Transmission	[ ]	[ ]	[ ]
Audio	[ ]	[ ]	[ ]
Images	[ ]	[ ]	[ ]
Others	[ ]	[ ]	[ ]

INDICATIONS

[ ]

NEXT VISIT

[ ]

Fig. 27.6. Physician/patient satisfaction survey forms

a video conferencing consultation mode. Several important issues must be taken into account when deciding which application or tool is best for dealing with these types of images: image acquisition, transmission (bandwidth and compression), and reception.

27.3.1.1 Image Acquisition

The following issues must be taken into account when considering image acquisition:

- Ophthalmic peripherals and their accessories are valuable tools used in our daily practice, which enhance our view of the eye and its internal components. The slit lamp permits

Fig. 27.6. Continued

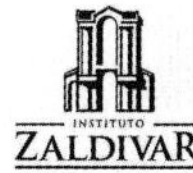

VC PATIENT SATISFACTION SURVEY

I. DOCTOR-PATIENT INTERACTION

1- Did you feel comfortable during the VC? Yes ☐ No ☐

2- In general terms, how was your experience?

____

3- Would you repeat the VC, or do you prefer a face-to-face consult? Yes ☐ No ☐

II. TECHNICAL & PHYSICAL ASPECTS

1- Were you able to see well the Consultant? Yes ☐ No ☐

2- Were you able to hear clearly? Yes ☐ No ☐

3- Were you comfortable in the VC room? Yes ☐ No ☐

III. CONVENIENCES

1- Was it convenient to have a VC? Yes ☐ No ☐

2- Why?

☐ **Easy Access to the Consultant**
☐ **Saved Money in traveling to see the Consultant**
☐ **Saved Time (work, school, etc)**
☐ **Others (please specify)**

IV. SUGGESTIONS

Would you like to add or suggest something? Yes ☐ No ☐

a biomicroscopic view of the eye with different magnifications (×5, ×10), which may be further enlarged with the additional use of contact or non-contact diagnostic lenses (×57, ×78, ×90, etc.). Although the resolution of the images is usually good, glare artifacts are very common and require skill and experience to overcome in order to capture a high quality image for diagnostic purposes. Underexposed or overexposed pictures are unsuitable, especially if transmitted remotely where other limiting factors such as compression ratio, frame grabbers, and monitors play an important role in the final viewing of the image by the consultant stationed at the hub [3, 4].

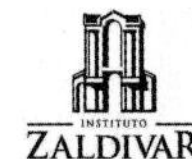

INSTITUTO ZALDIVAR

VIRTUAL CONSULT

INFORMED CONSENT

Date [ ] **Time** [ ] **Medical Record** [ ]

Patient [ ]

Referring Physician [ ]

Consulting Physician [ ]

MOTIVE

27

[ ]

OBSERVATIONS

You have solicited or you have been advised to perform a Virtual Consult, with one of the Consulting Physicians of the Instituto Zaldivar S. A. in the city of Mendoza, Argentina.

This innovative service utilizes video-conferencing equipment (monitors with incorporated microphones) installed in ophthalmic examining rooms designed specifically for these purposes, and linked to Mendoza thru a secure –private- digital telephone network (ISDN).

You will be able to see, hear and talk with the Consultant. You will also be accompanied at all times by your Referring Physician, who will coordinate and present your eye exam to the Consultant.

Although remote diagnoses equipment will be used in your exam, your consult will be as private and secure as it would be face-to-face. The only personnel authorized to be present during your examination are the Referring and Consulting Physicians.

I have read and fully understood the above explanation.

Signature [ ] **Date** [ ]

Fig. 27.7. Teleconsultation consent form

- Other variables affecting acquisition are the splitters and the cameras used for capturing the images. The digital era has blessed us with new, but costly, digital technology. Both photographic and video cameras have undergone intense development enabling high resolution and low noise digital images. Three-chip CCD video cameras have demonstrated excellent performance in our experience and are considered very appropriate for these purposes. With the aid of beam splitters, depending on the type used, the amount of light going into the photographic or video camera is enhanced or reduced and therefore improves or degrades the quality of the image capture [3, 4, 20].
- Our project involved capturing images from the corneal surface, which is relatively trouble-free due to its simple visual access when compared to funduscopic imaging. Since we decided to implement a real-time mode for the teleconsultation, we used video cameras attached to the slit lamp as our primary acquisition tool. These enabled the consultant to actually view the motion of the slit lamp as it crosses the corneal surface and thickness

Table 27.1. Standard operating procedures for duties and responsibilities

Buenos Aires project coordinator	– Scheduling appointments one month post-op, unless anticipated or specified by the referring physician – Confirming to Instituto Zaldivar's project coordinator, via e-mail or private radio network, the time frames for the teleconsultation – Ensuring the pertinent medical files have been scanned, sent by courier, or faxed to Instituto Zaldivar before the teleconsultation – Accompanying the patient to the examining room, while briefly going over the instructions and explanations required – Notifying the referring physician that all is set to go – Troubleshooting with the technicians, if any problems are adverted before beginning the teleconsultation – Making the opening call to Instituto Zaldivar – Scheduling the next follow-up visit as indicated at the conclusion of the teleconsultation – Plotting all the proceedings on the protocol sheet and recollecting the patient satisfaction surveys – Inputting all the data collected in an Excel Spreadsheet, and e-mail copy to Instituto
Instituto Zaldivar project coordinato	– Verifying, via e-mail or private radio network, the scheduling of the virtual appointments made previously in Buenos Aires – Allocating the pertinent medical files in the consultant's office – Setting up the connections in Instituto Zaldivar and waiting for the opening call – Ensuring that the patient is sitting at the slit lamp with the Buenos Aires physician, before the consultant is notified – Troubleshooting with the technicians, if any problems are adverted before beginning the teleconsultation – Cross-checking all the data that arrives from Buenos Aires after the teleconsultation has concluded
Referring physician	– Once the patient is in the examining office, the referring physician proceeds with visual acuity verification, automated keratorefactive readings, and corneal topography (Orbscan II) – Concludes the eye examination under slit lamp and authorizes the opening call to the central hub Instituto Zaldivar – Aids the consultant through the examination and takes notes of the indications or prescriptions if performed – All the proceedings are plotted on the protocol sheet and the patient satisfaction survey is given to the patient
Consulting physician	– The consultant is advised of the time frames for the teleconsultation by the project coordinator – Once the teleconsultation has initiated, he/she will go over the slit lamp examination with the aid of the referring physician and discuss the progress made with both the patient and the physician – New indications or prescriptions are made at this point and the next follow-up visit is agreed upon mutually

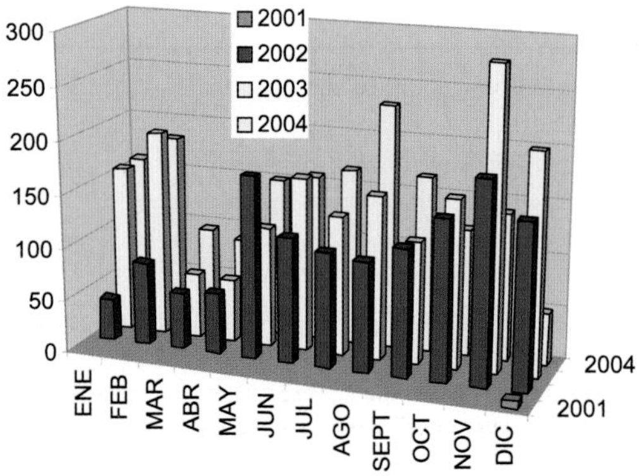

Fig. 27.8. Consultations made through the institutional web site, from December 2001 to December 2004. n = 4,860 online consults

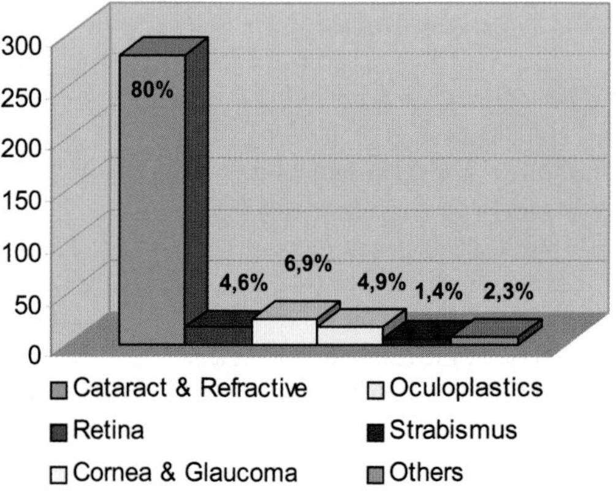

Fig. 27.9. Teleophthalmology consultations performed with the hybrid teleophthalmology model. n = 349 teleconsults

with optimum contrast and spatial image resolution. Otherwise, digital photographic cameras provide excellent still images, which are best for store-and-forward consultations.

27.3.1.2 Image Transmission: Bandwidth and Compression

The following issues must be taken into account when considering image transmission:

- High speed telecommunications (large bandwidth) with low rate compression permit high quality information transmission, essential for proper diagnostic purposes, especially when analyzing moving images. When choosing high speed services, a wide variety of options are currently available (asynchronous transfer mode (ATM), T1, cable modem, ADSL, ISDN), and the choice should depend on the type and quality of images that will be transmitted, as well as on the cost of transmission. The use of ISDN lines offers many benefits, primarily high bandwidth and interoperability with analog phone and digital services, capability to improve the speed of Internet access, and a wide geographical distribution at a relatively low cost. Therefore, it has proved its cost-effectiveness as a telecommunication tool in telemedicine [3, 4, 21–23].
- Considering the compression algorithms coded into current hardware, most reports have established a minimum bandwidth of 384 Kb/s as a crucial requirement for real-time telemedicine consultations. The video quality provided at this bandwidth has been proven adequate for most telemedicine applications, including slit lamp examinations but not cine-angiograms and ultrasounds [21–26].
- Although much progress has been made, standardization of all these parameters still needs to be developed and endorsed globally.
- In our case, the use of a VPN linked by six ISDN lines (International Telecommunication Union Standard H.320) permitted an adequate transmission of video-captured corneal biomicroscopy images (NTSC video format) at a relatively low compression rate at 30 frames per second. While most of the common post-operative conditions were assessed correctly, (e.g., in refractive surgery post-operative management: dry eye syndrome, flap displacement or misalignment, folds, epithelial ingrowth, intraocular contact lens vaulting), larger bandwidth is necessary to adequately capture subtle changes such as striae or minor corneal edema (Figs. 27.10, 27.11, and 27.12).

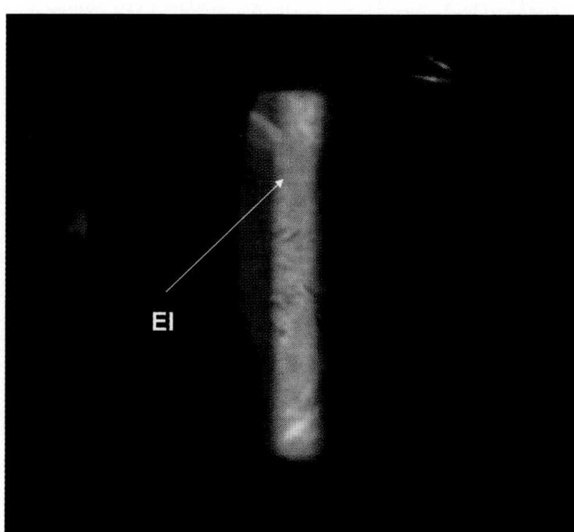

Fig. 27.10. Anterior segment video-captured image with the Tanberg 500 video conference system at the consultant's site. Epithelial ingrowth on the upper edge of the corneal flap of a LASIK case

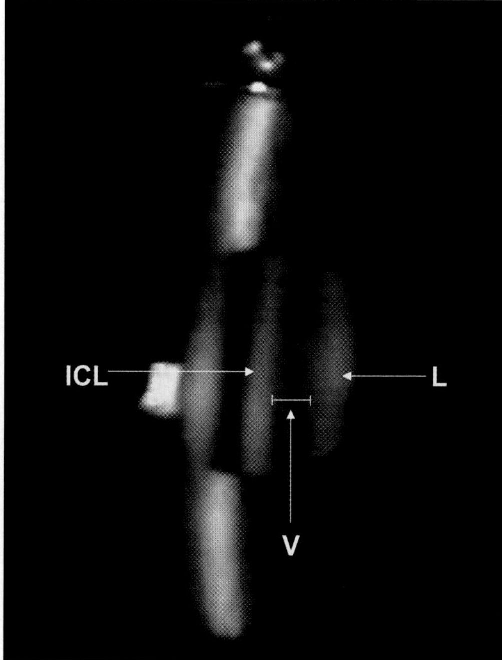

Fig. 27.11. Anterior segment video-captured image with the Tanberg 500 video conference system at the consultant's site. ICL = Intraocular Contact Lens, V = Vault, L = Crystalline Lens

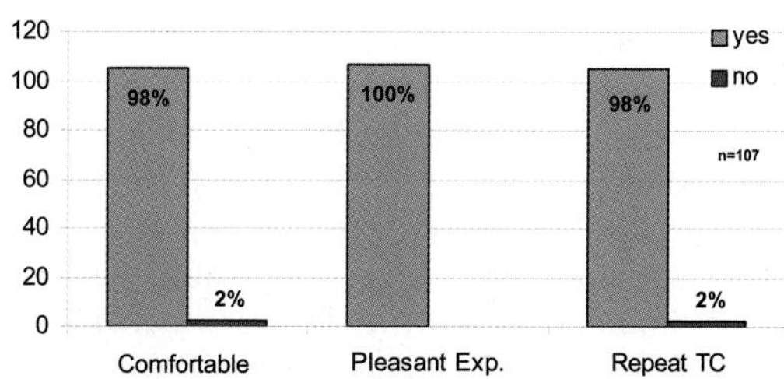

Fig. 27.12. Physician-patient encounter. This graphic reflects how the patient felt during the teleconsult. Three basic questions were asked: Were you comfortable? Was it a pleasant experience? Would you repeat the experience?

27.3.1.3 Image Reception

The use of CRT monitors versus LCD will not be discussed here since our project utilized only CRT video and television monitors for the reception of images transmitted via the Tandberg video conferencing system.

The following issues must be taken into account when considering image reception:

- In order to ensure proper color management (essential for diagnostic purposes), monitor calibration was accomplished by the audio-video technicians at both sites.
- A standard color placard was created with the aid of the digital video camera, and the monitors were calibrated using this placard, taking the precaution of warming up the display before performing the calibration, and avoiding shining lights or glare reflecting on the monitor [25, 26].
- All colored diagnostic charts, such as corneal topographies and wavefront analyses, were also scanned and forwarded as JPEG images by e-mail.
- Attention was also paid to the frequency of the monitor (+85 Hz) in order to enhance the optical perception of the image and avoid visual fatigue.

27.3.2 Physician-Patient Satisfaction

Another milestone in real-time telemedicine applications is the physician/patient satisfaction issue. Innovative consultation modalities imply the need for open-minded actors. Both the physicians' and patients' perception of this new environment is crucial when it comes to adopting emerging technologies that will eventually facilitate the usual means of consultation [27].

Regardless of the tools used, however, the basic fundamentals of the physician-patient relationship have not changed. Privacy, confidentiality, and security must be assured in order to sustain a *healthy* relationship. One must bear in mind that face-to-face consultations offer a traditional emotional experience for all intervening parties. When facing non-traditional settings, the advantages and disadvantages must be taken into account, in order to avoid dissatisfaction of one or both parties, as summarized in Table 27.2. Teleconsultations are ordinary consultations, physically different, but ethically the same.

Overall, a review of the literature reveals high rates of satisfaction with telemedicine encounters, due to clear advantages, such as improved access to health care and cost reduction of both time and money [28–30]. In our model, satisfaction surveys were given out during the first year of implementation to both the physicians and patients. An easy-to-fill-in questionnaire was provided together with the consent form, and patients completed the surveys voluntarily. A total of 107 surveys were completed and processed, revealing general acceptance of this innovative consultation modality (Figs. 27.12, 27.13, and 27.14). Therefore, physician/patient satisfaction in a non-traditional consultation scenario (teleconsultation) can be used as one of the indicators of quality of care and acceptance of this new consultation modality.

27.3.3 Sustainability

Sustainability is one of the key issues to any successful enterprise. Health care costs are not the only ones soaring. In the Latin American region, telecommunications, hardware, software and overheads are all cost limiting, and they constitute one of the most important impairments when it comes to planning a sustainable telemedicine program [31]. With time, as the market demand increases, prices will eventually decrease and access to these technologies will be universal, a key success factor in telemedicine [32, 33].

In our case, private funding was used to design and implement the program. Once the patient population was educated and accepted this

Table 27.2. Physician and patient satisfaction

Traditional consultations offer:	
To the physician	**To the patient**
Face-to-face interaction Possibility of hands-on examination Privacy, confidentiality User friendly language (verbal and body language) Non-dependent on time frames	Face-to-face interaction Privacy, intimacy Confidentiality, sense of security Traditional emotional experience
Virtual consultations offer:	
Advantages	**Disadvantages**
Increased access to highly qualified medical services Possibility of seeing and speaking remotely to the specialist (consultant) Costs less time and money Enthusiasm in adopting emerging technologies	Nervousness when using new technologies Difficulties in expressing themselves in front of a television monitor Tendency to be less spontaneous during the exam Distant emotional experience

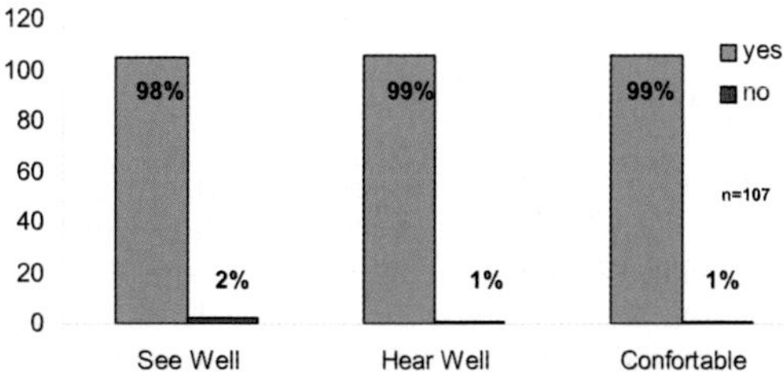

Fig. 27.13. Physician-patient encounter. This graphic reflects how the patient felt, concerning the technical and environmental aspects of the teleconsult. Three basic questions were asked: Could you see well the consultant? Could you hear him/her well? Was it a comfortable experience?

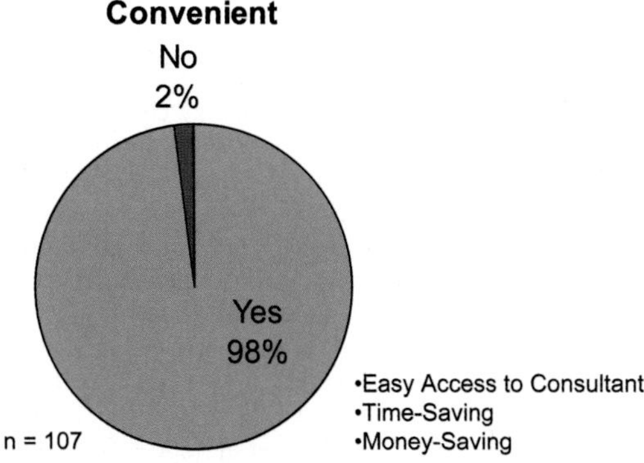

Fig. 27.14. Physician-patient encounter. This graphic reflects how the patient felt, concerning the conveniences of accepting a teleconsult instead of a face-to-face consultation

new consultation modality, their demand for it increased substantially, making it possible to offer it as a pay-per-view service. At present, our service is paid for by our patients privately, since health care insurance companies have not yet addressed the reimbursement issues.

27.4 Conclusions

From the physician's point of view, high speed connections were crucial when adequately assessing eye conditions, thus avoiding unnecessary pre-operative services at the hub site, saving both time and money. Although the new digital era allows for faster communications and digital imagery, enhancing the possibility of remote diagnoses, it also presents a new scenario with new challenges: insufficient bandwidth, noisy transmissions, hackers, electrical faults, unknown or equivocal users, etc. Therefore, there is a real need for standards and legislation to protect a teleconsultation and to help guarantee the proper use of medical information, as well as its adequate transmission, safe processing, storage, and timely delivery.

From the patient's point of view, it has turned out to be an innovative physician-patient relationship. The majority expressed their satisfaction at being able to see and talk with their attending surgeon. Time-consuming and costly expenses of traveling back and forth to Mendoza were avoided.

From both the physician's and patient's point of view, teleconsultations demand privacy, confidentiality, and security. These parameters are essential and mandatory in any type of consultation. Although a teleconsultation is performed in a virtual environment, in essence it represents an ordinary consultation. Therefore we must all strive toward a satisfactory physician/patient relationship. This is a key factor for all successful consultations, whether virtual or not.

What does the near future hold? Perhaps it has already arrived. At present, the Instituto Zaldivar has designed a full-scale integration project called *Focus* that will include a high speed (E1) VPN with on-line electronic medical records between all its affiliated centers (including its new center in Asunción, Paraguay), Wi-Fi connectivity within each facility, a new mobile clinic, and is opening its doors in search of new international collaborative projects.

References

1. Tang R, Hearst J (2001) Teleophthalmology across the miles. OMIC Digest, http://www.omic.com/new/digest/10_3/teleo.html. Cited 6 Nov 2001
2. Bashshur R (2001) Where we are in telemedicine/telehealth, and where we go from here? Editorial. Telemed J E Health 7(4):273–277
3. Schiffman JS, Tang RA (2000) Telemedicine consultation in ophthalmology. Ophthalmol Clin North Am 13:197–212
4. Li HK (1999) Telemedicine and ophthalmology. Surv Ophthalmol 44(1):61–72

27

5. Cuzzani O (2000) Teleophthalmology, present and future. Arch Soc Esp Oftalmol 75(1):1–2
6. Telehealth Practice Recommendations for Diabetic Retinopathy. http://www.atmeda.org/ICOT/diabeticretionpathy. FINAL.pdf. Cited 28 Feb 2005
7. Baker CF, et al. (2004) JPEG compression of stereoscopic digital images for the diagnosis of diabetic retinopathy via teleophthalmology. Can J Ophthalmol 39(7):746–754
8. Al Sabti K, Raizada S, Wani VB, Al Ajmi M, Gayed I, Sugathan TN (2003) Efficacy and reliability of fundus digital camera as a screening tool for diabetic retinopathy in Kuwait. J Diabetes Complications 17(4):229–233
9. Aoki N, Dunn K, Fukui T, Beck JR, Schull WJ, Li HK (2004) Cost-effectiveness analysis of telemedicine to evaluate diabetic retinopathy in a prison population. Diabetes Care 27(5):1095–1101
10. Soto-Pedre E, Hernaez-Ortega MC, Vasquez JA (2003) Digital retinal images and teleophthalmology for detecting and grading diabetic retinopathy. Diabetes Care 26(3):963–964
11. Gomez-Ulla F, Fernandez MI, Gonzalez F, et al. (2002) Digital retinal images and teleophthalmology for detecting and grading diabetic retinopathy. Diabetes Care 25(8):1384–1389
12. Tennant MT, Greve MD, Rudinsky CJ, Hillson TR, Hinz BJ (2001) Identification of diabetic retinopathy by stereoscopic digital imaging via teleophthalmology: a comparison to slide film. Can J Ophthalmol 36(4):187–196
13. Tennant MT, Rudinsky CJ, Hinz BJ, MacDonald IM, Greve MD (2000) Teleophthalmology via stereoscopic digital imaging: a pilot project. Diabetes Technol Ther 2(4):583–587
14. Li HK, Tang RA, Oschner K, Koplos C, Grady J, Crump WJ (1999) Telemedicine screening of glaucoma. Telemedicine J 5(3):283–290
15. Tuulonen A, Ohinmaa T, Alanko HI, Hyytinen P, Juutinen A, Toppinen E (1999) The application of teleophthalmology in examining patients with glaucoma: a pilot study. J Glaucoma 8(6):367–373
16. Yogesan K, Constable IJ, Barry CJ, et al. (1999) Evaluation of a portable fundus camera for use in the teleophthalmologic diagnosis of glaucoma. J Glaucoma 8(5):297–301
17. Boyanovsky C (2001) La calidad en riesgo. Revista MO Médico Oftalmólogo 14(2): http://www.oftalmologos.org.ar/mo/mo142-1.html#calidad. Cited 20 May 2005
18. Sosa-Iudicissa M, Monteagudo Peña JL, Ferrer-Roca O (2001) Standards and telemedicine. Telemedicine, Editorial Médica Panamericana, Madrid, Spain, pp 216–227
19. American Academy of Ophthalmology (2005) Digital Imaging Standards. http://www.aao.org/aao/education/library/memberalert/digital.cfm. Cited 18 Mar 2005
20. Ferrer-Roca O, Sousa Pereira A (2001) Minimum technical requirements. Telemedicine, Editorial Médica Panamericana, Madrid, Spain, pp 58–65
21. Ferrer-Roca O, Sousa Pereira A (2001) Minimum technical requirements. Telemedicine, Editorial Médica Panamericana, Madrid, Spain, pp 36–57
22. ECU Advance Telemedicine Training Centre Training Manual (2000) Bandwidth and compression and systems integration. ECU, Brody School of Medicine
23. Morin JE, Klein SA, et al. (2005) Introduction of new telemedicine applications to ophthalmology: standardized evaluation of transmission modalities. http://www.i-med.com/mi/teleop.html. Cited 10 Mar 2005
24. ECU Advance Telemedicine Training Centre Training Manual (1996) Ophthalmology clinic: clinical service protocols for telemedicine; standard operating procedure manual. Copyright Telemedicine Center, ECU, Brody School of Medicine 1996:38
25. Burgis S, Sprang R, Tracey J (2005) Telehealth technology and guidelines. http://telehealth.hrsa.gov/pubs/tech/optha.htm. Cited 15 Feb 2005
26. Ferrer-Roca O (2001) Color theory. Telemedicine. Editorial, Médica Panamericana, Madrid, Spain, pp 237–245
27. Broderick TJ, Harnett BM, et al. (2003) Impact of varying transmission bandwidth on image quality. Telemed J E Health 7(1):47–53
28. Gustke S, Balch D, et al. (2000) Patient satisfaction with telemedicine. Telemed J 6(1):5–13
29. Williams TL, May CR, Esmail A (2001) Limitations of patient satisfaction studies in telehealthcare: a systematic review of the literature. Telemed J E Health 7(4):293–303
30. Whitten PS, Mair F (2000) Telemedicine and patient satisfaction: current status and future directions. Telemed J 6(4):417–423
31. Rodrígues R (ed) e-Salud en Latinoamérica y el Caribe (2003) Tendencias y temas emergentes. Organización Panamericana de Salud, Washington, DC
32. Strobel V, Ferrer-Roca O (2001) Economy and strategic planning. Telemedicine, Editorial Médica Panamericana, Madrid, Spain, pp 185–197
33. Ferrer-Roca O (2001) Quality assurance in telemedicine. Telemedicine, Editorial Médica Panamericana, Madrid, Spain, pp 127–134

Chapter 28

Teleophthalmology in the United States Army

28

Michael J. Mines, Kraig S. Bower, Thomas P. Ward

DISCLAIMER: The opinions expressed in this manuscript are those solely of the authors and do not represent the views or official policies of the United States Army or Department of Defense.

This chapter addresses the following

Key Concepts:

- Teleophthalmology has the potential to increase access to medical care, extend valuable resources, and decrease the cost of care, allowing a limited number of ophthalmologists to better serve a geographically diverse beneficiary population.
- In a military environment, bandwidth is a finite resource that is allocated based on the needs of the mission and the organization.
- Given bandwidth and logistical support constraints while deployed, straightforward, non-resource intensive solutions are the key to smooth implementation, quick acceptance, and productive results.
- Teleophthalmology screening and remote diagnosis of anterior segment pathology and diabetic retinopathy is reliable and reproducible.
- To be clinically useful, these systems require a minimum level of sophistication, including high resolution, stereopsis, and magnification, as well as outcomes that must be validated.
- Ophthalmic robotic microsurgery is possible, and could ultimately serve as a helpful adjunct, as well as provide new functionality while performing ocular microsurgery.
- Digital image manipulation can enhance pre-operative planning to better guide the surgeon and inform the patient.

28.1 Introduction

The United States (US) Army Medical Command employs 60 active duty Army ophthalmologists in 26 locations world-wide, whose primary mission is to provide state-of-the-art eye care to our troops in garrison, in the field, and in the theater of combat. This currently includes ophthalmologists deployed in Afghanistan, Kuwait, and Iraq in support of Operations Enduring Freedom and Iraqi Freedom. Moreover, Army ophthalmologists provide care for a beneficiary population of over 8.1 million people located in 59 different countries and territories around the globe [1]. In addition to soldiers serving on active duty, this population includes their spouses and children, and retired service members and their spouses.

Unlike the widely dispersed beneficiary population, ophthalmic resources are predominantly located at a limited number of medical centers and regional hospitals in the continental US, Europe, and Asia. Approximately 30% of eligible beneficiaries are located greater than 40 miles (65 km) from one of these facilities [2]. This number continues to grow as US military bases are closed or consolidated as a result of the end of the Cold War. In fact, during the decade from 1987 to 1997, 35% of US Department of Defense medical facilities closed [3].

These expanding distances between patient and hospital and the resultant travel-related expenses become prohibitive, preventing many beneficiaries from seeking health care in the military system. Instead, they must rely on civilian medical care, which increases cost. For active duty patients, this cost is paid for by the government. For family members and retirees, a portion of the cost is subsidized by the government. The remainder is the responsibility of the patient in the form of deductibles and co-payments. Similar challenges arise when providing care for our deployed population.

While a robust medical system accompanies units in the field, it is not feasible or preferable to place all medical assets in far-forward positions. Likewise, some military units must operate at great distances from their nearest medical support. Therefore, an evacuation system is required where patients in need of specialized diagnostic or therapeutic care are evacuated to other facilities when not available locally. This places a financial and logistical cost on the organization as a whole, and a cost in manpower to the unit losing a soldier. For both the deployed soldier in the field and the family member or retiree located in the US, strategically implemented and easily accessible teleophthalmology services could improve their ability to obtain care while decreasing the cost to them and our tax payers. The following discussion outlines a number of the US Army ophthalmology initiatives currently in use or in development to advance those goals.

28.2 Teleconsultation in Practice

During past military operations the ability to provide medical support has necessarily been constrained by logistical realities. Moving manpower and military supplies is of paramount importance to be successful on the battlefield. Medical care is well supported by the command structure and considered an essential element to a successful military, but it will not supplant tactical or strategic considerations in the resource intensive environment of military activities. In effect, those resources are competed for, and allocated based on the needs of the organization and its mission. During today's deployments, whether they are to the battlefield, or in support of humanitarian missions, an additional resource is competed for – bandwidth. In operational terms, this is also a finite resource and is allocated to support the group as a whole. Our task therefore, is to make the case for our need of this resource and to maximize the amount given to its full effect. This necessitates an approach that focuses on easy to use, resource efficient technology that provides what the user needs in a timely fashion.

28.2.1 The Kosovo–Bosnia Experience

One such system is e-mail based consultation. In a deployed environment, the typical civilian referral paradigm is often unfeasible. Due to mission requirements, excessive distances, limited transportation assets or hostile action, patient transport for specialty evaluation may not be practical. E-mail consultation eliminates these challenges and in fact can speed health care delivery. Since the early 1990s, e-mail equipped computer systems have been readily accessible in military theaters. From the Kosovo–Bosnia conflict, enterprising deployed providers began sending the first e-mail consultations to distant ophthalmology sub-specialists located in Germany and the US (Fig. 28.1). Responses could be sent back in time to help manage patients or recommend evacuation to larger medical facilities.

28.2.2 Teleconsultation

Since that time a formal e-mail consultation system has been designed and implemented, the Tele-Ocular Consultation system. It is a secure e-mail communication system deployed worldwide. Military providers anywhere on the globe can consult an ophthalmologist by e-mailing a single e-mail address. The system is monitored by both a clinical and technical manager. Specific ophthalmologists are identified to respond to consultation requests. Due to the global na-

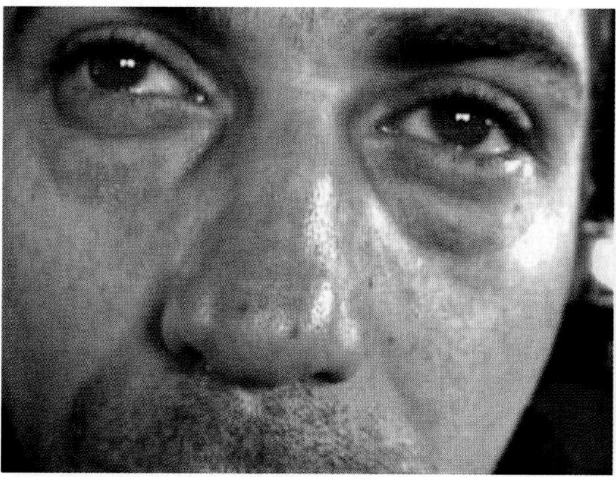

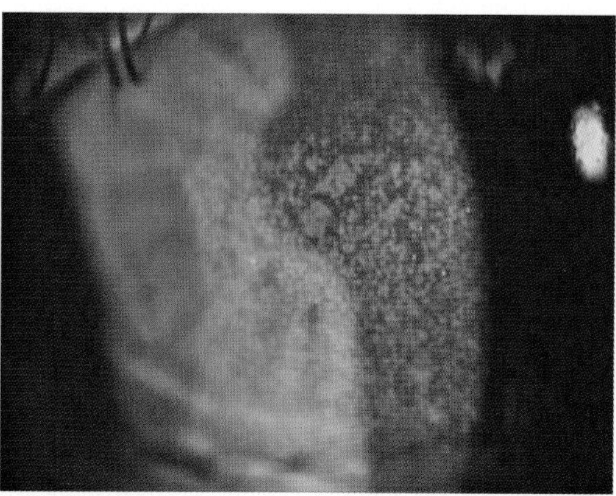

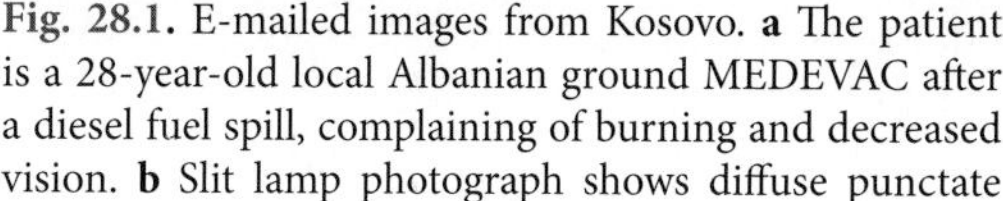

Fig. 28.1. E-mailed images from Kosovo. **a** The patient is a 28-year-old local Albanian ground MEDEVAC after a diesel fuel spill, complaining of burning and decreased vision. **b** Slit lamp photograph shows diffuse punctate epithelial staining. Based on these images and the history given, the ophthalmologist recommended treatment with topical lubricants and antibiotics with successful resolution of the condition

ture of the Army mission, deployed providers may not be in the same time zone as consultants. These differing time zones were considered in the design of the system. Ophthalmology consultants are located in various locations around the world ensuring that whenever a consult is initiated a consultant is available. The local provider obtains history and other pertinent data from the patient. Digital images are captured focusing on the area of interest. Since consultation information is de-identified by the local provider to ensure patient confidentiality, a unique patient code is generated and maintained by the submitting provider. The information and images are sent as an e-mail to a central e-mail address. The date and time of the consult are recorded by the technical manager and reminders sent if the consult is not responded to in 24 h.

The system began accepting consultations in July 2004. From July through to December of that year, 13 consultations were addressed. In the first quarter of 2005, 11 consultations were reviewed. The majority of these consultations have originated in Iraq and Afghanistan. Five patients were recommended for evacuation out of the country. The remainder were managed by the consulting physician or referred to local eye care assets. Calculating an exact cost of an evacuation is difficult at best, but rough estimates suggest approximately 20,000 USD per patient. The non-monetary expense of losing a soldier to evacuation and the resultant unit degradation, however, cannot be underestimated.

28.2.3 Screening and Remote Diagnosis

The following subsections provide insights into treatment teleconsultation technology.

28.2.3.1 Ocular Trauma

Ocular injuries comprise approximately 13% of all injuries during combat, and the first treatment available may be given by a non-ophthalmologist [4]. Technology that allows teleconsultation with an ophthalmologist can enable the first responder, a front line medic or general medical officer, to assist in triage and determine who needs evacuation and with what priority. To evaluate the role of teleophthalmology in the assessment of anterior segment and ocular adnexal trauma, Army ophthalmologist Dr David Simon and colleagues evaluated the ability of four camera systems to image eight ocular injuries created in an animal model [5]. The images were transmitted via the Internet and reviewed by 83 ophthalmologists masked as to the injury, camera and photographer. The correct diagnoses were made most consistently for full-thickness eyelid laceration (96%), corneoscleral laceration with uveal prolapse (92%), partial-thickness eyelid laceration (86%) and hyphema (80%), and less frequently for intraocular foreign body (10%) and corneal foreign body (46%). Dr Simon's group felt that while teleophthalmology offered the potential to remotely diagnose certain ocular injuries, improvements in technology would be necessary before the diagnosis of most intraocular injuries would be possible on a consistent basis.

28.2.3.2 Anterior Segment

The slit lamp is one of the primary tools of the ophthalmologist, and is essential for examination and diagnosis of patients with disorders of the anterior segment. Understanding that the acquisition of high resolution *stereo* images would be essential for successful remote diagnosis and management of anterior segment problems, the John A Moran Eye Center at the University of Utah partnered with the Army's Telemedicine and Advanced Technology Research Center (TATRC) and the Walter Reed Army Medical Center (WRAMC) Ophthalmology Service to develop and test a prototype high-resolution digitized stereo slit lamp for use in teleophthalmology. In a study comparing the clinical diagnostic performance of the stereo video slit lamp with in-person examination, 64 adult patients (127 eyes) with common anterior segment findings were recruited from the patients presenting to the ophthalmology clinics at the University of Utah and WRAMC. The digital exam protocol used a set of 16 high-resolution digital still images (Fig. 28.2) and 16 fields of dynamic stereo imagery. With the reviewers at both institutions masked to all patient history and in reviewing only the standard set of images, this system proved effective in screening for common anterior segment pathology. Using the face-to-face exam as the gold standard, the sensitivity of the digitized exams ranged from 60% (anterior chamber findings, n = 5) to 92% (lens findings, n = 27). Specificity of diagnoses made from digital exams ranged from 76% (lens findings, n = 27) to 100% (anterior chamber findings, n = 5). This particular system provides some of the best imagery available in teleophthalmology to date, and is the first that we know of to provide dynamic stereo imagery.

28.3 Diabetes Mellitus

Diabetes mellitus (DM) is the leading cause of new cases of blindness in the US among adults aged 20–74 years with diabetic retinopathy causing as many as 40,000 new cases of blindness per year. Currently only 54% of the Army health care beneficiaries with DM receive annual retinal examination. Barriers to a regular eye exam are multifactorial and include lack of transportation, lack of clinic availability, and a shortage of eye care professionals. Teleophthalmology could assist in this area of critical need. To that end, Army ophthalmologists are exploring the potential use of digital retinal imaging to overcome some of these barriers.

In a technology evaluation for diabetic screening, researchers at WRAMC assessed the level of agreement between dilated fundus examination by a retina specialist and 45° non-mydriatic digital fundus photographs taken using a Canon CR6-45NM OIS system (Ophthalmic Imaging Systems, Inc., Sacramento, CA) with video capture via a Sony DXC390 3CCD video camera (Sony Electronics, Inc., New York, NY). In a prospective, comparative, observational case series in 231 eyes of 120 patients, the level of agreement between digital photos and dilated fundus examination was moderate for diabetic retinopathy ($\kappa = 0.44$), macular edema ($\kappa = 0.60$), and recommended follow-up interval ($\kappa = 0.38$). Our investigators concluded that due to its low sensitivity and relatively low level of agreement with clinical exams, remote review of a single 45° non-mydriatic digital fundus photograph cannot be relied upon as the sole modality for diabetic retinopathy screening at this time. However, there may be a role in populations where ophthalmoscopy by an experienced ophthalmologist is not an option.

In a separate but related project in collaboration with the Joslin Diabetes Center of Harvard Medical School and the Joslin Vision Network, a disease management program was established in

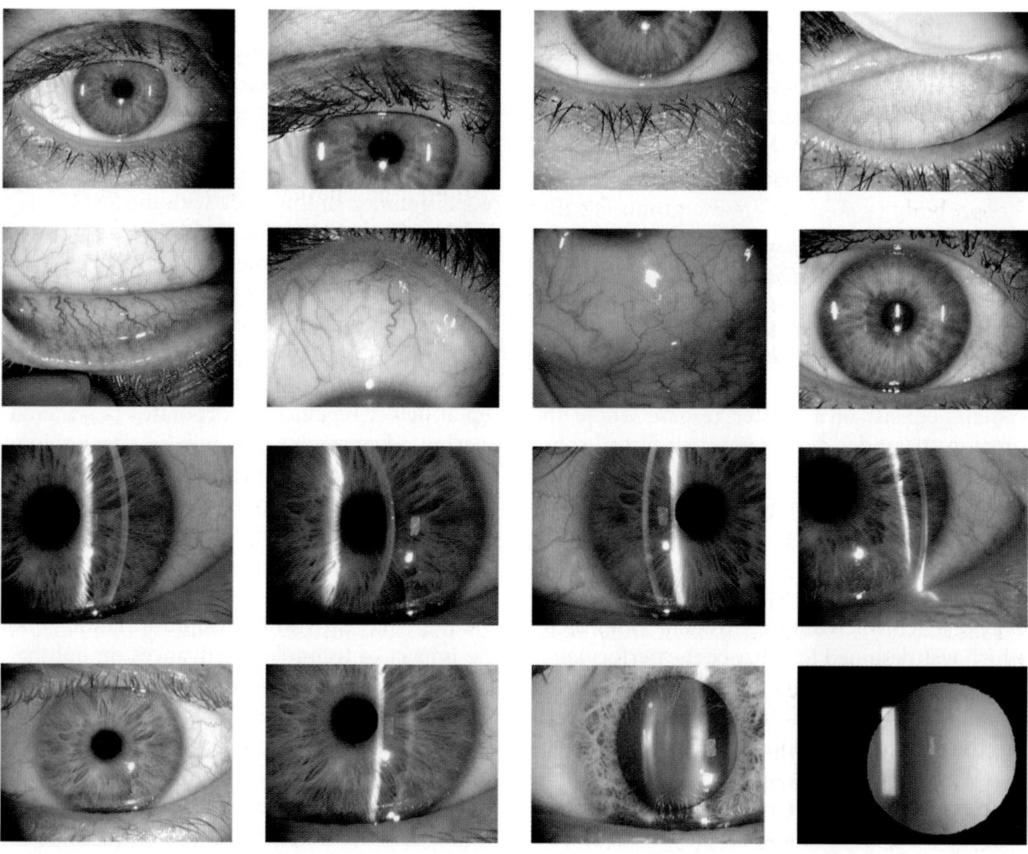

Fig. 28.2. Video slit lamp 16-field photo protocol. The examination is performed in a standardized fashion with consistent magnification and illumination. The sequence allows examination of the ocular surface, tear film, lids, lashes, conjunctiva, sclera, cornea, anterior chamber, iris, and lens

the Walter Reed Health Care System in 2000 to improve compliance with the process and quality measures established by the Diabetes Quality Improvement Project. As part of this program, patients underwent Non-Mydriatic Digital Stereoscopic Retinal Imaging (NMDSRI) at the time of their routine diabetes clinic appointment at four locations in the metropolitan Washington, DC area. The image acquisition system used in the study has been previously described [6]. In brief, a Topcon TRC NW6S non-mydriatic stereoscopic digital camera was used to obtain three 45° retinal fields images that collectively encompass a significant portion of the retina imaged by the ETDRS seven standard field stereoscopic retinal photography. Images were typically compressed to 15:1 before sending via local area network to a central reading location in the Ophthalmology Service at WRAMC, where they were diagnosed and graded by a single retinal specialist. Images of 484 eyes from 244 patients were evaluated, and of the 313 eyes considered gradable there was an 85% agreement in the grading between NMDSRI and dilated fundus examination. All of the NMDSRI gradable images were either exactly or within one grade of the dilated fundus examination, though retinal thickness could not be assessed in 21% of the eyes with diabetic retinopathy. There was 100% agreement for macular edema in the gradable eyes. Investigators concluded that the Joslin Vision Network imaging system is a sensitive and specific method for screening and diagnosis of diabetic retinopathy and may help improve compliance with the standards of eye care for patients with DM. Its simplicity and convenience make this technology suitable for incorporation into a diabetes disease management program facilitating improved compliance with the standard care for retinopathy screening in diabetics.

28.4 Robotic Eye Surgery

Since 1990, SRI International, Inc has conducted an active program in the development of remotely operated surgical robotic systems. These systems consist of a master *console* where the surgeon sits and a *slave station*, a surgical robot that follows the movements of the surgeon. The motivation for developing these systems was to provide surgeons with an interface that enhances their surgical abilities yet remains intuitive and easy to use. One of the systems developed is the Telepresence Microsurgical System (Fig. 28.3), which was designed to enhance the performance of surgeons during microsurgery operations. Among other features, the system allows scaling the surgeon's movements and tremor filtering. With TATRC funding from 2000–2001, SRI adapted the system for remote ophthalmic microsurgical operations and developed the Robotic Slave Micromanipulator Unit (RSMU), which is currently deployed at the Uniformed Services University of the Health Sciences in Bethesda, Maryland.

In a recent protocol we demonstrated the feasibility of using the RSMU to remotely repair a 5 mm central full-thickness corneal laceration in enucleated rabbit eyes. Ability to complete a watertight surgical repair, leak pressure, repair time, and histological analysis of wounds repaired with the RSMU were compared to eyes repaired with a standard *by-hand* surgical technique. All eyes in both groups maintained an IOP of 25 mm Hg without leaking. Mean repair time was 80 min (range 50–130 min) with the RSMU, compared to 10.8 min (range 7–35 min) by hand [Mines, unpublished data]. A watertight repair was then successfully performed in an anesthetized goat eye. We concluded that remote robotic surgery to repair a corneal wound is possible using the RSMU. In enucleated rabbit eyes, RSMU closure took longer, but surgical times trended lower as familiarity with the device developed. Corneal wound closure is also possible in a live animal model. While limitations currently exist, this technology holds promise and warrants further exploration.

A newly funded project will serve as a natural progression of this work with the RSMU. The da Vinci Surgical System, developed by Intuitive Surgical Inc., is a commercially available robotic surgical platform that is approved by the US Food and Drug Administration for various surgical procedures including laparoscopy, thoracoscopically assisted mitral valve surgery and atrial septal defect repair. It incorporates many engineering advances beyond previous technology, including increased degrees of freedom, an improved imaging system, and enhanced surgeon interface. This study will evaluate the impact of these technological advances on a surgeon's ability to robotically close a corneal laceration and will hopefully provide critical information about the impact of technologic advances on ophthalmic microsurgical robotics. We also anticipate that it will help identify strengths and weaknesses of existing technologies and provide direction for future work that will be required to make robotic ophthalmic microsurgery a reality.

28.5 Laser Tissue Welding

Laser tissue welding techniques present a promising alternative to microsutures and have been used by various researchers in ophthalmic as well as in other surgical applications. Most of the current techniques use a solder medium, which can be composed of fibrin, albumin or collagen. The strength of the repair is dependent upon reaching a precise temperature, determined by the choice of laser and the solder composition, to obtain protein polymerization at the solder/tissue interface with minimal damage to peripheral tissue. In fact, temperature feedback control on the laser has been demonstrated to improve the outcome of bonds.

In ongoing research, WRAMC ophthalmologists are collaborating with SRI, Inc and Conversion Energy Enterprises to investigate the use of robotic assistance to more precisely guide laser tissue welding. Development of custom robotic

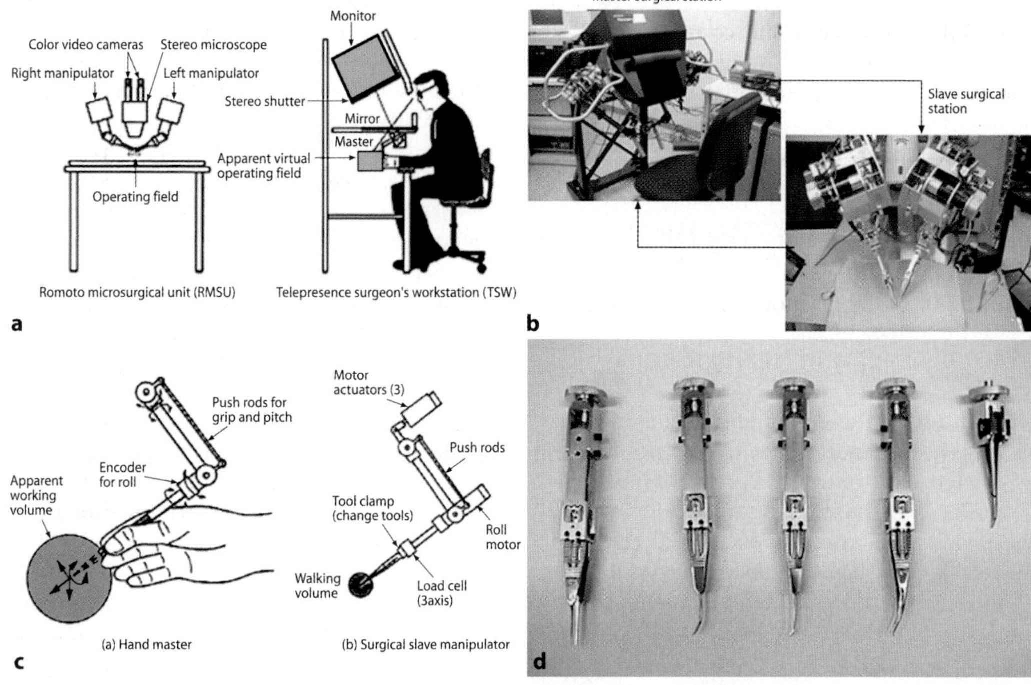

Fig. 28.3. Telepresence Microsurgical System. **a** SRI Telepresence principle applies to microsurgery. **b** SRI Telepresence Surgical System (TeSS). **c** SRI concept for microsurgical hand master and slave manipulators. **d** Quick connect-disconnect interchangeable microsurgical instruments

end effectors to appose tissue and to deliver and cure the solder aims to improve the quality and consistency of the laser tissue welding bonds. Incorporating laser tissue welding into the Telepresence Microsurgical System platform would allow greater precision of tissue apposition, accurate solder delivery and consistent laser power, all important parameters that are critical for a successful outcome of the bonds.

28.6 Digital Images in Evaluation and Management

As imaging and information technology continue to improve, digital photography is becoming more popular in eye care offices. Digital imaging allows convenient documentation and tracking of diseases. Photographs provide not only a better qualitative documentation of eye conditions than hand drawings, but images can now be used to compare *quantitative* aspects of ocular pathology with greater accuracy and reproducibility. WRAMC ophthalmologists use image processing software such as Adobe Photoshop® to accurately measure the surface area of lesions and to compare the lesion at each visit over time. This is routinely used in clinical practice as well as in research protocols where precise measurements are important.

Moreover, digital imaging can be used to assist in preoperative planning. For example, we have employed this in an 18-month-old child with a central corneal scar who underwent a corneal rotational autograft with the objective of moving the scar out of his visual axis. This was accomplished through eccentric trephination and 180° rotation of the central cornea. An image of the patient's cornea was manipulated digitally using Adobe Photoshop prior to surgery (Fig.28.4). This allowed for accurate prediction of the needed trephine size to within 0.2 mm, and greatly assisted in planning the best location for trephination. Digital imaging has many uses in ophthalmology. Although it is most commonly used in diagnosis and clinical monitoring, we demonstrate here another use – as an important tool in preoperative surgical planning.

28.7 Information Management

The following subsections review key systems for managing e-information.

28.7.1 Electronic Health Record

Since the advent of computer systems in maintaining clinical information, the development of an efficient electronic medical record has been a goal. One such system developed and in use in the US Army is a secure Web-based electronic medical record (EMR), *Health e Forces*. It began as an electronic documentation system utilizing the standard subjective, objective, assessment, plan (SOAP)format.

Army optometrists began adapting the electronic note for ocular examination documentation. The utility of a combined ocular electronic medical record with specific optometric and ophthalmic sections quickly became evident, and Army ophthalmologists and optometrists collaborated in refining the system for each specialty. Common aspects of the system include documentation of visual acuity, manifest refraction, ocular deviations, IOP, anterior and posterior segment examination and documentation, common diagnoses, and clinical plans.

Specific ophthalmic areas include means to document neuro-ophthalmic, oculoplastic, pediatric ophthalmic, corneal, glaucoma, and vitreo-retinal examinations. The system also allows for importing, storing, and viewing electronic images, updating the current visit note with information from prior visits including history,

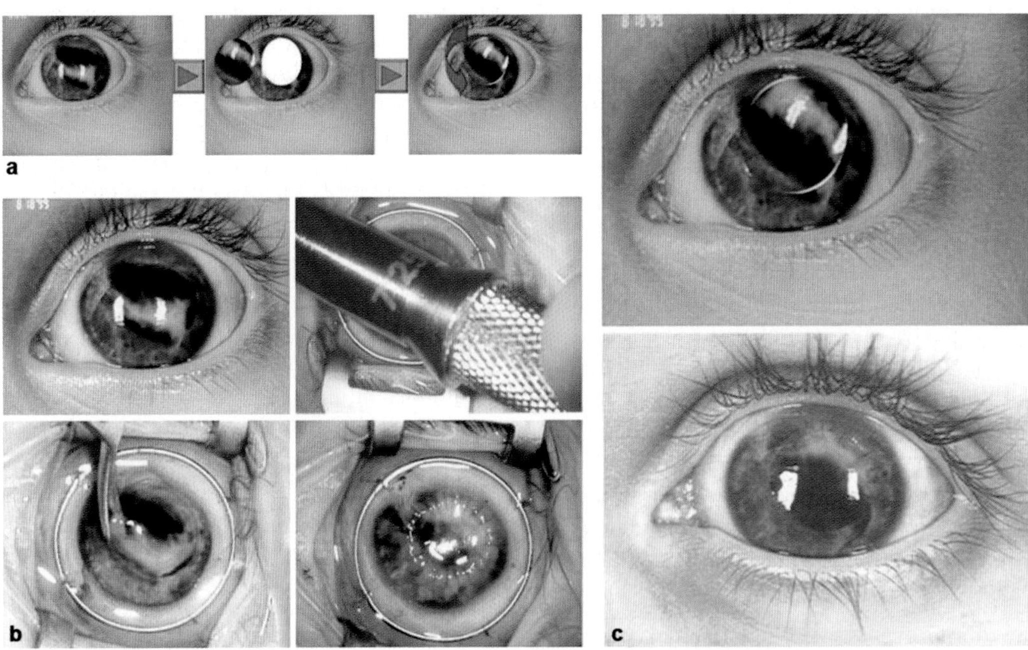

Fig. 28.4. Digital images are used in pre-operative planning for corneal autograft. The pre-operative digital image shows a vascularized corneal scar running through the visual axis (**a** *left*). The digital cornea is trephined using the *free transform* tool on Adobe Photoshop 7.0 (**a** *center*). The selected section is then rotated approx 180° showing a clear visual axis (**a** *right*). Intraoperatively, the appropriate corneal trephine is selected, the corneal button removed and sutured into place with the scar rotated superiorly out of the visual axis (**b**). The *digital post-op* used in preoperative surgical planning (**c** *top*) compares nicely to the six month post-op results (**c** *bottom*)

visual acuity, refractions, IOP, pachymetry, and incorporating pre-formatted patient education files in patient records. A current limitation of the system is the lack of color drawing capability organic to the application. This is an ongoing area of research and evaluation and refinement continues to occur.

An enterprise-wide electronic medical record solution is also being fielded. Called the Composite Health Care System II, it was created to provide secure, Department of Defense-wide interoperability for patient record management. This system is expected to be fully fielded in 2005.

28.7.2 Refractive Surgery Information System

The Army Warfighter Refractive Eye Surgery Program (WRESP) was established to reduce the limitations posed by corrective eyewear in combat arms soldiers. Between May 2000 and 30 September 2003, 32,068 eyes of 16,111 soldiers were treated, and the program currently plans on treating 12,000 or more new soldiers each year [7]. Optimal operation of the WRESP requires the ability to analyze outcomes and track complications and adverse events.

The Army has a rapidly mobile, geographically diverse population at risk of becoming lost to follow-up, despite the best of efforts. This is especially true in the current era of conflict with the global war on terrorism. The Army has recently completed beta testing of a Web-enabled database system for the WRESP, and is working to develop robust data mining and outcomes analysis tools. This refractive surgery information system will provide a complete database for all WRESP patients located world-wide, as well as an electronic record that will follow them throughout the Army. In this way Army ophthalmology can improve the efficacy and safety of the program and continue to provide the highest quality of care to our soldiers.

28.7.3 WRESP Web Portal

Currently in development is a web-enabled portal that will allow potential and current WRESP patients to access informational services describing the application process, eligibility criteria, Army WRESP policies, and supporting educational material. The initial release will query the user's basic military occupational status through a simple graphical interface. These data are presented to an appropriately structured database that will allow applicants to immediately establish their eligibility in the WRESP. Qualified candidates will be presented with downloadable registration forms and given additional information concerning the likely treatment timetable and scheduling requirements should they decide to proceed with surgery.

The second phase of web portal development will fully automate the application process. It will automate the management of pre- and post-surgical patient communications and track the timeliness of post-operative patient examination. A personal, password protected, page for each qualified candidate will include their appointment schedule, preoperative requirements, medication regimen and other relevant information. In addition, health care professionals distant from WRAMC who are providing post-operative follow-up care will be able to obtain information on the current state of the art treatment protocols supported by an extensive image library of material specific to the management of post-operative outcomes following refractive surgery.

28.8 Multimedia Repository and Remote Education

Army ophthalmologists, like their civilian counterparts, complete an internship and a three-year residency program accredited by the Accreditation Council for Graduate Medical Education (ACGME). Over 90% of Army ophthalmologists are trained in one of the three Army GME programs, where approximately 50% of staff time is directed toward GME activities including lectures, conferences, grand rounds, specialty courses, and presentations at local, regional and national meetings. These, as well as most peer-reviewed publications, have transitioned or are transitioning to an electronic format.

To support diagnosis and documentation of disease, most ophthalmology training programs are equipped with ophthalmic photography departments. These departments, however, likely began before digital imaging was possible. As a result, a vast amount of archived material currently exists on file, primarily as 35 mm transparencies or photographic prints, necessitating conversion of analog sources to digital files. Newer digital technologies address this shortcoming; however, while these images may exist in digital image format ready for multipurpose use, they are not archived for easy accessibility.

One solution being explored is MedPix™. Hosted by the Uniformed Services University, it is a fully Web-enabled cross-platform database that integrates images and textual information. Its primary target audience includes physicians and nurses, allied health professionals, medical students, graduate nursing students, and other postgraduate trainees. The content material is organized by disease location (organ system), pathology category, patient profiles, and by image classification and caption. MedPix™ can be searched through multiple internal image and text search engines. MedPix™ search formulations may be linked directly to PubMed and other outside search engines with a single click. Additional features, including Category 1 Continuing Medical Education (CME) and Continuing Nursing Education (CNE) credits, quizzes, uploading, and editing, are available to registered users.

We have also proposed an archive of ophthalmic images, illustrations, and videos that will be accessible via the World-Wide Web for educational purposes, and that will serve as a resource to medical personnel. A primary objective is to provide controlled access to archived images in a searchable, relational database with well-defined metadata, standardized multimedia file formats, and HTML and XML content.

This metadata will adhere to Department of Defense sharable content object reference model specifications [8], and allow resources to be repurposed for a variety of digital and traditional media publishing efforts. Consequently, the repository will serve not only ophthalmologists, but other audiences as well, such as emergency medical personnel and training organizations. Such a repository would have significant added value in remote ophthalmic consultation, i.e., providers faced with a challenging patient would be able to review images of similar findings to aid in diagnosis and management.

28.9 Conclusions

Delivering timely, cost-effective, quality care to beneficiaries and consultation partners is the goal of all health care systems. The particular challenges of distance, geography, and logistics faced by US Army ophthalmologists as they deliver this care attest to the ever-increasing relevance of telemedicine. Research and implementation of teleophthalmology solutions are providing opportunities to improve care, expand knowledge through training and distance learning, and provide services that were not possible a few short years before. Many of these applications, which are in use today, enable Army ophthalmologists both to assist other health care providers, and to deliver care directly to a geographically diverse beneficiary population. US Army ophthalmologists continue to develop and research new technologies in an effort to shorten the distance between the injured soldier or ill retiree and the ophthalmologist's exam chair, thereby speeding interventions to preserve ocular health.

References

1. Magdoff H, Foster JB, McChesney RW, Sweezy P (2002) US Military Bases and Empire. Monthly Review 53(10):8–9
2. Congressional Budget Office (1995) Restructuring military medical care, July 1995
3. Congressional Research Service Issue Brief for Congress (2001) Military medical care services: questions and answers. Congressional Research Service, Library of Congress
4. Mader TH, Aragones JV, Chandler AC, et al. (1993) Ocular and ocular adnexal injuries treated by United States military ophthalmologists during Operations Desert Shield and Desert Storm. Ophthalmology 100:1462–1467

5. Simon DP, Thach AB, Bower KS (2003) Teleophthalmology in the evaluation of ocular trauma. Mil Med 168:205–211
6. Aiello L, Cavallerano J, Bursell S (2000) The Joslin Vision Network innovative telemedicine care for diabetes, Preserving human vision. Ophthalmol Clin North Am 13:213–224
7. Hammond MD, Madigan WP, Bower KS (2005) Refractive surgery in the US Army: 2000–2003. Ophthalmology 112:184–190
8. Advanced Distributed Learning (2005) http://.www.adlnet.org/index-cfm?fuseaction=SCORMDown&listing=Specifications. Arch Soc Esp Oftalmol, Cited 4 Oct 2005

Part IV

Looking Into the Future – Current Experiments and Future Directions

IV

Chapter 29

Digital Imaging to Characterize Retinal Vascular Topography

29

Niall Patton, Tariq Aslam

This chapter addresses the following

Key Concepts:

- Digital image analysis has transformed the ability to obtain more accurate and reliable measurements from retinal photographs.
- The majority of techniques used to quantify retinal vasculature rely on accurate measurement of retinal vessel widths and vessel branching angles.
- Digital (and automated) imaging analysis can be used to quantify different aspects of retinal vasculature.
- Associations identified with the arteriovenous ratio include hypertension, atherosclerosis, diabetes, risk of stroke, cardiovascular mortality, risk of coronary heart dise ase, and smoking.
- In the future, digital image analysis of retinal photographs may offer an independent marker of risk for systemic disease for any individual.

29.1 Introduction

Fundal examination offers a unique opportunity to non-invasively visualize, photograph, and subsequently analyze images of the retinal vasculature in vivo. Technology has developed rapidly, permitting retinal digital image analysis to be readily accessible to both researchers and practicing clinicians via commercial software. Over the past five years, large epidemiological studies have utilized retinal image analysis to help to characterize the influence of cardiovascular disease on retinal vascular topography.

In this chapter, we describe the use of imaging analysis to measure blood vessel widths using microdensitometry. We provide an overview of the concept of *optimization* of a branching vascular structure, and the evidence that retinal circulation conforms to such optimization principals. We review how researchers have employed digital image analysis to characterize retinal vasculature in terms of these optimization principles, and how this has proved useful in providing quantitative measurements from retinal images that are more objective and less observer-driven than previous manual techniques. We speculate on a future application of telescreening of fundal images for individual cardiovascular risk stratification based on retinal vascular topography.

29.2 Measuring Retinal Blood Vessel Widths From Retinal Photography

The majority of techniques that have been used to quantify retinal vascular topography, such as the (original and revised) arteriovenous ratio (AVR) junctional exponents, and optimality parameters, rely on an accurate measurement of retinal vessel widths. No other measurements are recorded and the only difference between these entities is what vessels' widths are measured, and how they are formulated to measure different aspects of vascular topography.

Retinal arterioles are often small, and require high-resolution images to obtain accurate measurements (which may be as small as 10 to 15 pixels). In addition, to enhance the contrast between the retinal arteriole and the background, red-free images are often preferred to color fundal images. Alternatively, the green channel from the RGB image can be used. Further image processing can be used to enhance contrast between the vessels and background retina, such as adaptive histogram equalization.

29.2.1 Micrometry

Originally, before the widespread use of digital imaging systems, micrometric techniques were used to measure retinal vessel widths. Retinal photographs were taken using conventional film processing techniques. After processing, the films were projected onto a screen with some entity of known dimension. Using this as a reference, calculations using micrometric screws or calipers were performed in order to determine measurements of individual blood vessels. Indeed, micrometric techniques were originally used by Parr and colleagues to develop the Central Retinal Artery Equivalent (CRAE) measurement [1]. However, with the development of digital imaging systems, newer techniques based on intensity profiles of retinal blood vessels (microdensitometry) and edge detection programs have superseded micrometric techniques.

29.2.2 Microdensitometry

Digitalized image analysis techniques are more reliable than previous micrometric techniques [2–4]. In addition, they are subject to less observer bias and are less time consuming. However, microdensitometry techniques are semi-automated, requiring some observer input to designate what cross-section of blood vessel to measure. A cross-section of a retinal blood vessel will have a typical intensity profile, resulting from its grey level at each pixel point. The location of each pixel can be identified with spatial coordinates and each has a defined intensity, also known as its grey value. This profile typically has a similar configuration to a Gaussian profile, and can be described by the equation,

$$f(x) = a_1 e^{-\left(\frac{x-a_2}{a_3}\right)^2} + a_4$$

where a_1 is the amplitude of the peak of the profile, a_2 is the position of the peak, a_3 is a specific parameter of Gaussian function that controls the width of profile, and a_4 is the background retinal intensity.

The profile can also be expressed as a double-Gaussian function, with a smaller central Gaussian curve subtracted from the main profile to account for the central bright reflex.

The Gaussian profile (or double-Gaussian) can then be analyzed using image analysis techniques to obtain a measure of the width of the corresponding arteriole. The most common technique for acquiring the vessel width is to estimate the width of the vessel at half the height of the peak of the intensity profile of the double-Gaussian curve (half-height method) (Fig. 29.1). This strategy minimizes any effect of de-focusing at image acquisition [5], which may be caused by medial opacities, such as cataracts.

29.3 Other Image Analysis Techniques

Other techniques of automated vessel width measurement have included the use of edge detection masks [6], and sliding linear regression filters [7, 8]. Rassam et al., [9] have used *kick-points* on the image histogram, which, although appearing to be more accurate in determining vessel width for good quality images, are more prone to errors due to de-focus.

Chapman et al. [7] compared three different automated strategies to measure retinal vessel widths (double-Gaussian intensity profiles, Sobel edge detector, and sliding regression linear filter) with manual measurement in red-free images. The Sobel edge detector uses a pair of 3×3 convolution masks, one estimating the gradient in the x-direction (columns), and the other estimating the gradient in the y-direction (rows). The sliding linear regression filter method is based upon the fitting of a line by linear regression, relating image intensity against distance across the vessel cross-section. They found the most reliable of the three techniques was the sliding linear regression

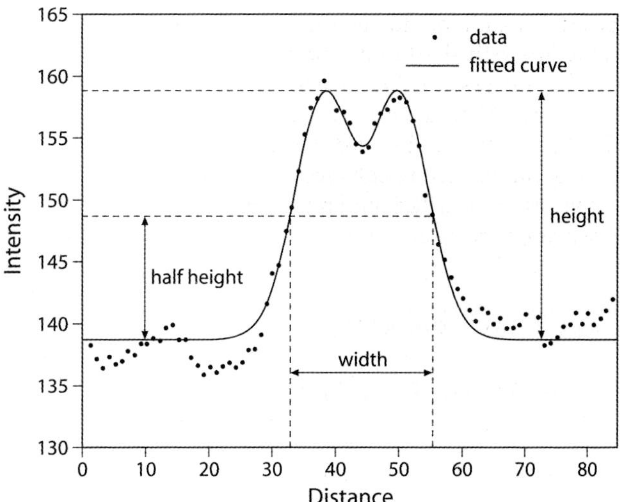

Fig. 29.1. Estimation of vessel width at half-height of the peak of the intensity profile

filter. Sobel edge detection was found to be the most inconsistent, possibly due to the program identifying the central light reflex from the blood vessel as an edge. The Canny edge detection program has been used in neural networks to automatically localize retinal blood vessels in fundal RGB images [10].

Using the algorithms described above, digital image analysis allows us to record individual measurements of retinal vessel widths and particular features of vascular junctions. However, to be able to obtain measures of overall retinal topography that can be compared from one individual to another, researchers have combined vessel measurements based on the principles of an optimized retinal vascular network.

29.4 An "Optimized" Branching Vasculature

While accepting the inevitable random scatter in any biological tissue with over a billion vascular branching points, it has long been known that a vascular structure in a healthy state conforms, to a degree, to an idealized optimal structure in order to minimize the costs involved across the vascular network. These *costs* include the shear stress experienced by the blood vessel due to vascular blood flow, volume of the vascular tree, power across the vascular network, and surface area. An optimal circulation can be considered when these costs are minimized. Features of a branching network that will determine the degree to which it is optimized include the angle between daughter blood vessels as they branch from the parent vessel, and the relationship between the widths of the trunk and branch vessels.

29.4.1 Branching Coefficient

One of the first parameters of vascular junctions to be considered was the branching coefficient. This was first considered by Young in 1809 [11] as a means of expressing the ratio of the area of the blood circulation before and after a vascular dichotomous junction:

Branching coefficient $(\omega) = (D_1^2 + D_2^2) / D_0^2$, where $D_1$is the width of branch vessel 1, D_2 is width of branch vessel 2, and D_0 is the width of the trunk vessel (Fig. 29.2).

Young (1809) [11] produced a value of 1.26 for the theoretical optimum value for ω, although the origin of this derived value is unclear [12]. However, the value of 1.26 was later explained by Murray (see Section 29.3.2, below) in 1926, in his seminal work on the relationship between parent and daughter vessel widths at vascular junctions [12].

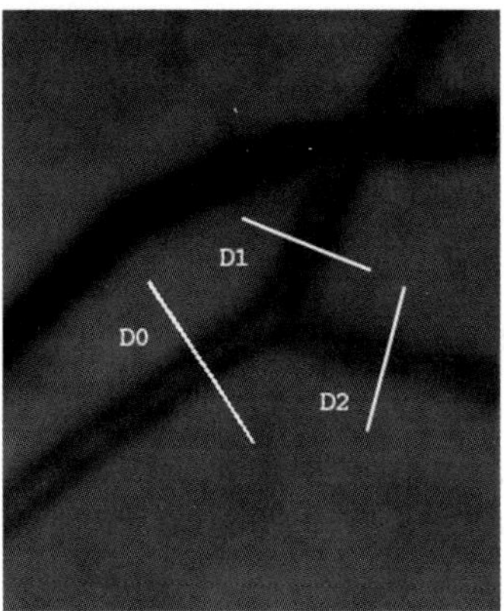

Fig. 29.2. Calculation of branching coefficient at a vascular dichotomous junction

29.4.2 Junctional Exponent

29

In 1926, Murray published his work on the design of an optimal branching vascular system [12], which minimizes the power required to overcome viscous drag in a fluid and the energy metabolically required to maintain the volume of blood and vessel tissue involved in blood flow. Murray's law relates the diameter of the trunk and branch vessels at a vascular junction in an optimal circulation, such that the cube of a diameter of the trunk vessel equals the sum of the cubes of the branch diameters. This can be expressed as $D_0^3 = D_1^3 + D_2^3$, where D_0 is the diameter of the trunk vessel and D_1 and D_2 are the diameters of the branch vessels. For a derivation of Murray's law, see Sherman [13]. For the situation where $D_1 = D_2$ (a symmetrical, dichotomous junction), this can be reduced to $D_0^3 = 2D_1^3$ and it can be shown that the area ratio of

$$(D_1^2 + D_2^2) / D_0^2 = 2^{1/3} \quad (\approx 1.26)$$

(The value of the optimum branching coefficient as given by Young [11]).

29.4.3 Vascular Bifurcation Angles

In addition to junctional exponents fitting theoretical values in an *optimized* vascular network, the angle subtended between two daughter vessels at a vascular junction has also been found to be associated with an optimal value, approximately 75°, depending on which costs (surface, volume, drag or power) [14, 15] are considered, and the degree of asymmetry between the two daughter vessels [16].

29.4.4 Image Analysis to Characterize Retinal Vascular Topography

Image analysis has been able to quantify different aspects of retinal vascular topography by measuring retinal vessel widths and angles at bifurcations, and employing the concept of an optimal circulation to obtain measures of generalized arteriolar attenuation and idealized vessel junctions. In order to obtain quantitative measurements from retinal photographs, any magnification effect resulting from retinal photography must be considered. The effect of magnification relates to both camera and ocular factors, and complex and simplified formulae based on Gullstrand's schematic eye exist in order to calculate true object size from image size [17]. However, the most common approach in quantifying retinal vascular topography has been the use of dimensionless measurements that are independent of any magnification effect. The most commonly performed measure used in large epidemiological studies has been the AVR.

29.4.5 Arteriovenous Ratio (AVR)

First considered by Stokoe and Turner in 1966 as representing a good dimensionless measure of generalized arteriolar attenuation [18], the AVR has been frequently employed to examine the relationship between the retinal vasculature and systemic disease. It was developed as a general measure of the ratio between the average diameters of the arterioles with respect to the venules and comprises two components, the CRAE and the Central Retinal Vein Equivalent (CRVE), expressed as a quotient. Rather than measuring a single retinal blood vessel, the AVR incorporates a measure of the width of all retinal blood vessels (arterioles and venules), usually measured at half to one disc diameter from the optic disc margin.

This location has been chosen as it is felt that at this location, the vessels have arteriolar rather than arterial properties, and thus may better reflect small vessel changes related to systemic factors such as blood pressure, age, etc. The AVR is felt to be a good measure of generalized arteriolar attenuation, as there is evidence that arterioles are much more affected by narrowing in response to cardiovascular disease than corresponding venules [19, 20].

29.4.5.1 CRAE and CRVE Calculations

The calculations used to derive the CRAE and CRVE were developed by Parr et al. in 1974 [1] and Hubbard et al., in 1992 [22], respectively. Both groups examined retinal photographs from a young, healthy normotensive population. By calculating the widths at numerous vascular junctions in this population, they employed a least squares method to calculate a formula that would minimize the differences between that observed and calculated for the width of the trunk vessel from the widths of the two branch vessels. The AVR was the ratio of the CRAE/CRVE.

Although in the original Parr technique, individual blood vessels were carefully traced out until all blood vessels were incorporated into the CRAE, Hubbard et al., used a process whereby the largest and smallest arteriole (or venule) were paired, followed by the second largest and second smallest, and so on. Thus the pairing all blood vessels in this arbitrary fashion were continued as an iterative process. If there were an odd number of vessels, the residual vessel was merely carried over into the next iteration. In such a fashion, values for the CRAE and CRVE could be calculated with greater speed and without the need for careful tracing of each individual blood vessel course.

29.4.5.2 AVR Calculation

The AVR requires a calculation of the width of individual arterioles and venules from retinal photography. When Parr and colleagues developed the calculations for the CRAE in 1974, digital image analysis was not yet available, and they relied on using *micrometric* techniques to formulate their calculations. This relied on the projection of fundal images onto illuminated screens and the use of micrometric screws to calculate projected widths. However, digital image analysis has transformed the ability to obtain more accurate and reliable measurements from retinal photographs.

29.5 AVR and Systemic Disease

The AVR has proved to be of great use in studies exploring generalized arteriolar attenuation as a marker of systemic vascular changes in a variety of conditions, and has been used in a large number of epidemiological studies, such as the Atherosclerosis Risk in Communities Study (ARIC), the Blue Mountains Eye Study (BMES), the Wisconsin Epidemiologic Study of Diabetic Retinopathy (WESDR), the Cardiovascular Health Study (CHS), the Beaver Dam Eye Study (BDES), and the Rotterdam Study (RS). Ailments identified with the AVR from these studies include hypertension [19–26], atherosclerosis [21, 25, 27–30], diabetes [22, 31], risk of stroke [32], cardiovascular mortality [33], risk of coronary heart disease [27, 29], and smoking [21, 28].

However, while the AVR has proved an extremely useful tool to explore the influence of systemic factors on retinal vascular topography, it has several limitations. For instance, the Parr–Hubbard formula contains constants that necessitate using measurements scaled only in micrometers. Therefore, to be able to use this formula, a conversion from pixel to micrometers needs to be performed, which will be an inexact summarized conversion. For example in the ARIC study, a value of 1850 μm was assumed to represent the average diameter of the optic disc, and therefore the mean width (in pixels) of the optic disc was used to derive this conversion ratio. In addition, the value of the AVR is dependent on the number of vessels measured. Thus, to overcome these difficulties and to try to improve the AVR as a measure of generalized arteriolar attenuation, in 2003, Knudtson et al. [34] devised a revised formula for the AVR.

29.6 Revised AVR

Knudston et al., returned to the concept of the branching coefficient mentioned previously to devise a new model for AVR [34]. They sought to find a technique that would incorporate measuring only the major arterioles and venules in the same predefined concentric zone around the disc, and to find a calculation that would be independent of the number of vessels measured.

29

In addition, by omitting any constants in the equation, they sought to make the formula independent of any scale. Based on the previous formula for the branching coefficient, they calculated the observed branching coefficient in a young normotensive healthy population (against a theoretical value of 1.26 for arterioles). Measuring a total of 187 arteriolar junctions, the branching coefficient was found to be 1.28 (95% confidence intervals from 1.25–1.32). From 151 venular junctions, the branching coefficient was calculated as 1.11 (95% confidence intervals from 1.08–1.14). Thus, by placing the calculated values into the *branching coefficient* formula, they calculated that:

For arterioles:

$$D_0 = 0.88 * (D_1^2 + D_2^2)$$

$$[0.88 = \sqrt{(1/1.28)}]$$

For venules:

$$D_0 = 0.95 * (D_1^2 + D_2^2)$$

$$[0.95 = \sqrt{(1/1.11)}]$$

The revised AVR is independent of the number of vessels measured, based on the fact that a total of 12 vessels are measured for all individuals. In addition, the absence of any constants allows measurements to be recorded at any scale, including a direct measurement of pixels. Also, greater accuracy in calculating the revised AVR may be expected from measuring only the six major arterioles and venules, as smaller vessels can be difficult to measure. Knudston et al. [34] undertook reanalysis of some of the previously published analyses using the revised formulae, and noted overall associations were still detected but with tighter confidence intervals. Based on these findings, the revised Parr–Hubbard formula should be regarded as the new reference standard for the measurement of AVR.

29.7 Junctional Exponent and Optimality Parameter

Image analysis is used to calculate junctional exponents by measuring the widths of the trunk and branch vessels as described previously. An iterative technique is then used to calculate the value of the junction exponent. The use of calculated junctional exponents to characterize retinal vascular topography is limited, as it is unclear how many vessel junctions are to be measured and how to summarize these individual exponents into a value that represents an individual. However, using the median junctional exponent from the five most proximal major arteriolar junctions on fluorescein angiography, Stanton et al., have shown that junctional exponents decrease with increasing age, but are similar in normotensive and hypertensive populations [35, 36].

Another limitation of junctional exponents is that a true value cannot be calculated if the diameter of the trunk vessel is less than either of the two branch vessels, which is a not-infrequent event in diseased circulations. In addition, the junctional exponent has been calculated to be extremely sensitive to small measurement errors, which may be expected to occur with small peripheral blood vessels. Hence, Chapman et al. [37] developed the *optimality parameter* as a measure of how much the junctional exponent deviates from an optimum value of three. This new calculation was found to be less sensitive to errors in vessel measurement than calculating the junctional exponent. In addition, for circumstances where the diameter of either of the branch vessels is greater than the diameter of the trunk vessel, a value for the optimality parameter can still be calculated. Using this new optimality parameter, Chapman et al., found that there was a significant difference in the *optimality* of retinal vascular junctions between healthy individuals and those with peripheral vascular disease [37].

29.8 Retinal Vascular Bifurcation Angles

Image analysis has been used to calculate the angles between branch retinal arterioles at vascular junctions. A Region Of Interest (ROI) can be selected to highlight and magnify the vascular junction. Plotting a line continuous with the trunk vessel, mapping the line of one of the branch vessels so that it intersects the trunk vessel at the junction and marking one other point on the other branch vessel will enable calculation of the total bifurcation angle between the two branch vessels using the cosine rule. Retinal arteriolar bifurcation angles are known to be reduced with hypertension [36], increasing age [35] and low birth weight males [38]. Reduced angles at vascular junctions are associated with less dense vascular networks [39]. In addition, vascular responsiveness to high oxygen saturation leads to a reduced angle at retinal vascular junctions, but this responsiveness is known to be reduced in hypertensives [40]. No relationship was reported between vascular bifurcation angles and peripheral vascular disease, compared with normal healthy controls [41].

29.9 Vascular Tortuosity

The degree of tortuosity of a vessel can be summarized as the ratio between the distance a vessel travels from A to B, and the shortest distance between points A and B drawn by a straight line. Indices of vascular tortuosity have been used as a measure of retinopathy of prematurity (ROP) [41–43]. Freedman et al., [44] used computer-aided analysis of fundus photographs from eyes with a wide range of ROP severity, and traced the posterior pole blood vessels' diameter and tortuosity. Swanson et al. [43] describe a semi-automated retinal vascular image analysis system (retinal image scale-space analysis) to measure retinal diameters and tortuosity in preterm infants. The authors point out some potential advantages of using such a system rather than regular clinical examination in the screening of ROP. Visualizing the posterior pole alone with the aim of diagnosing *plus disease* would considerably reduce the duration and trauma of examination and may allow health care professionals other than ophthalmologists to undertake screening. They point out the potential of telescreening to further improve the cost-effectiveness of the scheme, and the future potential of automated diagnosis (or grading) based on the captured fundal images.

29.10 Fractal Geometrical Analysis of Retinal Vascular Tree

The idea of using fractal geometry to describe branching patterns was first proposed by Mandelbrot [45, 46]. Fractal patterns exist when they exhibit self-similarity over a range of scale or magnification. Thus, a magnified view of a third of fourth order division of an arteriole would have a similar branching pattern to a first order arteriolar junction. Fractal patterns can also be considered as a measure of how well branching patterns fill the available two-dimensional space. Thus fractals are described in terms of a *fractal dimension*, which is a non-integer value between one and two. A value of two indicates that the fractal almost completely covers the available space.

29.10.1 Diffusion Limited Aggregation Model

Different models for the formation of fractals have been developed, but the one most commonly used to describe vascular branching patterns is the *diffusion limited aggregation model*, developed by Witten and Sander [47]. The basic principal involves a particle that moves in a random fashion until it gets close to part of the existing structure, at which point it becomes an adherent component of the structure. Such a model predicts a fractal dimension (D) of approximately 1.7, and studies of the retinal vasculature have found values for the fractal dimension remarkably close to this predicted value [48–52].

Performing fractal analysis of retinal vasculature is now possible using commercially available software. Initial studies utilized fluorescein images which clearly delineate the vasculature. However, modern imaging analysis using vascular segmentation and thresholding to produce a binary vessel/non-vessel image can be used to give a branching-analyzable image from conventional digital photography, and hence does not require angiography.

29.10.2 Clinical Studies

There are few clinical studies using retinal vascular fractal analysis. Quantitative region-based fractal analysis has been used in diabetic retinopathy [53, 54]. Non-proliferative diabetic retinal vasculature has been found to have a lower fractal dimension than normals within the macular region, using a region-based fractal analysis of retinal fluorescein angiograms.

29 It is currently unclear what the role of fractal analysis in characterizing retinal vascular topography is. Panico and Sterling [55] have questioned whether retinal vascular patterns are true fractals. Global fractal analysis of the retinal circulation may be too insensitive to detect subtle pathological changes of early disease [56]. Zamir has pointed out that fractal analysis of vascular systems must take into account the variability inherent within the arterial system [57]. This variability may be masked by a simple fractal dimension that is unable to differentiate two vasculatures that have the same space-filling properties, but widely different structures in their fluid dynamic design and function [58].

29.11 Future Directions

The use of digital image analysis of fundal images has allowed researchers to determine accurate, reliable measurements of retinal vessel widths and angles at retinal vascular junctions, and thus obtain measures of generalized arteriolar attenuation (AVR), optimal vascular junction branching patterns (junctional exponents, optimality parameter and angles at vascular junctions) and measures of how well the retinal vascular branching patterns fill the available two-dimensional space (fractal analysis).

While the AVR has been extensively used in studies, the other parameters of retinal vascular topography have been under-utilized, and further studies are needed to fully evaluate their contribution to retinal topography as markers of systemic factors. Other applications of retinal image analysis include image-based techniques to develop quantification of drusen area in age-related macular degeneration. New imaging modalities such as fundus autofluorescence offer further opportunities to employ digital image analysis for the objective, quantitative measurements of fundal characteristics [59].

Having characterized retinal vascular topography, digital image analysis of retinal photographs may offer in the future an independent marker of risk for cardiovascular disease for any individual, particularly for cerebrovascular risk [60]. For this potential to be realized requires further studies to show that retinal microvascular changes have additional predictive ability above current standardized clinical methods [61]. Also, techniques involved in characterizing retinal vascular topography are currently semi-automated, requiring significant observer input.

Further development of automated techniques used in image-based automated diagnostics may offer even faster, more practical strategies for widespread screening using store-and-forward methods. Digital compression of images may not be a realistic possibility for vessel measurement techniques, in view of the size of the vessels (15 to 20 μm). However, image compression algorithms are currently still evolving and with improved technology, it may be possible to transmit sufficiently high-resolution images to enable digital image analysis via teleophthalmology for the more widespread use of screening to determine individual risk stratification for systemic disease from retinal vascular topography.

References

1. Parr JC, Spears GF (1974) General calibre of the retinal arteries expressed as the equivalent width of the central retinal artery. Am J Ophthalmol 77:472–477
2. Delori FC, Fitch K, Feke G, Deupree D, Weiter J (1988) Evaluation of micrometric and microdensitometric methods for measuring the width of retinal vessel images on fundus photographs. Graefes Arch Clin Exp Ophthalmol 226:393–399

3. Newsom R, Sullivan P, Rassam S, Jagoe R, Kohner E (1992) Retinal vessel measurement: comparison between observer and computer driven methods. Graefes Arch Clin Exp Ophthalmol 230:221–225
4. Sherry LM, Wang JJ, Rochtchina E, Wong TY, Klein R, Hubbard LD, Mitchell P (2002) Reliability of computer-assisted retinal vessel measurement in a population. Clin Exp Ophthalmol 30:179–182
5. Brinchmann-Hansen O (1986) The light reflex on retinal arteries and veins: a theoretical study and a new technique for measuring width and intensity profiles across retinal vessels. Acta Ophthalmol Scand 179(Suppl):1–53
6. Gonzalez RC, Woods RE (1992) Digital image processing. Addison Wesley, Reading, MA, pp 418–420
7. Chapman N, Witt N, Gao X, Bharath AA, Stanton AV, Thom SA, Hughes AD (2001) Computer algorithms for the automated measurement of retinal arteriolar diameters. Brit J Ophthalmol 85:74–79
8. Gang L, Chutatape O, Krishnan SM (2002) Detection and measurement of retinal vessels in fundus images using amplitude modified second-order Gaussian filter. IEEE Trans Biomed Eng 49:168–172
9. Rassam S, Patel V, Brinchmann-Hansen O, Engvold O, Kohner E (1994) Accurate vessel width measurement from fundus photographs: a new concept. Brit J Ophthalmol 78:24–29
10. Sinthanayothin C, Boyce JF, Cook HL, Williamson TH (1999) Automated localisation of the optic disc, fovea, and retinal blood vessels from digital colour fundus images. Brit J Ophthalmol 83:902–910
11. Young T (1809) On the function of the heart and arteries. Philos Trans Royal Soc Lond 99:1–31
12. Murray C (1926) The physiological principle of minimum work: 1. The vascular system and the cost of blood volume. Proc Natl Acad Sci USA 12:207–214
13. Sherman T (1981) On connecting large vessels to small: the meaning of Murray's law. J Gen Physiol 78:431–453
14. Woldenberg MJ (1986) Relation of branching angles to optimality for four cost principles. J Theor Biol 122:187–204
15. Zamir M (1976) The role of shear forces in arterial branching. J Gen Physiol 67:213–222
16. Griffith T, Edwards D (1990) Basal EDRF activity helps to keep the geometrical configuration of arterial bifurcations close to the Murray optimum. J Theor Biol 146:545–573
17. Garway-Heath D, Rudnicka A, Lowe T, Foster P, Fitzke F, Hitchings R (1998) Measurement of optic disc size: equivalence of methods to correct for ocular magnification. Brit J Ophthalmol 82:643–649
18. Stokoe N, Turner R (1966) Normal retinal vascular pattern: arteriovenous ratio as a measure of arterial calibre. Brit J Ophthalmol 50:21–40
19. Hubbard LD, Brothers RJ, King WN, Clegg LX, Klein R, Cooper LS, Sharett AR, Davis MD, Cai J (1999) Methods for evaluation of retinal microvascular abnormalities associate with hypertension/sclerosis in the Atherosclerosis Risk in Communities Study. Ophthalmology 106:2269–2280
20. Leung H, Wang J, Rochtchina E, Tan A, Wong T, Klein R, Hubbard L, Mitchell P (2003) Relationships between age, blood pressure, and retinal vessel diameters in an older population. Invest Ophth Vis Sci 44:2900–2904
21. Ikram M, de Jong F, Vingerling J, Witteman J, Hofman A, Breteler M, de Jong P (2004) Are retinal arteriolar or venular diameters associated with markers for cardiovascular disorders? The Rotterdam Study. Invest Ophth Vis Sci 45:2129–2134
22. Klein R, Klein B, Moss S, Wong T, Hubbard L, Cruickshanks K, Palta M (2003) Retinal vascular abnormalities in persons with type 1 diabetes: the Wisconsin Epidemiologic Study of Diabetic Retinopathy: XVIII. Ophthalmology 110:2118–2125
23. Leung H, Wang J, Rochtchina E, Wong T, Klein R, Mitchell P (2004) Impact of current and past blood pressure on retinal arteriolar diameter in an older population. J Hypertens 22:1543–1549
24. Wang J, Mitchell P, Leung H, Rochtchina E, Wong T, Klein R (2003) Hypertensive retinal vessel wall signs in a general older population: the Blue Mountains Eye Study. Hypertension 42:534–541
25. Wong T, Klein R, Sharrett A, Manolio T, Hubbard L, Marino E, Kuller L, Burke G, Tracy R, Polak J, Gottdiener J, Siscovick D (2003) The prevalence and risk factors of microvascular abnormalities in older people: the Cardiovascular Health Study. Ophthalmology 110:658–666
26. Wong T, Wang J, Rochtchina E, Klein R, Mitchell P (2004) Does refractive error influence the association of blood pressure and retinal vessel diameters? The Blue Mountains Eye Study. Am J Ophthalmol 137:1050–1055
27. Klein B, Klein R, McBride P, Cruickshanks K, Palta M, Knudtson M, Moss S, Reinke J (2004) Cardiovascular disease, mortality, and retinal microvascular characteristics in type 1 diabetes: Wisconsin Epidemiologic Study of Diabetic Retinopathy. Arch Intern Med 164:1917–1924
28. Klein R, Sharrett A, Klein B, Chambless L, Cooper L, Hubbard L, Evans G (2000) Are retinal arteriolar abnormalities related to atherosclerosis? The Atherosclerosis Risk in Communities Study. Arterioscler Thromb Vasc Biol 20:1644–1650
29. Wong T, Klein R, Sharett A, Duncan B, Couper D, Tielsch J, Klein B, Hubbard L (2002) Retinal arteriolar narrowing and risk of coronary heart disease in men and women: the Atherosclerosis Risk in Communities Study. JAMA 287:1153–1159

30. Wong TY, Klein R, Klein BEK, Tielsch JM, Hubbard LD, Nieto FJ (2001) Retinal microvascular abnormalities and their relationship with hypertension, cardiovascular diseases and mortality. Surv Ophthalmol 46:59–80
31. Wong T, Klein R, Sharrett A, Schmidt M, Pankow J, Couper D, Klein B, Hubbard L, Duncan B, investigators A. (2002) Retinal arteriolar narrowing and risk of diabetes mellitus in middle-aged persons. JAMA 287:2528–2533
32. Wong TY, Klein R, Couper DJ, Cooper LS, Shaher E, Hubbard LD, Wofford MR, Sharrett AR (2001) Retinal microvascular abnormalities and incident stroke: the Atherosclerosis Risk in Communities Study. Lancet 358:1134–1140
33. Wong T, Klein R, Nieto F, Klein B, Sharett A, Meuer S, Hubbard L, Tielsch J (2003) Retinal microvascular abnormalities and ten-year cardiovascular mortality: a population-based case-control study. Ophthalmology 110:933–940
34. Knudston M, Lee K, Hubbard L, Wong T, Klein R, Klein B (2003) Revised formulas for summarizing retinal vessel diameters. Curr Eye Res 27:143–149
35. Stanton A, Mullaney P, Mee F, O'Brien E, O'Malley K (1995) A method for quantifying retinal microvascular alterations associated with blood pressure and age. J Hypertens 13:41–48
36. Stanton AV, Wasan B, Cerutti A, Ford S, Marsh R, Sever PP, Thom SA, Hughes AD (1995) Vascular network changes in the retina with age and hypertension. J Hypertens 13:1724–1728
37. Chapman N, Dell'omo G, Sartini MS, Witt N, Hughes A, Thom S, Pedrinelli R (2002) Peripheral vascular disease is associated with abnormal arteriolar diameter relationships at bifurcations in the human retina. Clin Sci 103:111–116
38. Chapman N, Mohamudally A, Cerutti A, Stanton A, Sayer A, Cooper C, Barker D, Rauf A, Evans J, Wormald R, Sever P, Hughes A, Thom S (1997) Retinal vascular network architecture in low birth weight males. J Hypertens 15:1449–1453
39. Kiani M, Hudetz A (1991) Computer simulation of growth of anastomosing microvascular networks. J Theor Biol 150:547–560
40. Chapman N, Haimes G, Stanton A, Thom S, Hughes A (2000) Acute effects of oxygen and carbon dioxide on retinal vascular network geometry in hypertensive and normotensive subjects. Clin Sci 99:483–488
41. Capowski J, Klystra J, Freedman S (1995) A numerical index based on spatial frequency for the tortuosity of retinal vessels and its application to plus disease in retinopathy of prematurity. Retina 15:490–500
42. Heneghan C, Flynn J, O'Keefe M (2002) Characterization of changes in blood vessel and tortuosity in retinopathy of prematurity using image analysis. Med Image Anal 6:407–429
43. Swanson C, Cocker K, Parker K (2002) Semi-automated computer analysis of vessel growth in preterm infants without and with ROP. Brit J Ophthalmol 87:1474–1477
44. Freedman S, Kylstra J, Capowski J, Realini T, Rich C, Hunt D (1996) Observer sensitivity to retinal vessel diameter and tortuosity in retinopathy of prematurity: a model system. J Pediat Ophth Strab 33:248–254
45. Mandelbrot B (1967) How long is the coast of Britain? Statistical self-similarity and fractional dimension. Science 156:636–638
46. Mandelbrot B (1982) The fractal geometry of nature. Freeman, San Francisco
47. Witten T, Sander L (1981) Diffusion-limited aggregation, a kinetic phenomena. Phys Rev Lett 47:1400–1403
48. Masters B, Platt D (1989) Development of human retinal vessels: a fractal analysis. Invest Ophth Vis Sci 30(Suppl):391
49. Daxer A (1992) Fractals and retinal vessels. Lancet 339:618
50. Family F, Masters B, Platt D (1989) Fractal pattern formation in human retinal vessels. Physica D 38:98–103
51. Landini G, Murray P, Misson G (1995) Local connected fractal dimensions and lacunarity analysis of 60° fluorescein angiograms. Invest Ophth Vis Sci 36:2749–2755
52. Mainster MA (1990) The fractal properties of retinal vessels: embryological and clinical implications. Eye 4:235–241
53. Avakian A, Kalina R, Sage E, Rambhia A, Elliott K, Chuang E, Clark J, Hwang JN, Parsons-Wingerter P (2002) Fractal analysis of region-based vascular change in the normal and non-proliferative diabetic retina. Curr Eye Res 24:274–280
54. Daxer A (1993) Fractal analysis of new vessels in diabetic retinopathy. Invest Ophth Vis Sci 34(Suppl):718
55. Panico J, Sterling P (1995) Retinal neurons and vessels are not fractal but space-filling. J Comp Neurol 361:479–490
56. Masters B (2004) Fractal analysis of the vascular tree in the human retina. Annu Rev Biomed Eng 6:427–452
57. Zamir M (1999) On fractal properties of arterial trees. J Theor Biol. 197:517–526
58. Zamir M (2001) Arterial branching within the confines of fractal L-system formalism. J Gen Physiol 118:267–275
59. Bellmann C, Rubin G, Kabanarou S, Bird A, Fizke F (2003) Fundus autofluorescence imaging compared with different confocal scanning laser ophthalmoscopes. Brit J Ophthalmol 87:1381–1386

60. Patton N, Aslam T, MacGillivray T, Pattie A, Deary I, Dhillon B (2005) Retinal vascular image analysis as a screening tool for cerebrovascular disease: a rationale based on homology between retinal and cerebral microvasculatures. J Anat 206:319–348

61. Wong TY (2004) Is retinal photography useful in the measurement of stroke risk? Lancet Neurol 3:179–183

Chapter 30

Emergency Telemedicine in Eye Care

30

Sotiris Pavlopoulos, Ilias Maglogiannis

This chapter addresses the following

Key Concepts:

- Wireless telemedicine systems and services are expected to enhance traditional emergency care provision, not only in the emergency department, but also in a variety of pre-hospital emergency care situations where geographically remote consultations and monitoring can be implemented.
- Although an emergency teleophthalmology system is not yet commercially available, one could take advantage of the experience gained from different emergency telemedicine systems and services and apply it to the ophthalmology sector.
- A potential application of telemedicine eye care is with emergency case management, and we propose that it would be effective for emergency teleophthalmology systems and services.
- The requirements of such a system are mobility, user friendliness, minimum user technical involvement, secure operation and reliability.

30.1 Introduction and Literature Review

The main focus of modern health care systems is to improve the health of the populations they serve. At present, there is a trend for decentralization of health care institutions with a move from institutional health care to primary and home care, and from inpatient care to outpatient settings. This results is an increased need for specialized care in outpatient settings and out-hospital environments.

Recent advances in telecommunications and information technologies have had a significant impact on health care service provision, and the emergency health services have been one of the sectors that have significantly benefited from these advances. In this chapter we present potential applications of telemedicine in eye care with an emphasis on emergency case management, along with a proposal for an emergency teleophthalmology system and service.

The term *emergency teleophthalmology* describes the real-time provision of medical eye care to patients who are at a distant location from specialized physicians (ophthalmologists) in accident and emergency conditions. The physicians use patient data that are acquired and transmitted by on-line telemedicine systems that utilize telematics technologies to assess the patient's condition and suggest appropriate pre-hospital patient care. Furthermore, using video conferencing with the transmission of images of the eye, specialists are able to provide secondary advice to general health practitioners at remote sites where transportation is not possible.

Since 1998, teleophthalmology has been used in trial sites within several countries and research centers to provide outreach services to primary care, support accident and emergency departments, and assess referrals. Two modes of eye image transmission may be found in the literature, namely, *real-time interactive video conference* mode and *store- and-forward* mode. Store-and-forward systems are simpler, cheaper and do not require synchronous communication between the two stations participating in a teleophthalmology session. Due to the asynchronous transmission of data, network delays are less important and thus lower bandwidth networks can be used. Furthermore, the examination procedure is quite easy to program, due to the fact that both sides (ophthalmologist and patient) can interact with the system independently. However, the majority of the surveyed applications found in the literature run in real-time mode. This is due to the inability of store-and-forward systems to cover emergency and accident situations, and the fact that real-time mode better simulates the clinical examination, because it allows the specialist to ask questions of the patient or general health practitioner – or even to request additional eye images and relevant medical data.

30.2 Telecommunications and Remote Consultation Models

An important part of teleophthalmology systems is the telecommunications infrastructure. Data transmission through the public telephone network is quite attractive due to high availability and low cost, but it suffers from low bandwidth and thus is inappropriate for the large amount of image and sound data that have to be transmitted.

30.2.1 ISDN Protocol

Many systems described in the literature use the ISDN protocol for the data link layer, while the introduction of faster DSL technologies is expected to improve the efficiency of such systems. For instance, Camara et al. [1] discussed how telemedicine technology may support real-time telemonitoring to teach ophthalmologists ophthalmologic surgical procedures in remote areas. To do so, they performed several tests over an ISDN line conveying information at a rate of 128 Kb/s. For the purpose of the tests, an endoscopic laser-assisted dacryocystorhinostomy, as well as live surgical and endoscopic images, were transmitted in real-time from the St. Francis Medical Center in Honolulu, Hawaii to ophthalmologists at the Makati Medical Center in Manila, Philippines.

30.2.2 Video Conferencing

In 1998, Moorfields Eye Hospital pioneered the use of video conferencing with the transmission of real-time slit lamp images at 384 kbits/s to support an outreach clinic [2].

Furthermore Holle and Zahlmann [3], after introducing a four-phase evaluation process, presented the results of that process obtained from the ophthalmological teleconsultation network established by the European Union (EU) project OPHTEL and the Bavarian state government. Medical data were exchanged through synchronous (ISDN video conferencing equipment) and asynchronous (encrypted e-mail) transmission modes. Their research proved that ophthalmological teleconsultations are very valuable, cost-effective and time saving, and that the learning effort required to handle the new technology is rather low.

30.2.3 TCP/IP Protocol

Many teleophthalmology applications also run over Internet-based transmission through the TCP/IP protocol with enhanced security features. Chew et al. [4] presented *OphthWeb*, a project related to a Web-based ophthalmic Electronic Medical Record implementation that can be accessed locally via the Internet. The paper reported a successful ophthalmologic data transmission trial between remote diagnostic centers, improving the holistic care of ophthalmic patients. All the text and image entries associated with a complete ophthalmic examination are stored in a database and forwarded at a subsequent stage. The system allows flexibility in the preparation of ophthalmic records, thus the physician may choose from the main categories of ophthalmic examinations available. Electronic Medical Record input is semi-automated; thus digital images are directly captured into the database; data entry is assisted by using pull-down screens; default descriptions of normal examination elements can be user-defined; and an entry from a prior examination can be accessed and edited. The presented store-and-forward implementation does not require high bandwidth and uses a PSTN/ISDN network.

30.2.4 Networking Image and Data

Warnicki et al. [5] describe a system of networking image and data acquisition areas in an ophthalmic department. These data are accessed throughout the local Internet or intranet from different working areas such as satellite offices and homes. The system presented collects and stores ophthalmologic data from many sources, and displays them in a common format. These data are accessible by anyone, in the form of World-Wide Web pages viewable by a web browser. The system offers immediate access and its ease of operation encourages its use. Furthermore, by using data encryption methods and password protection, the system achieves a satisfactory security level.

30.3 Screening for Diabetic Retinopathy

The transfer of still images has been studied in the context of screening for diabetic retinopathy [6, 7]. A plethora of studies also exist in the literature regarding the value of digital images in teleophthalmology. Bursell et al. [8] evaluated the ability to determine clinical levels of diabetic retinopathy using stereoscopic non-mydriatic digital video color retinal images. Their results validated that this imaging technique may be an effective telemedicine tool for remotely determining the level of diabetic retinopathy, suggesting timing of the next retinal evaluation, and identifying the need for prompt referral to ophthalmology specialists.

30.3.1 Fundus Digital Image and Clinical Examination

Sabtia et al. [9] assessed the correlation between fundus digital image and clinical examination for diabetic retinopathy. They also described a screening program for the early detection of sight-threatening diabetic retinopathy using a camera. In order to assess fundus digital image and clinical examination, they based their study on patients who had not been treated for diabetic retinopathy previosly. All patients underwent digital fundus photography, and the photographs were evaluated and compared with the clinical findings as recorded by retinal specialists. Diabetic retinopathy and macular edema were analyzed separately, and the correlation was measured statistically.

They concluded that digital images provide an efficient method for diagnosing and classifying sight-threatening diabetic retinopathy, particularly proliferative diabetic retinopathy (PDR). However, agreement between the digital fundus camera and clinical examination by an ophthalmologist for diabetic maculopathy detection, though statistically substantial, was not very satisfactory.

30.3.2 Video Conferencing Pictures

Lamminen et al. [10] proposed an estimate of the quality of video conferencing pictures in a real-time environment by means of resolution, contrast sensitivity, and color discrimination tests. Furthermore, a panel of different tests related to those three parameters was carried out via a PictureTel video conference system at ISDN line speed. Based on the results, it is argued that much still has to be done in the field of teleophthalmology, because although teleophthalmology is exceptionably valuable during diagnosis and treatment, many parameters, such as the system's quality and user's ability to use the equipment in an appropriate manner, have to be considered in order to achieve high quality teleconsultation services.

30.3.3 Artificial Intelligence Tools

Artificial intelligence tools, such as fuzzy logic applications, are used in conjunction with teleophthalmology systems. Taleb et al. [11] evaluated the patient's visual acuteness without the physician's actual presence, using Web-based medical advice. In order to achieve this, a number of tests were performed during which letters of different sizes were presented to the patient's screen.

The authors also proposed an algorithmic treatment of the binary answers, based on the use of fuzzy set functions, in order to eliminate the different mistakes that can be incurred. The application uses an automatic method for the medical examination. The examination is carried out directly by a system, so verification is automatic and assisted by computer. The patient answers the questions from the system, which then processes the results and asks new questions if necessary. The target of this project was to implement a ophthalmologic telemedicine network to handle several incidents, including emergency cases [12].

30.3.4 Assessment of Strabismus

Research effort is also concentrated regarding the assessment of strabismus via teleophthalmology systems. Helveston et al. [13] described a store-and-forward telemedicine program that uses digital imaging and e-mail transmission of medical images for consultation for patients with strabismus. The medical images captured by digital camera are sent to the consultant via e-mail, and the diagnosis and treatment are sent back to the doctor via e-mail. The authors demonstrated that the diagnosis and treatment plan determined by an ophthalmologist for several patients after the study of digital images sent by e-mail was the same as the diagnosis and treatment plan determined by the same doctor after an in-person examination of the patients.

Cheung et al. [14] assessed the quality of strabismus examinations using the audiovisual telecommunications of a telemedicine system in term of reliability and adequacy to permit assessment of typical ocular motor disorders.

Two studies were conducted: the first assessed the level of agreement of strabismus examination by telemedicine with standard face-to-face examination, and the second assessed the level of agreement of examination in person with a second independent examination in person. The authors concluded that a considerable level of agreement exists between telemedical and standard strabismus evaluations, indicating the potential application of telecommunication technologies for strabismus consultations. They also noted reduced reliability in the detection of small vertical deviations by inspection and in evaluating oblique muscle actions.

30.3.5 Performance of Telesurgical Operations

An emerging aspect of teleophthalmology is the performance of telesurgical operations. Camara et al. [15] demonstrated the feasibility of proctoring a complex ophthalmologic procedure from a distance with appropriate instrumentation and video conferencing technology. The teleophthalmology surgery session took place in real-time and was completed successfully via a 384 kb/s ISDN line. The success of the surgical procedure was comparable to traditional hands-on orbital surgery.

30.3.5.1 Telesimulation Service

Similarly, a prototype of a telesimulation service that can be used for training ophthalmologists performing phacoemulsification surgery has been described [16]. The system considers the network as a vital element for collaboration in virtual educational environments and is user friendly, as it can display graphic interaction elements, such as a stereoscopic visualization element, or educational aids, such as a video. Many tasks, including detailed implementation, and performance and usability measurements, are stated as future work in this article.

30.3.5.2 Transmission of Eye Images

While the technology is changing rapidly, the basic principles of the transfer of video, audio, and other data at high speed in either real-time or store-and-forward modalities in teleophthalmology remain applicable. The transmission of eye images has been shown to be effective in several studies. Johnston et al. [17] discussed the cost-effectiveness of teleophthalmology. The authors presented the cost-effectiveness and practitioner benefits associated with a technology transfer project using teleophthalmology to provide specialist advice to practitioners in South Africa. Although the technology transfer project itself was cost-increasing, it led to patient benefits and therefore to a reduction in the burden of eye disease.

Clearly from the above survey, an emergency teleophthalmology system and service are essential. Although such a system is not commercially available today, one could take advantage of the experience gained from different emergency telemedicine systems and services and apply it to the ophthalmology sector. In the following section such a system is proposed and presented in more detail.

30.4 An Emergency Teleophthalmology System

In a report prepared by the American College of Emergency Physicians in 1998 [18] there are specific references to current and future applications of emerging technologies in the practice of emergency medicine [19]. More specifically, it is anticipated that wireless communication technologies will greatly impact emergency care provision in the near future. It is also evident that wireless telemedicine systems and services are expected to enhance traditional emergency care provision, not only within the emergency department, but also in a variety of pre-hospital emergency care situations where geographically remote consultation and monitoring can be implemented. The existence of high bandwidth mobile communication links can ensure use of telemedicine resources to facilitate acute and non-acute care provision in the field, and to provide a direct link between field personnel and medical direction [20].

Many studies have demonstrated the potential benefits, based on patient survival, of early and specialized pre-hospital patient management [17, 19–23]. Emergency care requires that services are provided anywhere and any time; thus systems designed for emergency care should meet some very crucial requirements [24–26]. Specifically, it should:

- *Be transportable*, in order to be carried at the emergency site by a single person. In principle, if such a system were to be used by paramedics, it should not weigh more than 5 kg, including the image capturing device, the computing device, and the communication components. This is achievable, considering that a laptop, portable computer should not exceed 2.5 kg, with a camera around 0.5 kg, and the rest being consumed by the carrying cases and batteries.
- *Be easy to use*, ideally requiring minimum hand operation, in order to enable medical and paramedical personnel to handle the case. To meet this requirement, the application software should have automatic mechanisms to establish communication with the consultation unit, and to allow data collection and transmission without the need of complex operation. If for any reason the communication is interrupted, the system should enable automatic re-connection procedures, while data are stored locally (if needed) to be transferred when communication is re-established.
- *Be secure in operation*, especially under difficult environmental conditions. It is conceivable that there may be cases where the system would be used in outdoor environments or during patient transportation. This requirement indicates that at least the computing device should be designed for outdoor use (e.g., rugged case, operation on the move, etc.).
- *Be implementing wireless technologies*, thus enabling operation outdoors and in other environments where wired communication links are not available. This is in line with the current trend in health care provision wherein the "any where-any time" concept applies.

In Fig. 30.1, the architecture of an emergency teleophthalmology service is depicted. The service is implemented with the use of two separate systems, namely, the mobile system used at the emergency site, and the consultation system used at the emergency coordination center. It is clear however, that the system worth presenting

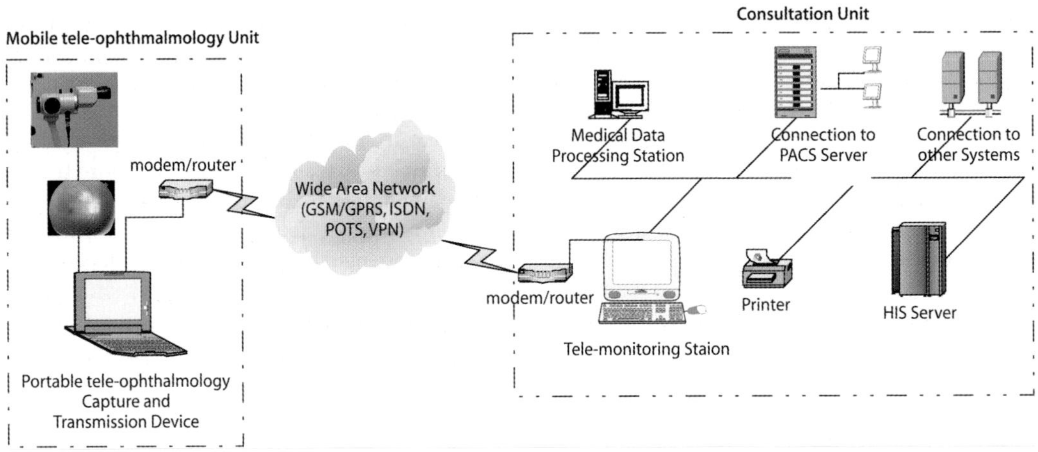

Fig. 30.1. Schematic representation of the proposed emergency teleophthalmology system

in more detail is the mobile system, which is responsible for collecting patient information at the emergency site.

30.4.1 Mobile Teleophthalmology Unit

The mobile unit is used to collect the ophthalmology study data, and to transmit them to the consultation center for the purpose of telemedicine support. Transmission could be done synchronously or asynchronously, depending on the clinical protocol and of course, on the available communication infrastructure. The mobile unit consists of three main subunits:

1. **Image capturing subunit.** In a teleophthalmology application, the image capturing subunit should be an ophthalmoscope. Of course, if the system is designed to be used outdoors (or on the move), a hand-held ophthalmoscope should be used, such as an AMD-2500p general examination camera (www.amdtelemedicine.com/).
2. **Computing subunit.** This subunit is responsible for digitizing, encoding, displaying, and storing the image data. Although a desktop personal computer could be used in cases of general purpose telemedicine, in cases of telemedicine on the move a tablet personal computer or a rugged portable computing device would be recommended. Examples can be found in www.getac.com.
3. **Communication subunit.** This subunit is responsible for transmitting the collected data to the coordination center. The communication subunit may be included in the computing subunit in the form of a modem. To maximize the potential use of the system, wireless communication means should be supported, such as GSM/GPRS (Global System for Mobile Communication/General Packet Radio Service), Wi-Fi, satellite communication links, etc. The TCP/IP protocol has been used in many cases to provide interoperability across communication links, given that the majority of currently available links support it. Furthermore, TCP/IP can support secure and reliable data transmission, which is usually a major requirement in medical data handling.

Currently third generation (3G) mobile communication technologies can be extremely useful for emergency telemedicine applications, since they provide high data rates (384 Kb/s or higher) on the move as well as an automatic switch to GPRS links when 3G is not available. In addition, 3G allows concurrent voice and data calls thus enabling vocal communication between the emergency site and the consultation site together with data exchange (images and medical data transmission).

30.4.2 Consultation Unit

The consultation unit is used to receive the study data and to provide the consulting physicians with the required tools and data to support the emergency case. Typically, it provides viewing stations to visualize the received images and data. The consulting physician is able to review the received case information, to assess the case severity, and to give instructions to the physician who is handling the case on how to deal with the case.

30.4.2.1 Communication

Most often, together with the data exchanged, the two practitioners also have vocal (telephone) communication. Furthermore, if such an option is available, consulting physicians would like to have access to the electronic patient record (EPR) through connections to a hospital information system (HIS). Usually such connections are implemented via standardized messaging schemes like the HL7 protocol (www.hl7.org). Additional functionalities provided to the consultation unit include the option to *remote control* the image collection process (e.g., magnification, rotation, etc.), provided that such options are supported by the image capturing device. Furthermore, the consultation unit should store all collected information, both for reporting needs and for legal purposes. The latter is considered a major issue in telemedicine, since many concerns arise around responsibilities when telemedical services are provided [27].

30.4.2.2 Potential Application

Although a system like the one described above has not been used in the past for teleophthalmology applications, it is evident that its use may have a significant impact for emergency ophthalmic care applications. Similar systems used in other emergency telemedicine application have demonstrated significant clinical benefits. Studies performed in Greece and Sweden using mobile telemedicine devices for emergency cardiology cases demonstrated that patient treatment (with supervision by specialists) can be initiated 25 to 35 min, on average, before patient arrival at the hospital [26]. This is extremely significant since in many emergency cases the *golden hour* rule applies, i.e., if proper treatment is provided within the first hour, then the case outcome is substantially improved. Since no relevant clinical studies have been performed for emergency ophthalmic care, it is essential that such concepts are first validated in practice. It is however, very important to note that no significant technology barriers presently exist to implement such a solution.

30.5 Conclusions and Suggestions

In this chapter we have (1) provided a state-of-the-art review on telemedicine applications in eye care with emphasis on emergency case management, (2) discussed the corresponding technologies, and (3) proposed an emergency teleophthalmology system, based on experience from other emergency telemedicine applications. The benefits of teleophthalmology for patients include (1) speed and accuracy of eye disease diagnosis, (2) avoidance of unnecessary transportation (and therefore low cost/high quality eye care services), and (3) efficient handling of emergency incidents. This is important for countries with dispersed populations in isolated areas (such as Greece, Sweden, Australia, etc.), where there are many regions where it is difficult to access medical services, and where there is unequal demographic distribution. Thus emergency teleophthalmology may be considered as an essential service.

The requirements of an emergency teleophthalmology ystem, as discussed above, are mobility, user friendliness, minimum user technical involvement, and secure operation and reliability. However, it remains necessary for such systems to be tested by expert ophthalmologists and relevant medical personnel in order to assess not only user acceptance and satisfaction, but also the impact on the quality of the provided eye care services, along with health economics. Also of significant importance are issues related to organization of such services, training, and the legal and ethical issues linked to telemedicine

30

applications. The fact, however, that emergency telemedicine has proved very successful in other health care areas is very promising for the ophthalmic care areas.

References

1. Camara JG, Rodriguez RE (1998) Real-time telementoring in ophthalmology. Telemed J 4(4):375–377
2. Murdoch I (1999) Telemedicine. Brit J Ophthalmol 83(11):1254–1256
3. Holle R, Zahlmann G (1999) Evaluation of telemedical services. IEEE Trans Inf Technol Biomed 3(2):84–91
4. Chew SJ, Cheng HM, Lam DSC, Cheng ACK, Leung ATS, Chua JKH, Yu CP, Balakrishnan V, Chan WK (1998) Ophth Web-cost-effective telemedicine for ophthalmology. Hong Kong Med J 4(3):300–304
5. Warnicki JW, Justice Jr J, Justice MK (2001) Digital database for clinical ophthalmology and telemedicine. Insight 26(3)
6. Lahtela JT, Lamminen H (2002) Telemedical devices in diabetes management. Ann Med 34:241–247
7. Owens D, Gibbins R, George L (1997)Telemedicine in screening/monitoring of diabetic eye disease. Healthc Comput Commun, pp 166–171
8. Bursell SE, Cavallerano JD, Cavallerano AA, Clermont AC, Birkmire-Peters D, Aiello LP, Aiello LM, and the Joslin Vision Network Research Team (2001) Stereo nonmydriatic digital-video color retinal imaging compared with early treatment diabetic retinopathy Study Seven Standard field 35-mm stereo color photos for determining level of diabetic retinopathy. Ophthalmology 108:572–585
9. Al Sabtia K, Raizadab S, Wanib VB, Al Ajmib M, Gayedb I, Sugathana TN (2003) Efficacy and reliability of fundus digital camera as a screening tool for diabetic retinopathy in Kuwait. J Diabetes Complications 17:229–233
10. Lamminen H, Ruohonen K, Uusitalo H (2001) Visual tests for measuring the picture quality of teleconsultations for medical purposes. Comput Meth Programs Biomed 65:95–110
11. Taleb-Ahmed A, Bigand A (2003) Telemedicine and fuzzy logic: application in ophthalmology. Pattern Recogn Lett 24:2731–2742
12. Taleb-Ahmed A, Bigand A, Lethuc V, Allioux PM (2004) Visual acuity of vision tested by fuzzy logic: An application in ophthalmology as a step towards a telemedicine project. Info Fusion 5:217–230
13. Helveston EM, Orge FH, Naranjo R, Hernandez L (2001) Telemedicine: strabismus e-consultation. J AAPOS 5(5):291–296
14. Cheung JC, Dick PT, Kraft SP, Yamada J, Macarthur C (2000) Strabismus examination by telemedicine. Ophthalmology 107(11):1999–2005
15. Camara JG, Zabala RRB, Henson RD, Senft SH (2000) The use of real-time telementoring to remove an orbital tumor. Ophthalmology 107:1468–1471
16. Newballa AAN, Velezb JA, Satizabalc JE, Munerad LE, Bernabee G (2003) Virtual surgical telesimulations in ophthalmology. Int Congr Ser 1256:145–150
17. Johnston K, Kennedy C, Murdoch I, Taylor P, Cook C (2004) The cost-effectiveness of technology transfer telemedicine. Oxford University Press, Health Policy Plan 19(5):302–309
18. Auer NJ (ed) (1998) The future of emergency medicine. American College of Emergency Physicians Sales and Services, USA
19. Weston CF, Penny WJ, Julian DG (1994) Guidelines for the early management of patients with myocardial infarction. Br Med J 308:767–771
20. Krohmer JR (1998) Emergency medical services of the future. In: Auer NJ (ed) The future of emergency medicine, American College of Emergency Physicians Sales and Services, USA, pp 5–9
21. Canto JG, Rogers WJ, Bowlby LJ, French WJ, Pearce JD, Douglas WW (1997) The prehospital electrocardiogram in acute myocardial infarction: is its full potential being recognized? J Am Coll Cardiol 29:498–505
22. Case RB (1998) The role of emerging technologies in the practice of emergency medicine, In: Auer NJ (ed) The future of emergency medicine, American College of Emergency Physicians Sales and Services, USA, pp 25–27
23. Sedgewick ML, Dalziel K, Watson J, Carrington DJ, Cobbe SM (1993) Performance of an established system of first responder out-of-hospital defibrillation :the results of the second year of the Heartstart Scotland Project in the utstein style. Resuscitation 26:75–88
24. Chan TC, Killeen J, Griswold W, Lenert L (2004) Information technology and emergency medical care during disasters. Acad Emerg Med 11(11):1229–1236
25. Kyriacou E, Pavlopoulos S, Berler A, Neophytou M, Bourka A, Georgoulas A, Anagnostaki A, Karayiannis D, Schizas C, Pattichis C, Andreou A, Koutsouris D (2003) Multi-purpose healthcare telemedicine systems with mobile communication link support. Biomed EngOnline 2(7)
26. Pavlopoulos S, Kyriakou E, Berler A, Dembeyiotis S, Koutsouris D (1998) A novel emergency telemedicine system based on wireless communication technology – ambulance. IEEE Trans Inf Technol Biomed 2(4):261–267
27. Stanberry B (2001) Legal ethical and risk issues in telemedicine. Comput Meth Programs Biomed 64(3):225–233

Chapter 31

Transcontinental Robot-Assisted Remote Telesurgery, Feasibility and Potential Applications

31

Jaques Marescaux, Francesco Rubino

This chapter addresses the following

Key Concepts:

- Technical limitations related to the problem of time delay for transmission of digitized information had prevented the development of remote surgery.
- Tests and research performed by our group suggest the use of a high speed terrestrial network (ATM service), rather than satellite connections to reduce the time lag for transmission of data.
- Through the use of ATM technology, our group demonstrated the feasibility of performing surgery across transoceanic distances by safely carrying out a laparoscopic cholecystectomy.
- Using ATM technology, the mean time lag for transmission of data and images was 155 ms, despite a total roundtrip distance of 14,000 km.
- Remote surgery ensures availability of surgical expertise in remote locations for difficult operations, and may improve surgical training world-wide.
- Several limitations remain, including the need to render ATM networks available to hospitals, the costs of technology, ethical and liability issues, and possible conflicts of jurisdictions between countries involved.

31.1 Introduction

The introduction of computer technology in surgery has made it possible to digitize images and surgical gestures. Digitized information can be transmitted to a distant location, within the same operating room or in another country.

Robot-assisted remote telesurgery was first developed by the United States (US) Department of Defense to allow performance of operations on wounded soldiers on the battlefield [1, 2]. However, technical limitations have for many years limited the application of remote surgery to interactive teaching of techniques, or to basic tasks rather than to the actual performance of a full surgical operation.

Remote transmission of simple manipulations, such as control of a robotically held laparoscope from a separate room [3] or of an electrocautery instrument between the US and Austria [4], as well as instruments for kidney biopsy between the US and Italy [5], were the first attempts to develop a real remote surgical operation, but technical limitations were still a major issue. Indeed, whereas an average delay of 1 s may not compromise execution of simple tasks, the complex manipulations required during any surgical operation are more difficult to carry out. For this reason, it had been suggested that remote surgery could be applied safely only for telementoring rather than for the performance of a full surgical operation [6].

Some investigations, including our experimental experience, suggest that the maximum time delay acceptable for performance of a safe surgical operation should not exceed 300 ms [7], a time delay that is unfeasible if using satellites for transmission of information between the two sites. Using terrestrial ATM telecommunications, our group at the European Institute of Telesurgery was able to decrease the time lag across transoceanic distances to less than 160 ms [7]. This allowed the performance of laparoscopic cholecystectomy on six pigs in July 2001 and, on 7 September 2001 the first long distance remote operation on a human being [8].

31.2 Technical Issues of Remote Surgery

Remote surgery requires the use of robotic systems. The robotic systems currently available consist of a surgeon's console wherein the surgeon's input is digitized and compressed in transmissible information, and a robot subsystem (located at the patient's side) wherein the information is translated into actual instrument manipulation and endoscopic camera control.

31.2.1 Time Lag

For the transmission of information, video images must be compressed with algorithms that require significant time and processing power [9]. The time lag is defined as the delay for an instruction to be locally encoded, propagated over a transmission line to a remote machine, decoded and executed. The propagation of data through a busy network with limited bandwidth may significantly increase time lag [10, 11] and deteriorate performance [12]. The speed of transmission and the issue of latency are influenced by three factors: the distance, the intrinsic speed of the transmission system and the speed of computer interfaces in compressing and decompressing data. Using satellites for teletransmission would cause delays of around 600 ms or more, which are definitely unsuitable for remote surgery.

31.2.2 Digital Phone Lines

Although low altitude satellites may potentially reduce this delay, digital phone lines appear more useful. At the European Institute of Telesurgery, we investigated the effect of using asynchronous transfer mode (ATM) networks as the communication link across transoceanic distances. ATM technology can merge robot commands, audio and video images in a single stream of ATM data packets and can allocate bandwidth on demand, enabling a guarantee of a certain and predefined quality of service.

31.2.2.1 Robotic-Assisted Laparoscopic Cholecystectomy

In an experimental study our group attempted remote robotic-assisted laparoscopic cholecystectomy in pigs between New York, NY (USA) and Strasbourg (France) for a 14,000 km roundtrip. The operator site was in New York and the animals in Strasbourg. The two sites were connected through an ATM network (France Telecom/Equant). A bandwidth of 10Mb/s was reserved through the network. Round trip delay by ATM transport ranged between 78 and 80 ms, which, adding 70 ms for video coding and decoding and a few milliseconds for rate adaptation and Ethernet to ATM packet conversion, accounted for a total roundtrip time delay of 155 ms.

Laparoscopic remote robotic cholecystectomy was successfully performed in all six pigs of the experiment with a mean operative time of 45 min (26–78 min); with no complications. In addition to cholecystectomy, other complex surgical tasks were tested during the experiment. During the operative procedures, reproduction of image details on the video monitor in the operative site was highly accurate, resulting in perfect visualization of structures with no interruptions or degradation of video signals. The short time lag facilitated adaptation of surgeons, as evidenced by the short operative time.

31.2.2.2 The Lindberg Operation

Based on the findings of the above experiment, we performed the first clinical application of remote surgery on a human being. The project was symbolically named *Lindberg*, based on the name of the first aviator traveling across the Atlantic Ocean. The patient, a 68-year-old female with a history of symptomatic cholelithiasis underwent a remote robotic-assisted laparoscopic cholecystectomy on 7 September 2001 [8].

We used the ZEUS robot system (Computer Motion, Galeta CA). The operator site was in New York City, and the patient's subsystem in Strasbourg. The telecommunication system was set up as described before. Camera movements were directed from the computer in New York, according to the operating surgeon's instructions. The laparoscopic cholecystectomy was performed in 54 min without complications, the post-operative course was uneventful and the patient discharged from the hospital within 48 h from the operation.

These two studies were the first demonstration of the feasibility and safety of performing a complete surgical operation from remote locations. In March 2003, Doctors Anvari and MacKinley also successfully performed a series of robot-assisted remote operations, including Nissen fundoplication and right colectomy, in Canada, across 400 miles using ASDN telecommunication lines.

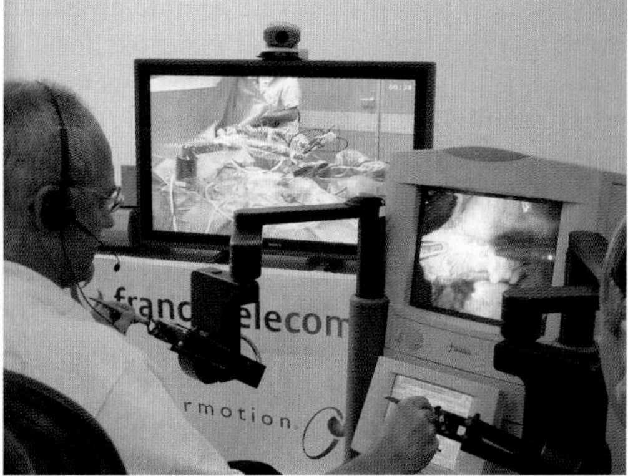

Fig. 31.1. The operator site in New York with the Zeus Surgeon's console

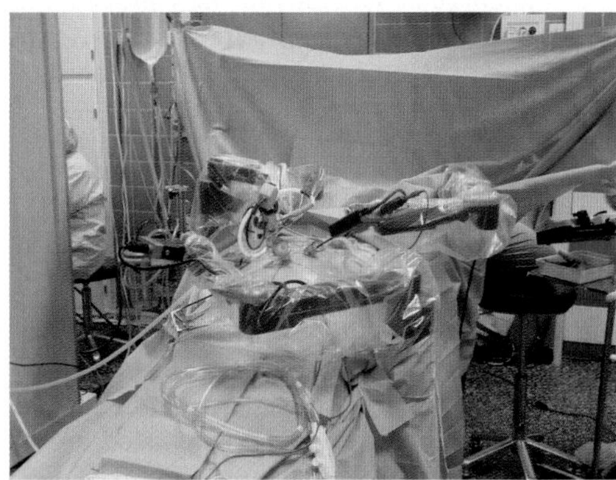

Fig. 31.2. The Zeus' robotic arms during the experimental Lindberg operation in Strasbourg

31.3 Current Limitations of Remote Surgery

Although an ATM fiber network is present in more than 200 countries world-wide, most hospitals are not equipped with ATM technology. ASDN lines may be easier and cheaper to use, but, so far, their reliability has been tested only within a few hundred miles. The costs of remote surgery are still formidable as they include the price of robotic machines, telecommunication lines, and human resources. However, if remote surgery will increase access to health care, improve training, and enhance outcomes, it may prove less costly than expected.

Other important issues include legal aspects, such as whether the surgeon should be liable for errors related to delays in transmission or equipment failure, and the impact of state and international borders, differences in legislations as well as in medical licensing. Until new international standards for licensure, reimbursement and other regulations are developed, remote surgery is unlikely to be performed by surgeons residing in one country on patients residing in another country. Moreover, the traditional surgeon–patient relationship is revolutionized due to the lack of direct contact between the patient and clinician, with potential implications for malpractice actions.

31.4 Potential Benefits of Remote Surgery

The most evident benefit of remote surgery is its ability for providers and patients to avoid the impact that geographic constraints might have on the type of treatment the patient receives. Indeed, the availability of expert assistance from outside local and/or rural and remote areas can overcome the lack of surgical expertise locally, especially for infrequently performed operations or new minimally invasive techniques.

As suggested by Ballantyne, an expert surgeon from a state university may perform operations for an entire region, or in areas with shortages of specialist surgeons [13]. In developing countries, where health care is often provided by volunteers that do not necessarily have expertise in all fields of medicine and surgery, this might be particularly valuable.

Besides benefits for patients, remote surgery might also prove beneficial for surgeons. In fact, real time assistance from an expert might help reduce errors related to the early phase of the learning curve of surgeons for new procedures, and encourage surgeons to embark themselves on learning and practicing new minimally invasive techniques.

31.5 Future Applications of Remote Surgery

Further developments in robotic and computer technologies may possibly expand the potentialities of remote surgery. Implementation of virtual reality technologies into robotic-assisted procedures may have the most significant impact. Prepracticed surgical procedures based on a virtual three-dimensional model of a specific patient may reduce the issue related to the lack of physical contact between the surgeon and the patient. Virtual reconstructions can be easily transmitted via Internet and allow real-time consultations. The operating surgeon may therefore have reliable information about the patient's anatomy as well as participate in the diagnostic process and discuss indications to surgery. Furthermore, the remote surgeon could train for the procedure in a virtual environment, using the patient's specific anatomical reconstruction, thus anticipating possible problems and perfecting solutions ahead of time.

Use of low-altitude satellites could overcome the limitation associated with the use of terrestrial cables, and enable performance of operations on ships or on space stations.

31.5.1 Telesurgery in Ophthalmology

An emerging aspect of teleophthalmology is the performance of telesurgical operations. Camara et al. [14] demonstrated the feasibility of proctoring a complex ophthalmologic procedure from a distance with appropriate instrumentation and video conferencing technology. The teleophthalmology surgery session took place in real time via a 384 kb/s ISDN line and was completed successfully. The success of the surgical procedure was comparable to traditional hands-on orbital surgery.

31.5.2 Telemonitoring as a Teaching Tool

Camara et al. [15] also discuss how telemedicine technology may support real-time telemonitoring to teach ophthalmologists ophthalmologic surgical procedures in remote areas. To do so, they performed several tests over an ISDN line conveying information at a rate of 128 kb/s. For the purpose of the tests, endoscopic laser-assisted dacryocystorhinostomy with live surgical and endoscopic images was transmitted in real-time from the St. Francis Medical Center in Honolulu, Hawaii to ophthalmologists at the Makati Medical Center in Manila, Philippines.

31.6 Conclusions

Remote robot-assisted telesurgery is feasible and safe using terrestrial telecommunication lines, even through transcontinental distances. In addition to several potential benefits for the patient, remote surgery might improve surgical training and education. Future developments of computer technology and their surgical applications, particularly in the field of virtual reality three-dimensional reconstructions of patient's specific anatomy and pathology, are the possible solutions to overcome the lack of direct patient–surgeon contact. Indeed, virtual reality systems may not only improve surgical performance by allowing preoperative simulations and rehearsal of surgical procedures ahead of time, but may also allow, thanks to real-time Internet teleconsultations, active intervention of the operating surgeon in the diagnostic process and in the evaluation of indications and contraindications to surgery.

References

1. Satava RM (1995) Virtual reality, telesurgery, and the new world order of medicine. J Image Guid Surg 1:12–16
2. Satava RM (1997) Virtual reality and telepresence for military medicine. Ann Acad Med Singap 26:118–120
3. Kavoussi LR, Moore RG, Partin AW, Bender JS, Zenilman ME, Satava RM (1994) Telerobotic assisted laparoscopic surgery: initial laboratory and clinical experience. Urology 44(1):15–19
4. Lee BR, Bishoff JT, Janetschek G, Bunyaratevej P, Kamolpronwijit W, Cadeddu JA, Ratchanon S, O'Kelley S, Kavoussi LR (1998) A novel method of surgical instruction: international telementoring. World J Urol 16(6):367–370
5. Micali S, Virgili G, Vannozzi E, Grassi N, Jarrett TW, Bauer JJ, Vespasiani G, Kavoussi LR (2000) Feasibility of telementoring between Baltimore (USA) and Rome (Italy): the first five cases. J Endourol 14(6):493–496
6. Mack MJ (2001) Minimally invasive and robotic surgery. JAMA 285:568–572
7. Marescaux J, Leroy J, Gagner M, Rubino F, Mutter D, Vix M, Butner SE, Smith MK (2001) Transatlantic robot-assisted telesurgery. Nature 413(6854):379–380
8. Marescaux J, Leroy J, Rubino F, Vix M, Simone M, Mutter D (2002) Transcontinental robot-assisted remote telesurgery: feasibility and potential applications. Ann Surg 235(4):487–492
9. Link RE, Schulam PG, Kavoussi LR (2001) Telesurgery: Remote monitoring and assistance during laparoscopy. Urol Clin North Am 28:177–187
10. Rosser J, Herman B, Ehrenwerth C (2001) An overview of videostreaming on the Internet and its application to surgical education. Surg Endosc 15(6):624–629
11. Schulam PG, et al. (1997) Telesurgical mentoring. Initial clinical experience. Surg Endosc 11:1001–1005
12. Sudarsan SP, Du LQ, Cobb PN, Yager ES, Jacobus CJ (1997) Influence of frame rate and image delay on virtual driving performance. Biomed Sci Instrum 33:203–208
13. Ballantyne GH (2002) Robotic surgery, telerobotic surgery, telepresence, and telementoring. Surg Endosc 16(10):1389–402
14. Camara JG, Rodriguez RE (1998) Real-time telementoring in ophthalmology. Telemed J 4(4):375–377
15. Camara JG, Zabala RRB, Henson RD, Senft SH (2000) The use of real-time telementoring to remove an orbital tumor. Ophthalmology 107:1468–1471

Chapter 32

Non-Invasive Monitoring of Ocular Health in Space

32

Rafat R. Ansari, J. Sebag

DISCLAIMER: The views and opinions expressed in this article are those of the authors and not those of NASA or the Government of the United States of America.

This chapter addresses the following

Key Concepts:

- Vision is the most relied on of the human senses, and one of the most critical tools used by astronauts in the performance of mission duties.
- The absence of gravity in space affects human physiology in a number of ways. Deep space travel will also expose astronauts to high levels of radiation for extended periods of time.
- The needs of astronaut health can be met by effective, non-invasive miniaturized systems for monitoring health via telemetry.
- The eye represents a useful site for non-invasive access to the body. It also contains structures that are representative of nearly every tissue type in the body, enabling broad-spectrum monitoring of ocular and systemic health.
- A head-mounted apparatus equipped with several non-invasive optical diagnostic technologies, and technologies based upon skin contact and proximity to the brain, is under development at NASA.

32.1 Introduction

Interest in space travel and planetary exploration is gaining momentum. On 13 October 2003, China successfully launched a man into space and it seems that Japan and India are not too far behind. On 4 October 2004, a non-governmental American civilian rocket (Space Ship One) entered the edge of space (100 km above the Earth's surface) for a short duration, winning the 10 million USD Ansari X-Prize [1].

On a larger scale, on 14 January 2004, United States President George Bush announced that the National Aeronautics and Space Administration (NASA) would revive efforts to send a manned mission to the Moon and Mars. It should be noted that a round-trip mission to Mars will take approximately three years to complete. This includes from nine months to one year travel time from Earth to Mars, a one-year stay, and another nine months to one year for return travel to Earth.

Maintaining good ocular health is essential to the completion of this mission. In spite of advanced automation in manned space exploration, vision is the most relied upon of all the human senses and one of the most critical tools used by astronauts in the performance of mission duties. For example, astronaut pilots land space shuttles with exacting precision nearly completely dependent upon vision.

32.2 Ocular Health and the Harsh Environment of Space

Both the Moon and Mars have extreme conditions for human survival. For example, the Moon has no atmosphere while Mars' atmosphere is highly rarefied (1/150th of Earth), with a composition of about 95% carbon dioxide, 3% nitrogen, 1.6% argon, 0.15% oxygen, and 0.03% water vapor. The surface temperature on the Moon can be as low as –240°C in the shade, with the average temperature on Mars around –60°C.

32.2.1 Environmental Factors

The amount of ultraviolet light on Mars is about 800 times greater than that on Earth. The gravity on the Moon is one sixth, and on Mars it is one third that of the Earth.

Recently the martian rovers Spirit and Opportunity recorded dust storms on the martian surface with wind speeds in excess of 100 miles per hour. Fine dust particles have been found to irritate the eyes and lungs of astronauts on the lunar surface during the 1970s short walks [2].

32.2.2. Gravity Concerns

In addition to these harsh environmental factors, the absence of gravity in space affects human physiology in a variety of ways. Immediately upon entering this environment, astronauts experience shifts in fluid distribution to upper parts of the body, and in the elimination of weight-bearing forces. This causes head congestion, face puffiness, and leg shrinkage. The only reliable way to sense motion is via the eyes since the otoliths in the inner ear respond differently to fluid motion. This altered sensory input confuses the brain, causing disorientation. Since weight-bearing forces are eliminated, the bones and muscles deteriorate and the kidney filtration rate increases, causing kidney stones.

32.2.3 Radiation

Lastly, but perhaps most importantly, deep space travel will expose astronauts to high levels of radiation for extended periods of time. As a result, long-duration space travel will likely prove to be rigorous for the human body. The long-term effects, which are hitherto unknown, may involve changes at the cellular and molecular levels due to all of the aforementioned conditions. Thus important systems such as the vestibular, cardiovascular, renal, musculo-skeletal, brain, and eye could be affected. Table 32.1 lists potential ocular risk factors. In two recent studies, relatively low doses of space radiation were found to cause an increased incidence and early appearance of cataracts in astronauts [3, 4].

32.2.4 Aging and Health

In the absence of effective countermeasures, the untoward effects of space travel could accelerate aging as well as introduce new pathologies. Assuring astronaut health is thus a major priority in planning missions to the Moon, Mars, and beyond. Constraints in available room onboard vessels such as the International Space Station and deep space voyage crafts, as well as limitations in the availability of in-flight medical expertise, add to the challenge of meeting health care needs during missions that will last years. These needs can, however, be met by effective, non-invasive miniaturized systems for monitoring astronaut health via telemetry.

32.3 Using the Eyes as a Window to the Body

The eye is a unique part of the body in that it is largely transparent and therefore represents a useful site for non-invasive access to the body using light that readily enters the eye. Since incident light is scattered back out of the eye, this organ represents a location where analysis of the back-scattered light could provide useful information regarding internal structures, fluids, and tissues.

The eye is further unique in that this relatively small organ contains structures that are representative of nearly every tissue type in the body. The cornea is a typical extracellular matrix composed primarily of collagen. Aqueous is an ultrafiltrate of blood, containing most of the molecules found in serum at concentrations that are reflective of systemic levels. The lens is a highly organized array of crystalline proteins. Vitreous is very similar in nature to fluid found in joints. The retina and optic nerves are in fact part of the central

Table 32.1. Potential ocular risk factors in long-duration space flight and on the Moon and Mars

Condition	Possible cause(s)	In-Flight	Moon	Mars
Cataract	Radiation	Yes	Yes	Yes
Ocular hypertension and glaucoma	Reduced gravity	Yes, particularly with borderline/pre-glaucoma astronauts	Likely	Likely
Transient vision changes of unknown etiology	Reduced gravity	Yes	Not known but likely	Not known but likely
Macular degeneration	Radiation (free radicals)	Possible	Possible	Possible
Keratoconjunctivitis	Air quality Fine dust	Yes (depending upon proper functioning of air-filtration systems)	Yes	Likely
Photopsia	Radiation (retinal light flashes)	Yes (but no known dangers on short-duration flights)	Likely	Likely
Choroidal engorgement	Reduced gravity	Likely	Likely	Likely
Macular nutrition (decrease in caretonoids levels)	Radiation and reduced gravity	Possible	Possible	Possible
Ocular ischemia	Reduced gravity	Possible	Possible	Possible
Trauma or physical injury	Foreign objects hitting or imbedded in the eye	Possible (bungee cord injury has occurred previously with serious consequence)	Possible	Possible

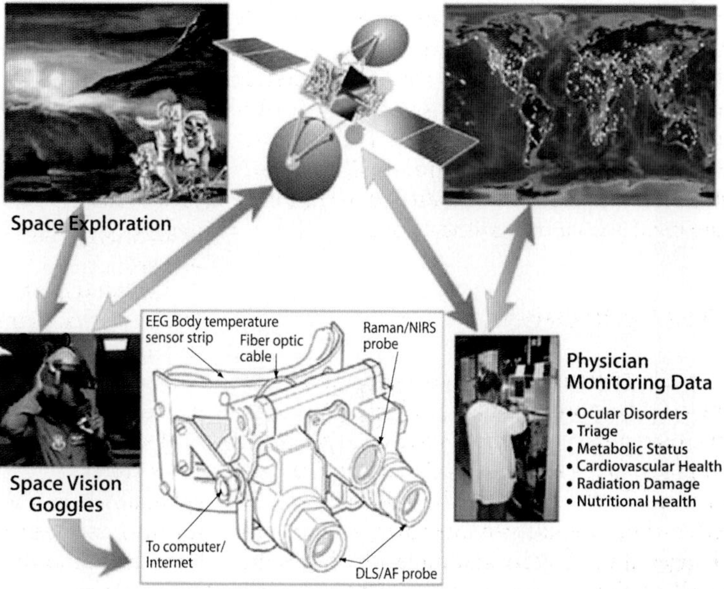

Fig. 32.1. Concept of a head-mounted goggles-like teleophthalmology apparatus

Table 32.2. Non-invasive optical technologies for monitoring astronaut health, early detection of ocular and systemic diseases and to enable early countermeasures

Technologies and readiness level	Diseases/studies	Instruments
Dynamic light scattering (DLS) in clinical/experimental use [8, 9]	– Corneal diseases and wound healing (LASIK) – Lens aging and cataract – Uveitis, glaucoma, Alzheimer's – Vitreous aging and lysis studies – Drug efficacy studies, cholesterol – Studies on effects of radiation, hyperbaric oxygen and other conditions on eye tissues – Diabetic vitreopathy	
Corneal/lens autofluoresence used in clinical study [10]	– Radiation induced biological effects – Diabetic retinopathy	
Laser-Doppler Flowmetry (LDF) Flown on KC-135- NASA's Microgravity airplane [11]	– Physiological circulatory changes – Hemodynamic response – Choroidal blood circulation – Age-related macular degeneration – Diabetic retinopathy	
Raman carotenoid pigment dispersion analysis used in clinical studies [12, 13]	– Lack of nutrition (luetin/xeaxanthin) – Age-related macular degeneration – Skin cancer – Stress status of living plants and plant products	
Ocular polarimetry in laboratory use; clinical system under development [14]	– Blood-glucose sensing	Glucose level reading Start button

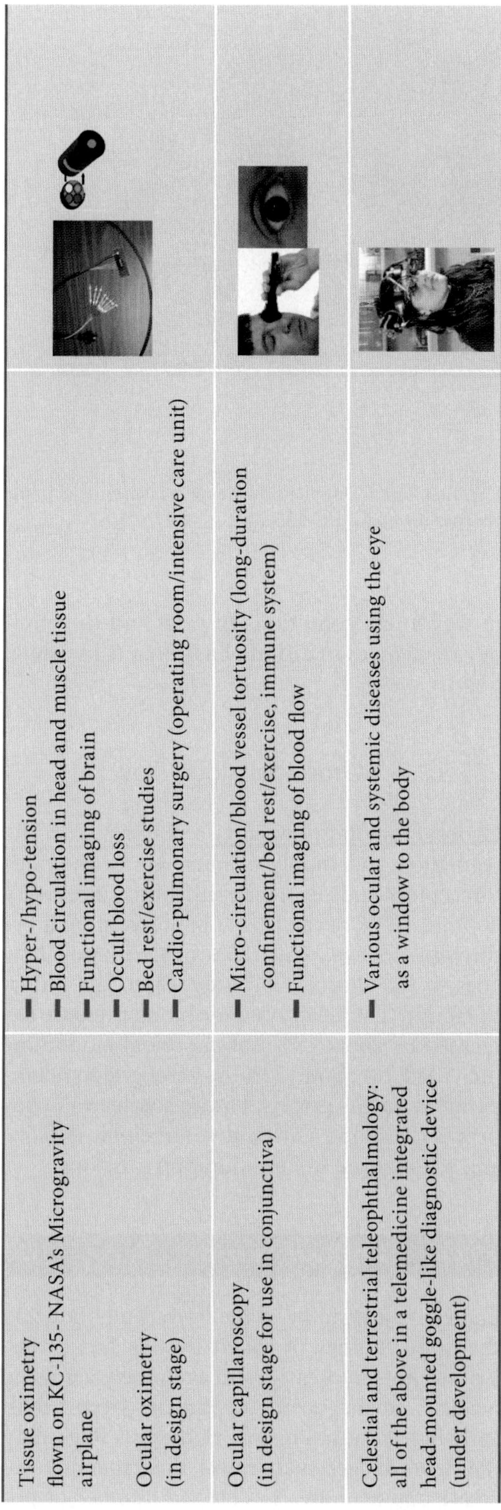

Tissue oximetry flown on KC-135- NASA's Microgravity airplane Ocular oximetry (in design stage)	■ Hyper-/hypo-tension ■ Blood circulation in head and muscle tissue ■ Functional imaging of brain ■ Occult blood loss ■ Bed rest/exercise studies ■ Cardio-pulmonary surgery (operating room/intensive care unit)	
Ocular capillaroscopy (in design stage for use in conjunctiva)	■ Micro-circulation/blood vessel tortuosity (long-duration confinement/bed rest/exercise, immune system) ■ Functional imaging of blood flow	
Celestial and terrestrial teleophthalmology: all of the above in a telemedicine integrated head-mounted goggle-like diagnostic device (under development)	■ Various ocular and systemic diseases using the eye as a window to the body	

nervous system. Within these two structures are neurons and blood vessels that can be directly visualized, the only place in the body where this can be done. Thus, neurophysiology and circulatory (blood flow, oxygenation, etc.) physiology can be evaluated non-invasively at this point, as well as in the conjunctiva, in the case of blood vessels. Because of these unique features, the eye can be considered a microcosm of the body that enables broad-spectrum monitoring of systemic and ocular health.

32.3.1 Head-Mounted, Goggle-Like Teleophthalmology Apparatus

A head-mounted apparatus equipped with several powerful non-invasive optical diagnostic technologies, as well as technologies based upon contact with skin and proximity to the brain, is under development at NASA. The concept shown in Fig. 32.1 has been discussed earlier [5]. Table 32.2 shows some of the capabilities that are being integrated into this apparatus to scan the various structures within the eye and skin. Other sensors mounted on the portion of the device in contact with periocular tissues will enable monitoring of body temperature, heart rate, electrolyte levels in sweat, and other health indices. One unique design feature is to integrate basic systems (lasers, detectors, correlator, spectrum analyzer) common to various technologies into a single unit that will subserve the technical requirements of all the different technologies. Due to space limitations, these technologies will not be discussed in detail here, but are cited in the pertinent references [9–15] in Table 32.2.

In terms of telemetry, the data transmission capacity from the Moon and Mars for a human mission is still a topic of further discussion and development. At present, a high rate downlink goes through the ku band on the international space station via a single access antenna, and is limited to 50 Mb/s. It may be upgraded to 150 Mb/s in the future. This data capacity is sufficient to download the ocular data from the apparatus back to Earth for evaluation by physicians.

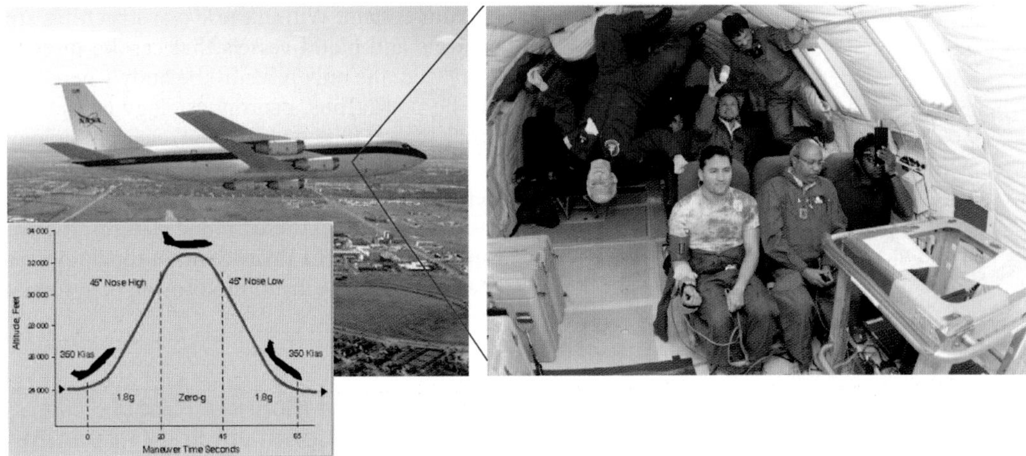

Fig. 32.2. NASA's KC-135 zero-gravity airplane and the parabolic flight trajectory

Fig. 32.3. Laser-Doppler flowmetry measurements in the choroid on-board KC-135

32.3.2 Changes in Vision

Over one third of astronauts who have flown in space have reported changes in their vision. The nature of these changes and the underlying cause(s) are yet to be determined. To do so will require the use of advanced non-invasive technologies in preparation for the use of such technologies during long-duration flights in space.

32.3.2.1 Proof-of-Concept Experiment

A proof-of-concept experiment, using a head-mounted compact laser Doppler flowmeter, was recently conducted on-board NASA's KC-135 airplane. This wide-body airplane, dubbed the vomit comet or weightless wonder, creates conditions of weightlessness or zero gravity during freefall lasting 25 to 30 s, and about twice the Earth's gravity during the climb phase of the parabolic flight trajectory shown in Fig. 32.2.

In this experiment, we measured choroidal blood flow in 25 volunteer human subjects. The experimental setup onboard KC-135 is shown in Fig. 32.3. The preliminary results can be found in previous papers [6, 7]; additionally, the detailed study is about to be published. The goal of this study was to evaluate choroidal blood flow in response to changing fluid levels in weightless conditions to help find the etiology of changes in vision of astronauts in orbital flight.

32.3.2.2 Choroidal Blood Flow

Choroidal blood flow plays a major role in the regulation and supply of nutrients to the photoreceptors and pigment epithelium since every 20 min, 100% of the body's blood volume flows through the eye, while 85% of that blood flow goes to the choroid and only 4% to the retina. We found that mean systemic blood pressure decreased by about 19% but choroidal blood flow increased by about 22% in zero gravity, compared to Earth's gravity. Future studies will confirm if the blood flow and volume will stabilize and self regulate in long-duration missions.

32.4 Conclusions

The eye is a window to the body. Fully utilizing the opportunities provided by this fact promises insights into easily and accurately assessing health, and diagnosing departures from health early in the natural history of disease. Regarding the rigors of deep space travel, this capability will create opportunities to detect a number of potentially debilitating diseases before the onset of irreversible damage.

We have presented the concept of an advanced instrument that integrates several non-invasive optical techniques that have been successfully demonstrated, or are currently under development in clinical and/or laboratory settings. These techniques are readily interfaced with the computer technology that by transmitting information from remote sites makes celestial teleophthalmology a reality.

Early diagnosis and prevention (rather than just cure) of disease is a critical direction for medicine in the 21st century. Technologies that are found to be useful in monitoring astronaut health in space may have great utility and value on Earth. In addition to the celestial teleophthalmic applications described above, it is possible that our compact, non-invasive, and multi-purpose diagnostic devices will be used for regular health monitoring by today's health-conscious consumers in settings of their choice, such as homes, offices, gymnasiums, drive-throughs, and shopping malls. Governments and health care agencies may further find useful applications for using such devices to extend health care to under-served areas of the world. This form of terrestrial teleophthalmology will also provide a powerful device for use in identifying diseases not adequately diagnosed and/or treated (e.g., diabetes in the US) in so-called advanced care settings.

References

1. Rutan B (2005) Rocket for the rest of us. National Geographic 207(4):28–35
2. Bell TE, Phillips T (2005) En route to Mars, the Moon; Why colonize the Moon before going to Mars? NASA scientists give their reasons. http://science.nasa.gov/headlines/y2005/18mar_Moonfirst.htm?list915919. Cited 4 Oct 2005
3. Cucinotta FA, et al. (2001) Space radiation and cataracts in astronauts. Radiat Res 156(5):460–466
4. Rastegar et al. (2002) Radiation induced cataract in astronauts and cosmonauts. Graefes Arch Clin Exp Ophthalmol 240(7):545
5. Ansari R, Singh B, Rovati L, Docchio F, Sebag J (2000) Monitoring astronaut health at the nanoscale cellular level through the eye. In: Proceedings of Nanospace 2000, Houston, TX
6. Ansari R, et al. (2003) Measurement of choroidal blood flow in zero gravity. Ophthalmic Technologies XII, In: Manns F, Soderberg PG, Ho A, (eds) Proc SPIE 4951:177–184
7. Hatcher M (2003) Flowmeter tests eyes in zero gravity; NASA scientists probe changes in astronauts' vision with a laser Doppler flowmeter. http://optics.org/articles/news/9/3/14/1. Cited 4 Oct 2005
8. Ansari RR (2004) Ocular static and dynamic light scattering: A noninvasive diagnostic tool for eye research and clinical practice. J Biomed Opt 9(1):22–37
9. Sebag J (2004) Seeing the invisible: the challenge of imaging vitreous. J Biomed Opt 9(1):38–46
10. Rovati L, Docchio F, Van Best J (2004) Autofluorescence methods in ophthalmology. J Biomed Opt 9(1):9–21
11. Geiser MH, Diermann U, Riva CE (1999) Compact laser doppler choroidal flowmeter. J Biomed Opt 4(4):459–464
12. Gellermann W, Bernstein P (2004) Noninvasive detection of macular pigments in the human eye. J Biomed Opt 9(1):75–85
13. Ermakov I, Ermakov M, Bernstein P (2004) Macular pigment Raman detector for clinical applications. J Biomed Opt 9(1):139–148
14. Ansari R, Bockle S, Rovati L (2004) New optical scheme for a polarimetric-based glucose sensor. J Biomed Opt 9(1):103–115

Chapter 33

Postscript

Kanagasingam Yogesan, Sajeesh Kumar,
Leonard Goldschmidt, Jorge Cuadros

33

While teleophthalmology is not yet a mainstream activity in eye care, the perspectives and activities presented in this book have demonstrated that it is not only feasible, but is an effective and sustainable way to provide eye care in diverse health care environments. Eye-care providers are now looking at teleophthalmology as a model for improving patient care.

In this book lie the guides and blueprints for widespread eye-care programs that are yet to be developed. By building on the experiences of the pioneers whose work is presented here, others can develop programs to provide eye care in areas that were previously unreachable. Programs were described in this book for providing eye care in such diverse environments from real-time consultations in remote towns in Argentina and villages in India, as we have seen in the Zaldivar and Aravind clinics, to intercontinental surgery and telemetry in space as was described by Drs. Marescaux and Ansari. These programs were developed for their particular situations, however, the methods that were created in all of the programs described in this book will increase timely and appropriate care not just for special populations but for everyone, regardless of their circumstances, ultimately contributing to the reduction of preventable blindness.

This book elaborates on many aspects of telemedicine in eye care, particularly its manifestations in various countries and its ability to provide images of high quality in the diagnosis of remote eye care. Authors in this volume have shown teleophthalmology to be practical, safe and effective. The technology depends on transfer of text, reports, voice, images and video between geographically separated locations. Success often relates to the efficiency and effectiveness of the transfer of information and translates to improved or enhanced patient care than would otherwise be possible.

The lessons learned in the development of these projects are valuable assets in the development of larger eye-care information systems. The future will surely bring a synthesis of telemedicine with other informatics endeavors, as store-and-forward telemedicine becomes as commonplace as email. Similarly, teleconferencing coupled with information sharing will become central elements in any clinical setting, just as it will in our day-to-day lives. The experiences that have been shared in this book will serve not only to develop new ways to care for patients, but also new ways to disseminate knowledge in the form of concepts, methods, clinical trials, and information. The author contributions in this book will help to form the next generation of solutions as many health care systems look for answers to what sometimes seems like intractable problems. These are professionals who have embraced evolving technologies, surely falling into the category of early adopters. The validation, assimilation, complementary innovations, and evolution associated with these methods will turn telemedicine simply into the routine practice of health care in the future that may seem unrecognizable to most of us now. In this context, the practice of "telemedicine" and "telehealth" simply becomes the practice of "medicine" and "health care."

We have reviewed many levels of technology, from simple Web-based image transmission in sparse technological environments, to the most sophisticated settings in outer space. In each of these settings it is clear that the major challenges faced are not only technological, but are also organizational and behavioral. Teleophthalmology may be viewed as a new tool, much like the keratome or laser that has the potential to transform the daily practice of eye care. The difference, however, is in the interactive nature of this new tool. Without interaction among colleagues and patients, teleophthalmology would be meaningless. It is because of the rapid increase in the demands for communication and interaction that teleophthalmology creates a rich and promising environment for new ways to communicate.

Available teleophthalmology technology still has considerable room for improvement. Rather, the challenge is why, where and how to implement which technology and at what costs. Asking the right clinical questions will drive the technologies. A needs assessment is critical before implementing a teleophthalmology project. Sometimes the technology drives the care model, rather than patient need taking precedence. Teleophthalmology as delineated in these pages may appear novel, but is rapidly coming into common and mundane usage through multiple applications.

The significance of the work that has been presented in this book should not be understated since these are the first steps toward the evolution of a new model for patient care delivery. The infrastructure that has been formed for the execution of the projects in this book will continue to form the basis for the realization of decades of theoretical work in computers and cognition as we remove the extraneous layers of traditional practice to arrive at the true nature of the health care encounter. The health care encounter can be viewed as the interaction of three components: data-gathering, decision-making, and patient communication (Fig. 33.1). The use of telemedicine allows health-care workers to provide expertise in the component where they are most effective. For example, highly trained experts may not need to gather data if someone else can provide it for them, and they may not be the most effective communicator to impart this knowledge to their patients.

Data gathering can be done by local individuals that are available where the patient is located and communication with the patient can be provided by patient educators or clinicians whose expertise lies in face-to-face intervention and interaction with patients. Communicators may be local primary care clinicians who are well-acquainted with the patient's complete health picture or they may even be community-based individuals with a deeper understanding of the social context in which they are interacting with the patient. Through telemedicine there is a potential to increase the efficiency of each component of the health care encounter, since they are no longer bound by time and location.

We may find that the doctor-patient relationship can evolve into a more communal activity involving doctors and patients as well as their families, allied health workers, educators, public health workers, and numerous others tightly woven into a matrix of information gatherers, information processors, and communicators.

Meanwhile, there is much work to be done in the allied areas of legal and policy making, reimbursement, image processing and knowledge management, decision support systems and information abstraction. Image processing for automated and human interpretation of images and data has been an active area of research and development. Research teams all over the world are developing computerized algorithms to extract meaning from digital images with increasing success. Similarly, systems that can abstract information from varied sources, such as laboratory data, clinical observations, and general patient health information are beginning to provide guidance to clinicians, from pop-up reminders on their computerized medical records to diagnostic interpretations that combine data that is too complex for a human to process. Our challenge will be to blend enhanced computation provided by image processing and decision support systems with enhanced communication provided by telehealth.

Time will tell whether teleophthalmology (to paraphrase Neil Armstrong) is: one small step

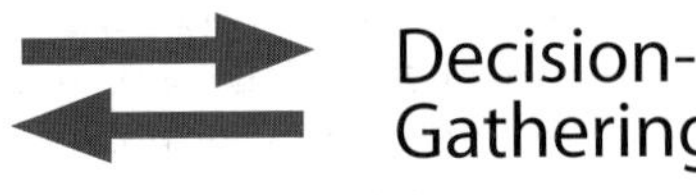

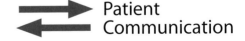

Fig. 33.1. Components of a health-care encounter

for information and communication technology but one giant leap for eye care. However, from the pages of this first book on teleophthalmology, the future promises to be exciting. Optimistically, the journey towards improved patient care will be well worth the wait for those benefiting from these technologies.

Appendix 1

Education and Training Opportunities

Country	Institute	Contact details
Argentina	Instituto Zaldivar	www.institutozaldivar.com
Australia	Center of Excellence in e-Medicine. Lions Eye Institute	www.lei.org.au www.emedicine.com.au
Brazil	Vision Institute/Ophthalmology Department, Federal University of São Paulo(UNIFESP)	www.unifesp.br http://www.oftalmo.epm.br
Canada	Department of Ophthalmology University of Alberta	http://www.ualberta.ca/~ophthalm/eye.html
Finland	University of Tampere	www.uta.fi
France	IRCAD-European Institute of Telesurgery EITS Institute	www.eits.org www.websurg.com
Germany	Department of Paediatric Ophthalmology, Strabismology and Ophthalmogenetics. University of Regensburg	www.uni-regensburg.de/
Greece	National Technical University of Athens, School of Electrical and Computer Engineering	www.biomed.ntua.gr
India	Aravind Eye Hospitals & Postgraduate Institute of Ophthalmology	www.aravind.org
India	Department of Teleophthalmology, Sankara Nethralaya	www.sankaranethralaya.org
Japan	Asahikawa Medical College Telemedicine Center	www. asahikawa-med.ac.jp
Lithuania	Telemedicine Center of Kaunas University of Medicine	http://tmc.kmu.lt
Spain	Department of Physiology, School of Medicine	www.usc.es/fspaco
Singapore	School of Electrical and Electronic Engineering Nanyang Technological University	http://www.ntu.edu.sg
UK	Institute of Ophthalmology	www.ucl.ac.uk/ioo/

Country	Institute	Contact details
USA	Inoveon Evaluation Center	http://www.inoveon.com
USA	Vanderbilt Ophthalmic Imaging Center	www.retinopathyscreening.org
USA	University of California	www.berkeley.edu
USA	ORBIS	http://telemedicine.orbis.org/bins/home.asp
USA	Ophthalmology Service, Department of Surgery, Walter Reed Army Medical Center	www.wramc.amedd.army.mil
USA	Wilmer Eye Institute, Johns Hopkins University	http://www.hopkinsmedicine.org/wilmer/
USA	University of Texas Medical Branch, Department of Ophthalmology and Visual Sciences	www.uth.tmc.edu
USA	United States Department of Veterans Affairs (VA) Palo Alto Health Care System	http://www1.va.gov/
USA	University of Southern California	www.usc.edu/

Appendix 2

Sample Protocol

The Lions Eye Institute Teleophthalmology Protocol

Store-and-forward/Videoconferencing teleconsultation

I. Introduction

This protocol gives the medical officers, coordinating health care professionals and nurses clear direction on how to make use of the teleophthalmology service provided by the Lions Eye Institute.

II. Aim

To provide specialist advice and a second opinion to health care providers in remote and rural areas.

III. Definitions

Teleophthalmology — Store-and-forward or interactive, real time television for eye care purposes.

Teleconsultant — Ophthalmologist whose expertise is requested via a teleophthalmology transaction.

Teleconsultation — Remote patient evaluation and consultation via a telecommunications system.
Originating Site/Remote Site Site where the patient is located at the time of the teleconsultation. A medical officer and/or a co-ordinating nurse also present here.

Consulting Site — Site where teleconsultant providing the teleconsultation is located at the time the service is provided via a telecommunications system.

Site Coordinator — Person designated to coordinate teleophthalmology activities.

IV. Teleophthalmology Consultation Criteria

The main service will be provided via store-and-forward techniques using a Web-based system. However, videoconferencing is also available for any emergency or acute ophthalmic conditions.

V. Requirements

A. Technical Requirements:

Store-and-forward
Slit lamp
Fundus camera
Desktop personal computer or laptop
Internet connection
Access to www.e-icare.com
E-icare software CD for image capture and advance imaging
Video conferencing
Video conferencing equipment
ISDN connection (128 kbps for face to face interview and 384 kbps for image reviewing from a slit lamp)

B. Training Requirements:

Training to operate the imaging device
Training on disease grading and image quality
Training to use the e-icare software package
Training to use the video conferencing equipment

C. Other Requirements:

Medical officers at the remote/originating site should be informed of the teleophthalmology and its benefits

VI. Responsibilities of the Originating/Remote Site Coordinating Nurse

A. Prior to Teleconsultation

1. Scheduling teleconsultation and connection time
2. Determining special needs or room arrangements
3. Contacting patient and referring provider with teleconsultation appointment time and location
4. Training users in the use of telemedicine equipment
5. Preparing patients for teleconsultation

B. During Teleconsultation

1. Setting up and operating telemedicine equipment
2. Ensuring privacy and confidentiality of the patient
3. Ensuring comfort and safety of the patient

C. After Teleconsultation

1. Distributing and collecting telemedicine evaluation forms
2. Logging telemedicine activities
3. Reporting telemedicine activity to the LEI

VII. Responsibilities of Teleconsultant(s)

A. Prior to Teleconsultation

1. Communicating special peripherals or room arrangements needed during teleconsultation to consulting site coordinator
2. Obtaining signed consent forms or medical records if applicable
3. Determining if interactive video teleconsultation is an appropriate means for providing the necessary services

B. During Teleconsultation

1. Ensuring privacy and confidentiality of the patient
2. Ensuring comfort and safety of the patient
3. Determining if the teleconsultation is of sufficient quality to diagnose or evaluate the patient appropriately
4. Determining if the teleconsultation is of sufficient quality to adequately convey necessary information to the patient and the referring Medical Officer

C. After Teleconsultation

1. Document teleconsultation and process resulting records appropriately

VIII. Rights and Responsibilities of Patients

A. Before Teleconsultation

1. Right to informed consent to use telemedicine
2. Responsibility to arrive on time for the teleconsultation
3. Responsibility to have identity information available

B. During Teconsultation

1. Right to terminate teleconsultation and request other mode of consultation
2. Right to have additional family members present during teleconsultation
3. Right to privacy and confidentiality

C. After Teconsultation

1. Right to have medical records or stored images maintained in a confidential manner

IX. Referral and Scheduling Process

1. Scheduling of video consultation – by originating site coordinating nurse
2. Scheduling information is recorded – by manual entry in a logbook
3. Information to be recorded in the logbook – beginning and ending time of teleconsultation, date, description of teleconsultation, individuals participating in teleconsultation
4. Hours during which video consultations scheduled – to be determined by coordinators at both locations
5. Contacting the consulting site at Perth – originating site coordinating nurse
6. Maintaining list of Perth consulting site contacts – Perth consulting site ophthalmologist/ teleconsultant.

X. Type of Referrals/Consultations

A. Ophthalmic Accident and Emergency

1. Coordinating nurse to collect relevant history from the patient or accompanying persons. Use the table below for relevant questions
2. Use video conferencing to consult an ophthalmologist or an ophthalmic registrar (on call) at Royal Perth Hospital before sending the patient to Perth
3. Or coordinating nurse can image the eye and send the high-resolution images to an ophthalmologist via the Web-based system. Then the specialist can be called for diagnostic advice and first aid based on the images/videos and history

B. Patient Referrals to Go to Perth for Any Ophthalmic Conditions

1. Medical officers to send the patients to the coordinating nurse for imaging
2. The coordinating nurse will image the eye and send the high-resolution images to an ophthalmologist via the Web-based system
3. Diagnostic advice/second opinion will be received within 24 h
4. Coordinating nurse to inform the patient and medical officer regarding the advice/second opinion received

C. Post-Operative Reviews, e.g., Cataract and Trabeculectomy

1. Medical officers to send the patients to coordinating nurse for imaging
2. Coordinating nurse will image the eye and send the high-resolution images/videos to an ophthalmologist via the Web-based system
3. Diagnostic advice/second opinion will be received within 24 h
4. Coordinating nurse to inform the patient and medical officer regarding the advice/second opinion received

D. All Diabetic Retinopathy, Glaucoma and Other Eye Screenings

1. Coordinating nurse to image the eyes and send the high-resolution images/videos to an ophthalmologist via Web-based system
2. Diagnostic advice will be received within 24 h
3. Coordinating nurse to inform the patient regarding the diagnostic opinion received

XI. Preparation of the Patient

Originating site coordinating nurse is responsible for preparing the patient for the teleconsultation. Preparation includes:

1. Informing patient, participating family member(s), or their legal guardians, about the teleophthalmology technology, capabilities, risks, benefits, and confidentiality issues
2. Reviewing patient rights and responsibilities, including informing participants that they may terminate the teleconsultation at any time

XII. Privacy and Confidentiality

1. Introduce all persons present at the originating and consulting sites during video consultation
2. Ensure privacy for patients by providing a private room for the teleconsulation and putting a "session in progress" sign on the door to the room
3. Obtaining patient consent form
4. Obtaining patient records if applicable
5. Archiving/protecting patient records or stored images if applicable

XIII. Documentation

1. Patient consent forms
2. Patient medical record
3. Teleconsultation logbook

XIV. Quality Control/Evaluation

Periodic review and evaluation of this protocol and teleconsultation for quality control.

Appendix 3

Sample Consent Form

Consent to Tele-imaging for Ophtalmology

Study Title: Tele-imaging for ophthalmology in Rural and Remote Western Australia

Specialist: Dr X
Dr Y

Health Providers: The Lions Eye Institute

Name of the Patient: ______________________________

I (the participant) have read or have had read to me the information concerning teleimaging and any questions I have asked have been answered to my satisfaction. I agree to participate in this activity, realising that I may withdraw at any time without reason and without prejudice. (Or where applicable - without prejudice to my future medical treatment).

I understand that all information provided is treated as strictly confidential and will not be released by the investigator unless required by law.

I understand that this programme is being developed to increase the efficiency of treatment in rural areas. I agree that research data gathered for the study may be published provided my name or other identifying information is not used.

______________	______________________	______________
Date	Name of Patient	Signature
______________	______________________	______________
Date	Name of Health Representative	Signature

The Human Research Ethics Committee at the University of Western Australia requires that all participants are informed that, if they have any complaint regarding the manner, in which a research project is conducted, it may be given to the researcher or, alternatively to the Secretary, Human Research Ethics Committee, Registrar's Office, University of Western Australia, 35 Stirling Highway, Crawley, WA 6009 (telephone number 9380-3703). All study participants will be provided with a copy of the Information Sheet and Consent Form for their personal records.
The Lions Eye Institute is an independent, non-profit organization established for the investigation, prevention and cure of eye disease.

Participant's Initials ____________

Appendix 4

Sample Information Sheet

Information Sheet for Patients

Study Title: Tele-imaging for ophthalmology
in Rural and Remote Western Australia

Specialist: Dr X
Dr Y

Health Providers: The Lions Eye Institute
The Health Department of WA

Many of the common diseases that affect the eyes and the teeth and gums can be readily analysed from photographs or digital pictures. Where eye specialists and dentists visit country areas rather than being present all the time, it is often difficult to make an appointment with them and particularly to have treatment carried out in an efficient and timely manner.

This programme allows medical support staff resident in your area to take images of your eyes transmit them securely and have the visiting specialist design the treatment and schedule it prior to visiting your area. This means that you will be treated where possible in a much more organised and efficient way with savings in time and cost to the whole system.

The images can only be read by authorised medical specialists involved in the programme and can only be transferred either back to you as a potential patient or your doctor.

You do not have to agree to have your eyes imaged and the records can be destroyed at any time if you change your mind.

This is not a clinical trial. Your records will be kept totally confidential and you will have access to them at any time. Your name and the digital records will only be released to authorized health personnel who will be looking after your treatment.

Your participation in this study does not prejudice any right to compensation, which you may have under statute or common law.

You are free at any time to withdraw consent to further participation without prejudice in any way. You do not need to give any reason nor justification for such a decision. In such case, your records will be destroyed, unless otherwise agreed by you.

The Human Research Ethics Committee at the University of Western Australia requires that all participants are informed that, if they have any complaint regarding the manner, in which a research project is conducted, it may be given to the researcher or, alternatively to the Secretary, Human Research Ethics Committee, Registrar's Office, University of Western Australia, 35 Stirling Highway, Crawley, WA 6009 (telephone number 9380-3703). All study participants will be provided with a copy of the Information Sheet and Consent Form for their personal records.

The Lions Eye Institute is an independent, non-profit organization
established for the investigation, prevention and cure of eye disease.

Appendix 5

Clinician Perception Evaluation

Clinician Perception Evaluation

				Excellent	Satisfactory	Poor
1.	Clinician rating of the following with regard to the application:	a)	Level of comfort with equipment & procedures			
		b)	Scheduling convenience			
		c)	Physical arrangements			
		d)	Location			
		e)	Timeliness of consultation			
		f)	Technical quality of service			
		g)	Patient/consultant communication level			
		h)	Functionality of equipment			
		i)	Overall satisfaction with the telemedicine session			
2.	Was the clinician satisfied with the telemedicine application compared to the alternatives?			Yes ☐		No ☐
3.	Did the clinician have patient privacy concerns?			Yes ☐		No ☐
4.	Did the clinician believe the application made a positive contribution to patient care?			Yes ☐		No ☐
5.	Was real-time visual contact with the other site essential?			Yes ☐		No ☐
6.	During the session was it more useful to have:	a)	Full motion video	Yes ☐		No ☐
		b)	Still images	Yes ☐		No ☐
7.	Would the clinician use the telemedicine service again?			Yes ☐		No ☐
8.	What was the alternative to the use of the telemedicine service?					
9.	Outline future care for the patient eg. Referral, admission…					

The Lions Eye Institute is an independent, non-profit organisation established for the investigation, prevention and cure of eye disease.

Appendix 6

Patient Questionnaire

Teleophthalmology, Western Australia
Patient Questionnaire

Please fill out this form for any single Telehealth session.
Patient participation in this evaluation is completely voluntary.
If you need more space, please use the back of the questionnaire to continue.

Part A: General Information

1. Site name (please circle): Carnarvon / Exmouth / Onslow / Burringurrah / Shark Bay

2. Date of Telehealth session : ______ / ______ / ______ (dd/mm/yy)

3. Starting time : ______ : ______ am/pm (estimate if not sure)

4. Ending time : ______ : ______ am/pm (estimate if not sure)

5. Person filling out questionnaire (1 = individual, 2 = health care provider, 3 = family)

6. Demographic data (please tick)

   a. Sex: ☐ male ☐ female

   b. Age: ☐ < 1-year ☐ child ☐ adolescent ☐ adult ☐ elderly

7. a. Type of service: ☐ screening ☐ treatment/care ☐ other

   b. If "other", please specify: ______________________________

8. Individual became aware of this Telehealth service from (** Tick as many as apply):

   ☐ Advertising (TV, Radio, Newspaper) ☐ Health professionals (GP, nurse, midwife etc)

   ☐ Another patient ☐ Family or Friend

   ☐ Other ______________________

Part B. Satisfaction Information

Self assessment having completed a Telehealth session	Yes	No*	N/A
This Telehealth service has given me access to health care faster than a traditional service			
This Telehealth service has provided a more convenient method for receiving this health service			
I am satisfied with the quality of service received for this Telehealth session compared to the alternatives			
I would choose to use Telehealth for future health services			
Did you have privacy concerns?			
Was the lack of direct physical contact with the distant clinician acceptable? (for videoconferencing only)			

*If "No", please explain why in space provided below

____

____

Patient rating of the following with regard to the service:	Poor	Satisfactory	Excellent
The comfort in the Eye Clinic area was			
The convenience of this service was			
The duration and timeliness of the consultation was			
The skills and attitude of attending personnel was			
The information provided was explained in a way that was			
The feedback I received about the consultation was			
The overall satisfaction I feel with the telemedicine session is			

* Comments / explanations:

____

____

Thank you for your participation in this survey – your comments will help improve our service. Please place this questionnaire in the envelope provided (no stamp required) and return to the nominated address.

Appendix 7

Teleophthalmology Logsheet

(see next page)

Teleophthalmology Project Evaluation
Weekly Logsheet

Location:

Week Starting ______________

Use this sheet for *Each Service Provision*. This logform is to be completed *during or immediately following* the telehealth service provision.

#	Pt. Identity Number	Date	Instru-ment used[1]	Consult Time start	Consult Time finish	Reason Review Requested[2]	Technical difficulties? (Y – N) (see other side)	Service[3]	Outcome Coding[4]	Image Quality Coding[5]	Follow-up[6]	Clinician ID
									Post Specialist Review			
1												
2												
3												
4												

[1] Instrument Coding

Videoconference	VDO
Email (Store and Forward)	WWW
Telephony	T
Slit Lamp	SL
Handheld Fundus Camera	FC
Tonometer	TN
Other	O

[2] Reason for Review Requested

Diabetic Retinopathy	DR
Glaucoma	G
Keratitis	K
Cataracts	C
Trachoma	T
Trauma	A&E
Other	O

[3] Service Coding

Primary / Preventative Care	1
Secondary Care	2
Emergency	3
Follow-up	4
Other	5

[4] Outcome Coding

No abnormality detected	N
Patient Transferred	T
Treatment at Receiving Site	R
Further follow-up	F
Other	O

[5] Image Quality Coding

Very Poor	1
Poor	2
Good	3
Excellent	4

[6] Follow-up Coding

None Required	0
Referral to local GP	1
Referral for diabetes coordinator services	2
Referral for visiting specialist (next available)	3
Referral to Perth or metropolitan-based Specialist	4
Routine repeat screening	5
Other	6

Technical Difficulties – please provide a brief explanation of the difficulty experienced and action, if any taken

1) ____

____

2) ____

____

3) ____

____

4) ____

____

Glossary

Adnexal. Attachments, such as arms or legs, which are appended to the body.

Amblyopia. Reduced vision in one eye that otherwise appears to be normal. Also called *lazy eye*.

Anaglyphs. Stereoimages that present monochromatic images to each eye, with different colors used for each image.

Angiography. Procedure used to image blood vessels, typically involving the administration of a contrast material and imaging the blood vessels. The contrast material is typically delivered into the body through a catheter placed into an appropriate blood vessel.

Arterioles. The smallest arterial vessels (about 0.2 mm or 1/125 inch in diameter) resulting from repeated branching of the arteries. They conduct the blood from the arteries to the capillaries.

Atherosclerosis. *Hardening of the arteries*, in which cholesterol and other deposits build up on the inner walls of the arteries, limiting the flow of blood.

Biomicroscopy. The examination of tissues on a microscopic level. Can refer to the specific examination of the cornea or lens of the eye, using a corneal microscope and a slit lamp.

Cardiovascular. Pertaining to the heart and blood vessels.

Cataract. Opacity or cloudiness of the crystalline lens, which may prevent a clear image from forming on the retina.

Cerebrovascular. Pertaining to the blood vessels of the cerebrum or brain.

Cholecystectomy. The surgical removal of the gallbladder.

Cine-angiogram. In an angiograph, as the dye travels down the branches of the coronary artery itself, continuous images are exposed onto movie film. The composite roll of images is known as a cine-angiogram.

Cytomegalovirus. A virus of the herpes family that, in the ophthalmic context, causes infection and inflammation of the retina in patients with AIDS (CMV Retinitis).

Conjunctiva. A thin, clear membrane that lines the inner surface of the eyelids and the outer surface of the eyeball, except for the cornea.

Cornea. The transparent, convex, anterior portion of the outer layer of the eyeball.

Current procedural terminology (CPT). Codes a systematic listing and coding of procedures and services performed by physicians. Each procedure or service is identified with a five-digit code maintained and copyrighted by the American Medical Association, and adopted by the US Department of Health and Human Services.

Cytology. The branch of science that deals with the structure and function of cells.

Diabetes Mellitus. Disorder that occurs when the body is not able to use sugar for growth and energy for daily activities. There are two main types of diabetes mellitus: insulin-dependent (Type 1) and noninsulin-dependent (Type 2).

Diabetic Retinopathy. Spectrum of retinal changes accompanying long-standing diabetes mellitus. Early stage is background retinopathy. May advance to proliferative retinopathy, which includes the growth of abnormal new blood vessels (neovascularization) and fibrous tissue.

Diabetologist. A doctor who sees and treats people with diabetes mellitus.

Dithering. The process of juxtaposing pixels of two colors to create the illusion that a third color is present. A simple example is an image with only black and white in the color palette.

By combining black and white pixels in complex patterns a graphics program can create the illusion of gray values. Dithering is the most common means of reducing the color range of images down to the 256 (or fewer) colors seen in 8-bit GIF images.

Drusen. Tiny, white hyaline deposits on Bruch's membrane (of the retinal pigment epithelium). Common after age 60; sometimes an early sign of macular degeneration.

Edema. Accumulation of fluid in organs and tissues of the body resulting in swelling.

Endophthalmitis. Inflammation of the interior of the eye, typically caused by an infection from eye surgery or trauma. Endophthalmitis is an ocular emergency. Symptoms include floaters, light sensitivity, eye pain or discomfort, a red or pink eye and vision loss.

Endothelium. The inner layer of cells on the inside surface of the cornea.

Esotropia. Cross-eyes. Eye misalignment in which one eye deviates inward (toward the nose) while the other fixates normally.

Etiology. A branch of knowledge concerned with the causes of particular phenomena, specifically a branch of medical science concerned with the causes and origins of diseases.

Exotropia. Wall-eyes. Eye misalignment in which one eye deviates outward (away from the nose) while the other fixates normally.

Exudation. The escape of fluid, cells, and cellular debris from blood vessels and their deposition in or on the tissues, usually as the result of inflammation.

Fluorescein. A harmless yellow dye used to outline the vessels of the eye.

Frequency doubling perimetry. Targets low redundancy ganglion cells; because these cells are sparsely populated, there is less compensation available to mask cell damage. By targeting these cells, these perimetry can detect glaucomatous damage early in the disease process.

Fundus. The larger part of a hollow organ that is farthest away from the organ's opening. The bladder, gallbladder, stomach, uterus, eye, and cavity of the middle ear all have a fundus.

Funduscope. Devices for examining the interior of the eye, permitting the clear visualization of the structures of the eye at any depth.

Gaussian. The bell shaped curve that is used to describe the distribution of quantities around some normal value. The distribution is uniquely determined by its mean and variance.

Ghosting. A shadowy or weak duplication of the original image. It can be the result of transmission conditions where secondary signals are created and then displayed earlier or later than the original.

Glaucoma. Group of diseases characterized by increased intraocular pressure resulting in damage to the optic nerve and retinal nerve fibers. A common cause of preventable vision loss. May be treated by prescription drugs or surgery.

Glaucomatous cupping glaucoma. Causes nerve fibers to die and this results in loss of vision. As nerve fibers die, the neuro-retinal rim of the optic nerve head thins and the optic cup enlarges.

Gonioscopy. Examination of the anterior chamber angle through a goniolens (special type of contact lens).

Hemoglobin A1c. A blood test for diabetics that reveals the average blood sugar values over the past 3 months. This test is used to monitor patients with diabetes and assess their level of disease control.

Histology. The study of the structure of cells and tissues; usually involves microscopic examination of tissue slices.

Hyperglycemia. A condition caused by greater than normal levels of glucose in the blood. Symptoms include thirst, frequent urination and fatigue.

Hypertensive. 1. Causing or marking a rise in blood pressure. 2. Denoting a person suffering from high blood pressure.

Hypertropias. One eye deviates upward relative to the opposite eye.

Hyphema. Bleeding into the interior chamber of the eye.

Informatics. The field of computer manipulation of scientific or medical data. Informatics is the part of the process that uses computer programs to capture, analyze, and transport data for the appropriate processing and analysis.

Interoperability. The ability of software and hardware on multiple machines from multiple vendors to communicate meaningfully.

Intraocular. Within the eye.

Iridocyclitis. Inflammation of the iris and of the ciliary body, anterior uveitis.

Keratitis. Inflammation of the cornea.

Laparoscopic. Performed using a laparoscope, a thin fiber-optic scope introduced into a body cavity for diagnostic and surgical purposes.

Laser-Assisted in situ Keratomileusis (LASIK). A surgical procedure intended to reduce a person's dependency on glasses or contact lenses.

Laser photocoagulation. Procedure in which a surgeon uses a laser to coagulate tissue, usually to seal leaking blood vessels and destroy new ones in diseases like macular degeneration and diabetic retinopathy.

Lenticular. Pertaining to the crystalline lens of the eye.

Licensure. The legal authority or formal permission from authorities to carry on certain activities which by law or regulation require such permission. It may be applied to licensure of institutions as well as individuals.

Macula. A small, highly sensitive part of the retina responsible for detailed central vision.

Macular degeneration. Degeneration in the macular region of the retina that results in decreased central vision and sometimes blindness.

Maculopathy. Any pathological condition of the macula lutea.

Metadata. About data, or information known about the image in order to provide access to the image. Usually includes information about the intellectual content of the image, digital representation data, and security or rights management information.

Microdensitometry. A procedure utilizing a densitometer.

Micrometry. The art of measuring with a micrometer.

Miosis. Constriction of the pupil.

Monochromatic. Light of a single wavelength. A color scheme that uses one color and all of the tones, tints, and shades that can be derived from it.

Monoscopic. When we normally look at objects, our two eyes see slightly different images (because they are located at different viewpoints). Our brain puts the images together to generate a stereoscopic viewpoint. For stereo, the left and right eye views need to be generated independently. Choosing only right or left eye produces only a right/left eye viewpoint (monoscopic).

Motility. The ability to move spontaneously.

Mydriatic. Dilating the pupil.

Mydriasis. A long-continued or excessive dilatation of the pupil of the eye.

Neovascularization. Abnormal formation of new blood vessels, usually in or under the retina or on the iris surface. May develop in diabetic retinopathy, blockage of the central retinal vein, or macular degeneration.

Neuro-ophthalmology. That branch of medicine concerned with the neurological aspects of the visual apparatus.

Normotensive. Characterized by normal tone, tension or pressure, as by normal blood pressure.

Nystagmus. Involuntary rapid movement of the eyes in the horizontal, vertical or rotary planes of the eyeball.

Pterygium. A fleshy growth that invades the cornea. It is an abnormal process in which the conjunctiva (a membrane that covers the white of the eye) grows into the cornea.

Ocular. Pertaining to or affecting the eye.

Oculoplastic. Deal with a wide variety of reconstructable disorders affecting the eyelids, eye sockets, and tear drainage systems.

Oculoplasty. Surgery to deal with a wide variety of reconstructable disorders affecting the eyelids, eye sockets, and tear drainage systems.

Ophthalmology. The branch of medicine that deals with the anatomy, functions, pathology and treatment of the eye.

Ophthalmoscopy. The examination of the interior of the eye with the ophthalmoscope.

Optic Disc. A small region of the retina where the fibers of the ganglion neurons exit from the eyeball to form the optic nerve, also called the blind spot.

Optometric. A specialty focusing on the diagnosis and nonsurgical treatment of disorders of the eye and vision care.

Otorynolaryngology. The division of medical science that includes otology (ear), rhinology (nose), and larynology (areas of the throat).

Otoliths. Small calcium carbonate crystals located within the maculae of the inner ear's utricle and saccule. The otoliths move in response to head movements, shifting their mass which distorts the hair cell processes. As a result, nerve impulses are generated to the brain for interpretation as head movements for static equilibrium.

Photocoagulation. Using a strong beam of light (laser) to seal off bleeding blood vessels such as in the eye. The laser can also burn away blood vessels that should not have grown in the eye. This is the main treatment for retinopathy.

Phacoemulsification. Also called "phako," this in-office cataract surgery procedure involves using a device with a vibrating, ultrasonic tip to break up the cataract, then suctioning the pieces out with a tiny needle.

Phaco-refractive. A procedure where refractive corrections are made at the crystalline lens inside the eye.

Photorefractive surgery. Is performed using an excimer laser in an attempt to correct refractive errors such as short-sightedness (myopia), astigmatism, and more recently long-sightedness (hypermetropia).

Pixel. Picture element. The smallest unit (point) of an image displayed on screen. The quality of an image depends on the number of pixels per inch that make up the image.

Pneumatic tonometry. The use of a puff-air device to measure the pressure within the eye.

Prophylaxis. Treatment that helps to prevent a disease or condition before it occurs or recurs.

Proximal. Nearest to, closer to any point of reference, opposed to distal.

Refraction. The bending of light rays as they pass from one medium (i.e., air) to another (i.e., glass), each with a different index of refraction.

Renal. Pertaining to the kidney, nephric.

Retina. Light sensitive nerve tissue in the eye that converts images from the eye's optical system into electrical impulses that are sent along the optic nerve to the brain. Forms a thin membranous lining of the rear two-thirds of the globe.

Retinitis. Inflammation of the retina. Symptoms include blurred vision, metamorphopsia, floaters and vision loss.

Retinoblastoma. An eye cancer that most often occurs in children younger than five years. It occurs in hereditary and nonhereditary (sporadic) forms.

Retinopathy. Any disease or disorder of the retina; usually refers to damage to the retina caused by high blood pressure or diabetes mellitus.

Stereo photograph. Has two images, one for each eye, that when viewed together provide three-dimensional information about the subject.

Stereopsis. Ability to see objects as three-dimensional and to judge their relative distance in space by putting together images from both eyes.

Stereoscopic. Relating to a stereoscope, or giving the appearance of three dimensions.

Strabismus. A misalignment of the eyes: they don't point at the same object. Crossed eyes are one type of strabismus.

Striae. Stretch marks on the skin with a silvery-white hue.

Systemic. Pertaining to or affecting the body as a whole.

T1 line. A telecommunications line made out of fiber-optics or copper. A T1 line can carry 24 digitized voice channels, or data at a rate of 1.544 Mb per second.

Telematics. Refers to the broad industry related to using computers in concert with telecommunications systems. This includes dial-up service to the Internet as well as all types of networks that rely on a telecommunications system to transport data.

Telemedicine. Use of telecommunications technology for medical diagnosis and patient care and education when the provider and client are separated by distance.

Thromboembolic. An acute septicemic disease characterized by fever, severe depression, ataxia, blindness, coma, and rapid death.

Tomography. Technique used to study the human body through the imaging of radiological slides of the organs.

Tonometer. Instrument used to measure internal eye pressure.

Topography. The accurate and detailed description or drawing of places or items and their surface details. Used to determine the corneal profile in order to program the computer for refractive correction as well as for post-operative corneal analysis.

Tortuositas. Abnormal twists or turns of retinal blood vessels.

Toxoplasmosis. A disease caused by the parasite Toxoplasma gondii; An infection that can cause inflammation of the retina.

Trachoma. A severe, chronic, contagious conjunctival and corneal infection.

Trephination. Is a form of surgery where a hole is drilled or scraped into the skull, leaving the membrane around the brain intact. It addresses health problems that relate to abnormal intracranial pressure.

Tunica vasculosa lentis. Blood vessels forming a network around the developing lens in the fetus (unborn child); a normal stage of development.

Uvea. The blood vessel-rich pigmented layers of the eye. It includes the iris, ciliary body and choroid. It contains the majority of the eye's blood vessels.

Uveitis. An inflammation of the uvea, the pigmented layer of the eye. Inflammation may occur suddenly, remain chronic, or recur. Symptoms include eye pain, sensitivity to light, blurred vision, tearing, and redness.

Vascular. Pertaining to blood vessels or indicative of a copious blood supply.

Vendor. Any individual, firm, or corporation from whom purchases are made.

Venules. Small veins that carry blood from the capillaries and join to form larger vessels known as veins.

Vestibular. Pertaining to the vestibular system in the middle ear and the brain which senses movements of the head.

Subject Index

P

R

S

T

V

The Swinfen Charitable Trust (SCT)

The Swinfen Charitable Trust (SCT) is a registered UK Charity whose aim is to "assist poor, sick, and disabled people in the developing world". The method by which it does so is Telemedicine, online advice to hospital doctors in remote situations. SCT operates in countries passing through conflict and post-conflict situations and disasters such as the Tsunami in South Asia, and the mighty Earthquake in Pakistan. www.swinfencharitabletrust.com

Since 2001 SCT has been approached with requests for Ophthalmology advice, and together with expert opinions from the Lions Eye Institute in Western Australia we have been able to supply TELEOPHTHALMOLOGY services to hospitals in the Solomon Islands, Uganda, Bangladesh, Pakistan, and Iraq.

Contact details: The Swinfen Charitable Trust, Dene House, Wingham, Canterbury, Kent. CT3 1NU, UK..
email: swinfencharitabletrust@btinternet.com

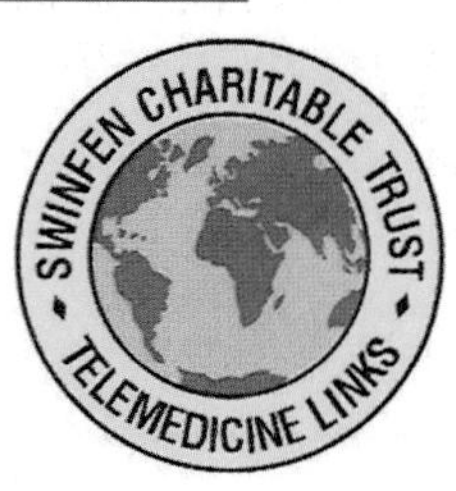

Printing: Krips bv, Meppel
Binding: Stürtz, Würzburg